# AGGRESSION, ANTISOCIAL BEHAVIOR, AND VIOLENCE AMONG GIRLS

## Duke Series in Child Development and Public Policy

Kenneth A. Dodge and Martha Putallaz, *Editors*

Aggression, Antisocial Behavior, and Violence among Girls:
A Developmental Perspective

*Martha Putallaz and Karen L. Bierman, Editors*

### Forthcoming

*Vonnie McLoyd, Nancy Hill, and Kenneth A. Dodge (Editors) on*
Emerging Issues in the Study of the African American Family

*Lisa J. Berlin, Yair Ziv, Lisa Amaya-Jackson,
and Mark Greenberg (Editors) on*
Enhancing Early Attachments

# Aggression, Antisocial Behavior, and Violence among Girls

## A Developmental Perspective

Edited by

MARTHA PUTALLAZ
KAREN L. BIERMAN

Foreword by JOHN B. REID

THE GUILFORD PRESS
NEW YORK   LONDON

© 2004 The Guilford Press
A Division of Guilford Publications, Inc.
72 Spring Street, New York, NY 10012
www.guilford.com

Printed in the United States of America

This book is printed on acid-free paper.

Last digit is print number:  9  8  7  6  5  4  3  2  1

**Library of Congress Cataloging-in-Publication Data**

Aggression, antisocial behavior, and violence among girls : a
developmental perspective / edited by Martha Putallaz, Karen L. Bierman.
    p. cm. — (Duke series in child development and public policy)
  Includes bibliographical references and index.
  ISBN 1-57230-994-6
  1. Girls—Psychology. 2. Aggressiveness in children. 3. Aggressiveness
in adolescence. 4. Conduct disorders in children. 5. Conduct disorders
in adolescence. 6. Child psychopathology. 7. Developmental psychology.
I. Putallaz, Martha. II. Bierman, Karen L. III. Series.
  HQ777.A45 2004
  305.23′082—dc22

                         2004002431

This volume is cosponsored by the Department of Psychology: Social and Health
Sciences, Center for Child and Family Policy, Child and Health Policy Initiative,
Duke University, and the Child, Youth, and Families Consortium, Pennsylvania
State University.

# About the Editors

**Martha Putallaz, PhD,** earned her undergraduate degree from Smith College and her doctoral degree in clinical and developmental psychology from the University of Illinois at Urbana–Champaign in 1982. She began her faculty career at the University of North Carolina at Chapel Hill, where she taught for 2 years. In 1983 she joined the faculty at Duke University, where she is now Professor of Psychology. Dr. Putallaz is a long-standing researcher in the field of children's social development and peer relationships. Most recently, she has been Principal Investigator of a comprehensive study of aggression and social rejection among middle childhood girls, funded by the National Institute of Mental Health. She is also a codirector of the Carolina Consortium on Human Development and the executive director of Duke's Talent Identification Program.

**Karen L. Bierman, PhD,** is Director of the Children, Youth, and Families Consortium and Distinguished Professor of Clinical Child Psychology at Pennsylvania State University. Her research has focused on understanding how peer relationships contribute to children's social–emotional development, social competence, and school adjustment. Dr. Bierman is particularly interested in the design and evaluation of programs that promote social competence and positive intergroup relations and that reduce aggression and violence. Currently, she is the director of the Pennsylvania site of the Fast Track project, a national, multisite prevention trial, funded by the National Institute of Mental Health (with additional funding from the National Institute on Drug Abuse [NIDA], and the U.S. Department of Education), which focuses on preventing antisocial behavior among high-risk youth. She is also coinvestigator of the newly funded PROSPER program, supported by NIDA, which involves the diffusion of empirically supported prevention programs to schools through the use of cooperative-extension-facilitated university–community partnerships.

# Contributors

**Karen Appleyard, MSW, MA,** Institute of Child Development, University of Minnesota, Minneapolis, Minnesota

**Rima Azar, PhD,** Department of Psychology and Research Institute for the Social Development of Youth, University of Montreal, Montreal, Quebec, Canada

**Joanne Belknap, PhD,** Department of Sociology, University of Colorado, Boulder, Colorado

**Karen L. Bierman, PhD,** Children, Youth, and Families Consortium, Pennsylvania State University, University Park, Pennsylvania

**Carole Bruschi, PhD,** Committee for Children, Seattle, Washington

**Deborah M. Capaldi, PhD,** Oregon Social Learning Center, Eugene, Oregon

**Juan F. Casas, PhD,** Department of Psychology, University of Nebraska, Omaha, Nebraska

**Stephen A. Cernkovich, PhD,** Department of Sociology, Bowling Green State University, Bowling Green, Ohio

**Meda Chesney-Lind, PhD,** Women's Studies Program, University of Hawaii at Manoa, Honolulu, Hawaii

**John D. Coie, PhD,** Department of Psychology, Duke University, Durham, North Carolina

**Jennifer Connolly, PhD,** Department of Psychology, York University, Toronto, Ontario, Canada

**Sylvana Côté, PhD,** School of Psychoeducation, University of Montreal, Montreal, Quebec, Canada

**Wendy Craig, PhD,** Department of Psychology, Queen's University, Kingston, Ontario, Canada

**Nicki R. Crick, PhD,** Institute of Child Development, University of Minnesota, Minneapolis, Minnesota

**Natacha De Genna, MA,** Department of Psychology, Concordia University, Montreal, Quebec, Canada

**Kenneth A. Dodge, PhD,** Center for Child and Family Policy, Duke University, Durham, North Carolina

**Celene Domitrovich, PhD,** Children, Youth, and Families Consortium, Pennsylvania State University, University Park, Pennsylvania

**Grace Yan Fang, MS,** Children, Youth, and Families Consortium, Pennsylvania State University, University Park, Pennsylvania

**Peggy C. Giordano, PhD,** Department of Sociology, Bowling Green State University, Bowling Green, Ohio

**Elana B. Gordis, PhD,** Department of Social Work and Psychology, University of Southern California, Los Angeles, California

**Christina L. Grimes, PhD,** Department of Psychology, University of North Carolina, Durham, North Carolina

**Naomi Grunzeweig, MA,** Department of Psychology, Concordia University, Montreal, Quebec, Canada

**Elizabeth A. Jansen, MA,** Institute of Child Development, University of Minnesota, Minneapolis, Minnesota

**Hyoun K. Kim, PhD,** Oregon Social Learning Center, Eugene, Oregon

**Janis B. Kupersmidt, PhD,** Department of Psychology, University of North Carolina, Chapel Hill, North Carolina

**Jane Ledingham, PhD,** School of Psychology, University of Ottawa, Ottawa, Ontario, Canada

**Allen R. Lowery, PhD,** School of Criminal Justice, Tiffin University, Tiffin, Ohio

**Eleanor E. Maccoby, PhD,** Department of Psychology, Stanford University, Stanford, California

**Kate McKnight, BA,** Department of Psychology, Duke University, Durham, North Carolina

**Shari Miller-Johnson, PhD,** Center for Child and Family Policy, Duke University, Durham, North Carolina

**Jamie M. Ostrov, PhD,** Institute of Child Development, University of Minnesota, Minneapolis, Minnesota

**Kathleen Pajer, MD,** Children's Research Institute, Columbus, Ohio

**Daniel Paquette, PhD,** Department of Psychology and Research Institute for the Social Development of Youth, University of Montreal, Montreal, Quebec, Canada

**Debra Pepler, PhD,** LaMarsh Centre for Research on Violence and Conflict Resolution, York University, and The Hospital for Sick Children, Toronto, Ontario, Canada

**Nicole Polanichka, AB,** Department of Psychology, Duke University, Durham, North Carolina

**Martha Putallaz, PhD,** Department of Psychology, Duke University, Durham, North Carolina

**Alex E. Schwartzman, PhD,** Department of Psychology, Concordia University, Montreal, Quebec, Canada

**Lisa A. Serbin, PhD,** Department of Psychology, Concordia University, Montreal, Quebec, Canada

**Joann Wu Shortt, PhD,** Oregon Social Learning Center, Eugene, Oregon

**Dale M. Stack, PhD,** Department of Psychology, Concordia University, Montreal, Quebec, Canada

**Elizabeth J. Susman, PhD,** Department of Biobehavioral Health, Pennsylvania State University, University Park, Pennsylvania

**Caroline E. Temcheff, MA,** Department of Psychology, Concordia University, Montreal, Quebec, Canada

**Richard Tremblay, PhD,** Department of Pediatrics, University of Montreal, Montreal, Quebec, Canada

**Penelope K. Trickett, PhD,** School of Social Work, University of Southern California, Los Angeles, California

**Marion K. Underwood, PhD,** School of Human Development, University of Texas at Dallas, Dallas, Texas

**Amy Yuile, MA,** LaMarsh Centre for Research on Violence and Conflict Resolution, York University, Toronto, Ontario, Canada

**Carolyn Zahn-Waxler, PhD,** Department of Psychology, University of Wisconsin–Madison, Madison, Wisconsin

**Mark Zoccolillo, MD,** Department of Psychiatry, Montreal Children's Hospital–McGill University, Montreal, Quebec, Canada

# Series Editors' Note

This volume is the first in the Duke Series in Child Development and Public Policy, an ongoing collection of edited volumes aimed at addressing the interface between research in child development and contemporary issues in public policy affecting children and families. The purpose of the series is to bring cutting-edge research and theory on social and behavioral development to bear on concerns for public policy making and application.

The needs of children and their families are receiving growing attention from the general populace. Issues such as youth violence, families in a culturally diverse society, education reform, and education policy have moved to the foreground of political debates. Mass school shootings have led to unprecedented funding for violence prevention in U.S. schools. Intranational conflicts worldwide have led to major dilemmas regarding the placement of homeless refugee children and families. Education reform now occupies a central place in U.S. presidential politics. Important decisions are being made with regard to public funding for programs and other public policies toward children. Unfortunately, these decisions are often made without regard to current scientific knowledge about child development.

At the same time, the scholarly field of child development is enjoying renewed vigor, funding, and discoveries. Advances are being made through interdisciplinary inquiry, novel methods for research design and data analysis, and access to a wealth of government data. Longitudinal studies with large samples that began in the early 1980s are yielding crucial data as the young participants now grow into adulthood. Computerized records of administrative, archival, and government data in education, public health, child welfare, and corrections afford the opportunity to understand children's development in a broader context than ever before. New data-analytic methods such as latent growth curve analysis, structural equation modeling, and hierarchical linear modeling are being applied to these data sets to enable scholars to draw conclusions that were not possible even 10 years ago. Large-scale experiments in prevention, public housing, and education are yielding crucial findings about the potential benefits that government programs can bring to children's lives. One of the most exciting innovations in child development today is the application of these novel findings to issues germane to public policy and contemporary society.

It is our goal that the Duke Series in Child Development and Public Policy be at the heart of this rapprochement between child development research and public policy. The advances made by individual contributors will be brought together in each volume to form a comprehensive picture aimed at developing a more complete understanding of the selected topic, spanning the domains of theory, research, and policy. By necessity, then, the contents of each volume are interdisciplinary, linking basic scientific knowledge of human development and functioning with knowledge of the process of public policy. It is our hope that each volume of the series will thus be of benefit not only to academic scholars in child development and public policy, but to practitioners and policy makers who serve children and families as well.

Inspiration for this series grew out of interactions among faculty members at the Duke Center for Child and Family Policy in the Terry Sanford Institute of Public Policy and the Duke Department of Psychology: Social and Health Sciences. These scholars—including Steven Asher, Susan Roth, and Bruce Jentleson, along with ourselves—recognized that important problems facing children and families in contemporary society could best be addressed by scholars working in an interdisciplinary environment. With generous support from the Duke Provost's Initiative in the Social Sciences, we began to plan an annual series of working conferences, each of which would lead to an edited volume.

Each conference brings together scholars from diverse disciplines, along with a participant audience of scientists, students, policy makers, and practitioners, who wrestle with a problem in contemporary society. Because each conference is defined by a broad current problem or issue, scholars are forced to depart from their individual disciplines' theories and methods in order to address the practice and policy issues that are germane to the particular problem. The solutions to vexing contemporary problems require the best efforts of this type.

This first conference and volume benefited greatly from the cosponsorship and collaboration of the Pennsylvania State University Consortium on Children, Youth, and Families (Karen L. Bierman, Director). It is our goal that many (but not all) of the conferences will be jointly sponsored with leading centers at other universities, and that the resulting volumes will be coedited by leading scholars from Duke University and these other universities.

KENNETH A. DODGE, PhD
MARTHA PUTALLAZ, PhD

# Foreword

This volume is definitely a benchmark in the systematic study of aggression and antisocial behavior. Taken together, the chapters in this volume describe the extremely recent and rapid development of theory, measurement strategies, and significant findings about the development and long-term outcomes of aggression in girls and adolescents. The contributors to this volume are the architects of this area of rigorous research that did not even exist a decade ago. The new knowledge about the forms and life-course development of girls' aggression described in each chapter now rivals that available for boys. In fact, the systematic integration of relational and physical aggression over the life course, articulated in this volume, places existing models for boys into a broader developmental context. The chapters present rich research contributions from different disciplines, methodologies, and perspectives. Each describes a critical piece in the development of this critical area.

An interdisciplinary perspective characterizes the volume, which brings together developmental studies of aggressive behavior displayed by girls in normative settings and studies of high-risk girls showing significant antisocial behaviors, along with later-life studies examining the romantic relationships and parenting of women with histories of significant conduct disorder and/or victimization.

The stage for understanding the development of gender differences in aggression and antisocial behavior is set in the first three chapters. In Chapter 1, Maccoby traces the evolution of research and conceptualizations of aggression in general, as well as the interrelated issues of gender, socialization, and development. The complex interplay of gender and early socialization leads her to the broad conclusion that a host of biological, social, and cultural factors contribute to the way individuals enact their gender. The dynamic interactions among such factors, and the early emerging gender differences, are illustrated both by examples of key developmental studies of children and nonhuman primates, and by an intensive and compelling description of systematic observations of classrooms of preschool boys and girls. Maccoby decribes the emerging scientific recognition of the importance of the different contexts, meanings, and topographies of aggression for boys and girls. She concludes that researchers must get beyond discovering sex differences in overt aggression in boys and girls; to study each gender in its own terms, examining differences and similarities in topography, development, context, and purpose; and to integrate both overt and relational aggression in models to other aspects of development.

Chapter 2, by Susman and Pajer, provides a conceptual framework for integrating biological variables and constructs into developmental models of aggression in girls. The current research and theoretical paradigms described are still in their infancy, with models and studies focusing for the most part on simple relationships between individual biological systems and one form of aggression (mainly overt, physical aggression), limiting their relevance to girls. The emerging conceptual framework is one that will articulate the reciprocal interactions and bidirectionality of several biological systems with each other, and with environmental and contextual factors, developmental changes, and behavioral and psychological factors involved in girls' aggression. Some important findings are reported in this chapter, particularly in research on the endocrine system, and are discussed in terms of relationships with environmental and developmental processes within the broad framework described above. Studies of the relationships of neurotransmitters, the neuroendocrine system, and aggression, as well as the relationships of physiological stress (e.g., attenuation of cortisol) with increased aggression, are also described. The discovery of biological processes that increase the odds of aggressive or other risky behaviors has important implications for prevention.

In Chapter 3, a developmental framework is described for examining environmental factors that affect the development of aggression and antisocial behavior in girls. Zahn-Waxler and Polanichka cover a lot of ground in this chapter. For example, studies reviewed show that girls are more receptive than boys to socialization efforts of their mothers, and that mothers, as well as teachers, tend to discourage physical aggression in girls and encourage it in boys. Other studies are beginning to indicate why some girls show high levels of physical aggression despite gender-based biological and environmental constraints. Although this chapter focuses on environmental processes, it is argued that they are firmly embedded in personality factors that are in part genetically determined. In addition to socialization factors associated with physical aggression, studies are reviewed that relate to girls' masking of anger, to their higher levels of submissiveness, and to the importance of relationships with girls who make relational, covert aggression a more common expression of anger. An important discussion describes the different assessment methodologies used by researchers in various disciplines concerned with girls' aggression.

These first three chapters thus provide an excellent overview of research on the development of aggressive behavior in girls, with an important consideration of the transactional influences of biological and socialization (family, peer, school) experiences that contribute to individual differences in aggressive propensities.

The three chapters in the second section, on aggression and victimization among girls in childhood, build upon the developmental framework, and break new ground in the conceptualization and measurement of aggressive behavior. Whereas aggression is now considered by most researchers to be a significant problem for females, it has until very recently been conceptualized as an adolescent problem for girls. The chapters in this section show clearly that early developmental trajectories leading to antisocial behavior are evident in girls as well as boys. In Chapter 4, Crick, Ostrov, Appleyard, Jansen, and Casas provide an overview of existing research on relational aggression in young children. Beginning with a review of theories prevalent in the mid-1990s that held that aggression in girls was not common, not serious, and developed only in adolescence, they describe three new and critical developments in the study of girls' aggression. The review of the literature clearly shows that the "relational" aggression most salient in girls is quite serious, has harmful short- and long-term effects on both perpetrator and victim, begins much earlier than originally assumed—at least as early as 3 years of age—and must be understood in terms of girls' overall social development. In addition to a review of empirical findings and theoretical developments, advances in the psychometric development of a wide variety of assessment strategies for young children are described. These strategies range from naturalistic observations of relational aggression and semi-structured observations designed to elicit specific interactions relevant to aggression in young children, to advances in peer, parent, teacher, and self-report strategies specific to young children. Crick and colleagues conclude by recommending that research be conducted on a number of social-cognitive factors relative to aggression in young girls and boys, specifically, attributional processes, perspective taking, language and gender role development, and peer, sibling, and parental influences.

In Chapter 5, Pepler, Craig, Yuile, and Connolly continue the themes emerging in previous chapters: that the definition of aggression be expanded to include nonphysical aggression and antisocial behavior, and that much can be learned by examining such behavior in a developmental context. Most studies of bullying have been conducted on preadolescent children. In this chapter, bullying is examined in three cross-sectional samples, including children in grades 1–12. Important issues concerning measurement of similar constructs in children from childhood through adolescence are dealt with systematically, and the analyses are informed by a broad range of developmental literatures. Important multimethod descriptive data on bullying are presented, showing, for example, that there are gender differences in the amount, type, and targets of bullying, but that there is also considerable overlap in the distributions. The developmental trajectories for bullying are also different for boys and girls, giving a number of clues to prevention strategies. As is the case with boys, girls who bully also report high rates of victimization by others, including sexual harassment and date aggression. Importantly, data from middle and high school students indicate that for girls, bullying is related to increased alienation and conflict, and lower levels of commitment in romantic relationships. Taken together, these and many other findings reported in this chapter strongly suggest that bullying by girls in middle and high school may set them up to select aggressive romantic partners, to engage in a number of forms of relationship aggression, and in short to put themselves at high risk for aggression in their romantic relationships.

Whereas systematic observations in both natural and analogue settings have played an important role in developmental models of boys' physical aggression, they have been used only rarely to study the types of aggression that girls more typically display. In Chapter 6, by Putallaz, Kupersmidt, Coie, McKnight, and Grimes, the research literature on gender differences and other central issues related to girls' aggression are reviewed. In reviewing the literature, a strong case is made that reports and ratings have been used almost exclusively to develop definitions, descriptions, and models of aggression in girls. Several serious concerns are raised about the vulnerability of such measures to gender biases or stereotypes, and the usefulness of such measures to provide detailed behavioral descriptions of the types of aggression used by girls. The authors describe an intricate observational study of the play interactions of fourth-grade girls. A behavioral code was developed to measure all direct physical and verbal acts of aggression, all indirect acts of aggression, and damage of others' possessions. Some rather surprising results are reported concerning the numbers of girls considered relationally aggressive, the relative rates of the three sorts of aggression, and the contextual determinants (e.g., twice the rate of aggression in the familiar groups). Extremely interesting transcripts and behavioral descriptions from the taped sessions are presented. Although only some preliminary analyses are available at this time, some exciting tidbits are described.

For example, the type of victim response to aggression had powerful effects on the probability of another aggressive act, or of a previously uninvolved girl joining the aggressor in another act. Such analyses will have powerful implications for prevention strategies, as well as for further theoretical development.

The studies in the second section thus focus on the social characteristics and dynamics of aggressive behaviors among girls as they emerge in the everyday contexts of preschool and elementary school peer interactions. They highlight the importance of a broad conceptualization of aggressive behavior and an understanding of the social functions and dynamics that support its development and display. They provide a foundation for the next set of chapters, which examine the more serious difficulties experienced by high-risk adolescent girls.

The third section includes four chapters focused on antisocial and related problem behaviors in adolescent girls who have already become engaged in, or are at high risk for becoming engaged in, violence, aggression, or delinquency. In Chapter 7, Bierman and colleagues argue that young boys and girls may show gender-specific developmental trajectories to serious delinquency and behavior problems in later childhood and adolescence. They conclude that whereas early-starting physical aggression may be the most common pathway to serious delinquency for boys, the pathway might be quite different for young girls, involving a broader range of disruptive behavior. To test this general proposition, they examined longitudinal data from a subgroup of high-risk boys and girls from the Fast Track Study. Using teacher ratings of aggressive and nonaggressive–disruptive behavior (oppositional or hyperactive–inattentive) for each child in kindergarten, they were able to create a narrow-band (aggressive/disruptive behavior only) and a wide-band (aggressive and nonaggressive combined) risk score. They next used the wide- and narrow-band scores to predict psychosocial and academic adjustment at grade 4 and self-reported delinquency at grade 7. This innovative analysis revealed some differences in early predictors for boys and girls. Perhaps most important is the finding that the narrow-band predictor underidentified girls who displayed maladjustment in grade 4 and self-reported delinquency at grade 7.

In Chapter 8, Trickett and Gordis address the development of aggressive and antisocial patterns in girls and adolescents with documented histories of sexual abuse. The somewhat sparse existing literature is reviewed to show that mothers of grade school girls who had been sexually abused consistently rate them as high in aggression. Similar data for sexually abused girls in adolescence are mixed and of limited quality. The results of a longitudinal study of sexually abused girls (ages 6–16 at time of abuse) and a control sample, including five waves of data collection, are reported. Although a large number of analyses of the data sets have been conducted over the last 10 years, the focus of this chapter is on the short- and long-term outcomes of sexual abuse and on the influence of the type of perpetrator on outcomes. Immediate and long-term levels of aggression after abuse for the abused girls in each perpetrator category are reported and discussed. A number of moderational and mediational analyses indicate that there may be a number of different developmental trajectories for girls after sexual abuse.

In Chapter 9, Giordano, Cernkovich, and Lowery examine the long-term outcomes for serious adolescent female offenders. Because there are very few adolescent girls who commit very serious or multiple offenses (i.e., 1–2%), population-based studies would have to have huge samples to permit powerful analyses. Because of the low prevalence, and because girls are thought to pose less of a threat to society than boys, there have been few studies, and the few that exist have been cross-sectional, which do not allow for life-course analyses. There are also very few data on these girls' transition to adulthood. The authors report results of a longitudinal study of over 100 serious female and 100 serious male offenders, interviewed when they were in training schools and again 12 years later. These data on the transition to adulthood are compared with identical data for a representative sample of adolescents in the same area. This unique data set, including qualitative interviews, systematic self-reports, and arrest data, is used to answer a number of important questions about the transition to adulthood for serious male and female offenders. A number of highly relevant outcomes are reported, including data on employment and marriage, school and occupational achievement, and psychological distress, and are discussed within a social control theory framework. Importantly, a number of hypothesized mediators are assessed, which account for variability in outcomes.

In Chapter 10, Chesney-Lind and Belknap present a critical examination of the widely publicized proposition that girls have become increasingly more violent over the past few decades. In reviewing the existing literature, many surprising findings and contradictions are described. For example, the huge increases in arrest rates for crimes such as "assault" by girls are not found in careful surveys using self-reports of delinquent and criminal behaviors. The self-report studies show decreases in violent aggression by girls over the last couple of decades. The authors describe their own careful work assessing the specific crimes that have led to the skyrocketing crime rates for youth and particularly for girls. The methodology is quite different from that used in other research reported in this volume, yet is uniquely suited to answer the questions posed. The analyses and details are fascinating. A major finding is that homicides by girls, the reporting of which cannot be much affected by police and prosecutor practices, fell by half in the period 1984–1993. The rates for less serious offenses have soared, due to factors such as zero tolerance and increased police presence in schools since the Columbine shootings in 1999. The conclusions are summarized in the context of a broader view of girls' antisocial behavior.

The fourth section examines the later-life experiences of aggressive girls as they move into adolescent romantic relationships and parenthood, illustrating mechanisms by which the behavioral and emotional vulnerabilities of these girls contribute to an ongoing spectrum of adult difficulties. Of particular note are the widespread risks these young women face in diverse areas of their lives, including compromised health status, difficult and tumultuous romantic relationships, and ineffective parenting. In Chapter 11, Capaldi, Kim, and Shortt review existing literature and theories relating to women's involvement in partner aggression in romantic relationships. As in Chapter 10, the popular images of adolescent and adult female aggression are critically examined and found to be based more on cultural stereotypes and feminist philosophy than on any rigorous data. In popular theory, women are described as inert victims of men's attempts to exploit and dominate, and much of the theory and research to date has been directed toward typologies of battering men, with the goal of fine-tuning interventions for dealing with the various types. More recent theoretical perspectives are described highlighting the developmental trajectories of both men and women leading to partner violence. The research and theoretical formulations expressed in this chapter challenge accepted feminist ideology and other models that portray women as passive victims rather than as being in potential control of their safety in heterosexual relationships. The authors report impressive findings from longitudinal studies that clearly demonstrate that adolescent and young adult women are not inert in aggressive-partner relationships. Analyses show that the developmental histories, conduct problems, and family experiences for both male and female romantic partners are powerful predictors of partner aggression. The longitudinal methodologies and analyses are state of the art and have clear implications for the design of preventive intervention strategies.

In Chapter 12, Zoccolillo, Paquette, Azar, Côté, and Tremblay examine parenting as an outcome of conduct disorder in girls. They review emerging findings of two of their ongoing studies: a large, population-based longitudinal study selected on the basis of birth certificates, and a sample of adolescent mothers. The studies use psychiatric diagnoses to identify and assess antisocial behavior, supplemented by clinical observations. Although the methodology and theoretical framework are somewhat different from those described in other chapters, the findings extend our knowledge of the life-course development of antisocial behavior in girls into parenthood. Importantly, the research reviewed provides findings relevant to transgenerational transmission of aggression and antisocial behavior, as well as a wide range of risks to physical health of the offspring of teenagers with conduct disorder. In addition to the broad review of parenting outcomes, the detailed discussion of four risk factors—assortative mating, adolescent motherhood, maternal sensitivity, and maternal irritability—provides powerful examples of the dynamic interplay between biological and environmental factors and the development and transmission of antisocial behavior. The strong implications of these risk factors for prevention and intervention are described.

The final chapter, by Serbin and colleagues, summarizes findings from an ongoing longitudinal study begun in 1976. The sample is population based, with groups of normative, extremely aggressive, extremely withdrawn boys and girls selected from a larger sample of first graders. The developmental trajectories of the sample are described, from first grade to adulthood and parenthood. Data for the offspring of the sample are also reported. The focus of this chapter is on the long-term trajectories and outcomes of girlhood aggression, emphasizing maternal and child health, parenting, and intergenerational transfer of risk to offspring. Analyses of data across elementary school, middle school, high school, and parenthood show a clear trajectory of increasing risk in both homotypic (e.g., delinquency) and heterotypic (e.g., drug use, early pregnancy) domains. The early outcomes for the children of aggressive girls are reported, showing clearly the generational transfer of early risk factors for aggression and antisocial behavior. Analyses of social interactions between mothers and their young children are described, and it is clear that the developmental trajectories of the mothers are being replicated by their children. These studies complete the developmental spectrum covered by this book, spanning from factors that contribute to the emergence of aggressive behavior problems and escalation to adolescent antisocial activity among girls, to the increased risk their children face for similar life-course difficulties.

Finally, two commentaries address the implications of this volume for prevention and public policy. Underwood and Coie highlight the need for early identification and intervention for girls. To achieve this, it is argued that the definition and assessment of aggression be broadened for girls to include both disruptiveness and relational aggression as well as physical aggression. Evidence is provided to show that some interventions that work well for boys also work well for girls. As relational aggression is a very serious problem for girls, and because it starts to develop before school entry, preventive interventions must be developed to sensitize parents and teachers to the need to deal with it early. Suggestions for the development of a range of specific interventions are offered.

In his commentary, Dodge makes a strong case for policy reform in youth violence. More girls are being inducted into the juvenile justice system because of increased prosecution for acts that have traditionally been treated as status offenses. Dodge uses data from various chapters in this volume to make the case that girls are not getting more violent, but they do have serious problems with aggression that are different from those of boys. Unfortunately, girls are squeezed into the same juvenile justice programs designed for boys. It is argued that policies must be changed to include relational as well as physical aggression in school prevention programs, and to educate policy makers about the serious long-term and transgenerational outcomes for girls with conduct problems that require early and effective interventions. Dodge cites the requirement that each state establish distinct intervention programs for boys and girls. He argues that the chapters in this volume provide sufficient data to begin the systematic development of a number of appropriate interventions.

These two commentaries integrate the diverse chapters and articulate important general implications of the groundbreaking research described in this book. As researchers from different disciplines study this volume, new studies certainly will be launched to further the specific lines of research described in each chapter. The advances in methodology, as well as the new data on the topography, the developmental trajectories of female aggression from early childhood through parenthood, and the discoveries relating to malleable antecedents and mediators, create a solid foundation for designing a new generation of randomized prevention and intervention trials. Specifically designed for girls, such trials will have the potential to result in powerful interventions and improved outcomes, and to provide rigorous experimental tests and extensions of the developmental models described in the individual chapters in this important volume.

JOHN B. REID, PHD
*Oregon Social Learning Center*

# Preface

Historically, much attention has been focused on understanding aggression and antisocial behavior among youth due to the deleterious effects of these behaviors on individuals and society as a whole. Research has focused on trying to understand the predictors and trajectories associated with youthful aggression and antisocial behavior, the most effective means of prevention and intervention, and the implications of these findings for policy makers. Almost exclusively this work has focused on understanding aggression and antisocial behavior among males. Recently, however, there has been an upsurge in research devoted to understanding the types of aggression and antisocial behaviors more characteristic of females. What before were best considered individual and infrequent investigative forays are now occurring with sufficient frequency that a body of research is developing, devoted to understanding aggression and antisocial behavior among females. Aggression is now being conceptualized more broadly than physical or overt aggression to also encompass more covert acts of aggression, variously labeled indirect, relational, or social aggression, directed at inflicting harm to social relationships. Although antisocial and violent behavior occurs less frequently among females than males, researchers have been searching to understand the reasons for its occurrence despite the presence of biological and societal constraints. Longitudinal data following aggressive and antisocial females are now available, allowing for the examination of developmental trajectories and intergenerational effects. Implications for violence in relationships are now being explored. Theoretical advances have been made as well, with an increased recognition of the importance of the developmental progression involved.

Despite these achievements in broadening our understanding of aggression and antisocial behavior among females, these studies have remained for the most part individual efforts. Little has been done to bring these research developments together to form a comprehensive picture aimed at developing an understanding of aggression and antisocial behavior in girls. This volume represents a compilation of some of these individual but complementary interdisciplinary efforts spanning the domains of theory, research, and policy. This effort dates to May 2002, when an interdisciplinary group of prominent scholars researching aggression, antisocial behavior, and violence among girls came together at Duke University for the first conference in the Duke Series in Child Development and Public Policy. The conference and ensuing volume were sponsored jointly by Duke University's Department of Psychology: Social and Health Sciences, Center for Child and Family Policy, and Child and Health Policy Initiative, as well as the Pennsylvania State University's Children, Youth, and Families Consortium. The perspective of the resulting volume is developmental in nature, tracking the progression of aggression and antisocial behavior in girls from early childhood through adulthood.

In designing the conference and subsequent book, an effort was made to bring together an interdisciplinary set of scholars whose work bridged the developmental phases of girls' aggression from early childhood through later romantic relationships, parenting, and intergenerational transmission. The authors represent a diverse set of disciplinary backgrounds, including psychology, psychiatry, sociology, and criminology. Within these disciplines, research tends to focus on different aspects of the phenomenon, from different perspectives, often using different methodologies. For example, childhood aggression has been studied primarily by developmental psychologists, typically focusing on school-based samples, using observational and questionnaire methods. Psychiatrists have more often targeted clinic samples in their research, focusing on the characteristics and life histories of individuals diagnosed with conduct disorder. Sociologists and criminologists studying juvenile delinquency have more often focused on broader population-based trends and characteristics, and delineated the roles of community and context factors. One goal of this book is to bring together these different perspectives in order to take a better look at "the whole elephant"—the phenomenon of female aggression and violence from a diversity of scholarly frameworks.

Integrating material across these different frameworks challenges the reader to attend carefully to the samples and methodology utilized by the various authors. For the most part, the chapters that cover developmental trends in early childhood to adolescence describe research conducted with normative samples in school-based peer contexts, focusing on girls in general or on at-risk girls who show elevated levels of various types of aggressive behaviors. In contrast, other chapters focus on "identified" samples of girls or women—individuals who have experienced particular trauma, been diagnosed with conduct disorder, or experienced incarceration. The results do not always map neatly onto each other, but the paradigms are complementary. Reflecting the approach of developmental psychopathology, the interfacing of developmental studies on normative samples with targeted studies on at-risk and disordered samples is designed to inform developmental, sociological, clinical, and forensic models, as well as speak to social–educational, clinical, and criminal justice system policies.

# Contents

## Part V. Implications for Policy and Intervention

# PART I

# SETTING THE STAGE

*Understanding the Development
of Gender Differences in
Aggression and Antisocial Behavior*

# CHAPTER 1

# Aggression in the Context of Gender Development

Eleanor E. Maccoby

This chapter begins with an overview of the role that gender plays in the development of social behavior and social relationships as children grow from infancy to adulthood. The chapter then focuses specifically on the gendered aspects of aggression in its various forms.

## CAN WE—SHOULD WE— DISTINGUISH "SEX" AND "GENDER"?

Over the past half-century there have been significant changes in the way we think about sex and gender. We have known for a very long time about the X and Y chromosomes, and their role in making the two sexes biologically distinct. And from the 1930s on, developmental psychologists were busy documenting the ways in which the two sexes differed in their behavior, abilities, temperament, and personality traits. As the feminist movement picked up momentum in the 1960s and 1970s, a countertheme came into play: People began emphasizing how much the distributions of scores on all these dimensions overlapped for the two sexes—that in fact, males and females were much alike in many respects (Maccoby & Jacklin, 1974). In addition, many people became concerned—and I think rightly so—about labeling such differences as *sex* differences, on the grounds that this terminology implied that any differences between male and female individuals were fundamentally biological in origin. The term "gender" was introduced to distinguish the social from the biological. The term "sex differences" would be used to refer to any differences, such as the secondary sex characteristics developing at puberty, that were clearly biological in origin. "Gender differences" would be used to refer to sex-linked characteristics that arose from the way children of the two sexes were socialized and the different roles assigned to them by the societies in which they grew up. Gender was said to be socially constructed, and it was widely believed that biological forces have very little to do with the way masculinity and femininity are defined in a given culture and the way in which gender is enacted in a cultural context.

This distinction between sex and gender has proved to be difficult to maintain. Indeed, in recent years these terms have come to be used pretty much synonymously. I believe it is hopeless to try to maintain a distinction between these terms, because biological and environmental factors interact from the moment of conception on, and also because as "sex" and "gender" are actually used in gender studies, the two terms are almost completely redundant. For example, in two recent textbooks on sex and gender, the texts no longer attempt to distinguish between the two terms, and in the subject-matter index, under the terms "sex differences" or "sex roles" one finds nothing except the direction: "See gender differences" or "gender roles." A recent book put out by the Institute of Medicine—a book called *Exploring the Biological Contributions to Human Health: Does Sex Matter?* (Weizmann & Pardue, 2001)—makes a valiant effort to maintain the distinction. They recommend: "In the study of human subjects, the term sex should be used as a classification, generally as male or female, according to the reproductive organs or functions that derive from the chromosomal complement. . . . The term *gender* should be used to refer to a person's self-representation as male or female, or how that person is responded to by social institutions on the basis of the person's self-presentation" (p. 8). To my mind, they are pointing to a distinction that seldom matters. Although there are a few people who are genetically of one sex but take up an identity and present themselves to the world as being of the other sex, for the vast majority of people their self-accepted gender identity, as well as the gender identity assigned to them by other people, is identical with their chromosomal sex. Both terms refer to a binary distinction—by either name, one is either a male or female person. Please note that I am talking about gender identity here, not sexual preference, which is not binary and admits of more distinctions. In current usage, the term *sex* has come to refer more specifically to sexual activity than it once did. Hence I usually follow the current trend and use the term *gender* in discussing the differentiation of the two sexes with respect to their psychological and social functioning.

My use of this term is not meant to imply that a gender effect is only or primarily social in origin.

## NATURE AND NURTURE

Whenever we study gender issues, then, we must always begin by classifying people into two categories. This in no way prevents us from studying the biological, cultural, and social conditions that contribute to the way in which individuals enact their gender. These things are not binary, the way sex and gender are. They vary widely from one individual to another, and from one culture or subculture to another, and even within the same individual from one context to another. Several of the chapters in this volume are directly concerned with questions such as how biology, sex roles, social customs, shared beliefs, and self-regulation work to differentiate people within each sex, or indeed sometimes to make the two sexes more alike.

It is extraordinarily difficult to make clear distinctions between what is biological and what is social in our gendered selves. Indeed, we must ask whether it is useful to try to do so. Let me illustrate some of the complexities of trying to make the sort of nature–nurture distinction that the early feminists hoped to make. I want to describe some studies by Ageliki Nicolopoulou (1997) with several classrooms of preschool children. The children were encouraged to make up little stories and dictate them to the teacher who was in charge of collecting stories. The teacher would write down the child's story as nearly as possible in the child's own words. At the end of each day, the teacher would read out to the class the stories the children had told during the day, and the author of each story would be invited to act out the story and to get other members of the class to take parts in the little drama if there was more than one character. Early in the school year, the stories were very simple. For example, one child's story was "There was a boy. And a girl. And a wedding." But as the year progressed, the children told more elaborate stories and became more enthusiastic and skillful in acting them out. Here is an example of a girl's story:

> Once upon a time there was a castle and a king, and a queen, and a prince and a princess and a unicorn and a pony lived in it. And they went for a walk. And they found a playground and they swang on the swings and they slide down the slide. And then they went back home. But they had some trouble finding the way. But then a dog came to them and said: "I'll help you find the way home." And he did. The end. (in Nicolopoulou, 1997, p. 166)

A boy's story:

> Once upon a time there was a wolf. And then a T-Rex came. And then
> Godzilla came. And then Pherodactyl came. Then they had a fight, and
> then T-Rex killed Godzilla. And then Godzilla came back alive again.
> Then there came a bunch of bad guys, and then the Godzilla knocked the
> bad guys down and they were trying to get him. Then a little superhero
> came. Then he was flying and he landed. Then he flipped, and then
> Godzilla realized it was Batman, so then he blowed fire at him, and then
> he falled down and he was dead. Then a Brontosaurus came and
> Godzilla jumped on him, and then he got squished. Then they had a ma-
> jor fight. Then they stopped the fight, and everyone looked at each other,
> and then they didn't do the fight anymore. The End. (in Nicolopoulou,
> 1997, p. 167)

Over the course of a preschool year, children would sometimes borrow
elements from stories told by other children, and elaborate on them. Occasionally, a boy would borrow a family theme from a girl's story, but
modify it in a male direction:

> Once upon a time there was a kingdom, and a prince and a king and a
> queen and Mutant Ninja Turtles in it. Then a wolf came. The prince and
> the wolf had a big battle. Then Knight in Shining Armor came. Then
> Batman came, and with his big weapon he killed the wolf. The End. (in
> Nicolopoulou, 1997, p. 177)

Even at the beginning of the preschool year, boys were already much
more likely to tell stories including themes of conflict, danger, heroism,
and aggressive violence, and the girls were more likely to tell stories with
romantic and family-oriented themes. But by the end of the year, the two
sexes had become even more polarized in terms of their story themes.
Notice how very strong these differences are: In the spring, 95% of the
stories told by boys included aggressive violence, compared to 27% of
the girls' stories. As for family themes, girls utilized them in 76% of their
stories, and boys in only 3% of theirs. It is worth noting that both boys
and girls drew on characters from TV and storybooks, but they drew
quite distinctively different elements from a corpus of media material
that was presumably equally available to both sexes.

The gender divide extended beyond the story themes. The boys
more often called on other boys to act in their stories, and the girls
mainly acted in girls' stories, and increasingly, children of each sex
would take only sex-congruent roles. As Nicolopoulou and colleagues
interpreted what was happening in these classrooms, two distinct subcultures were developing, in which boys more and more shared a corpus

of stories and story themes with other boys, and girls did likewise with other girls. One implication is that there is a kind of multiplier effect: A group of girls are more girl-like collectively than they are singly, and the same is perhaps even more true for a group of boys.

We should remember how unusual the situation is that was offered to children in these studies. Normally preschool children do not get an opportunity to invent their own stories and act them out with and for each other. In the classrooms studied by Nicolopoulou, both the researchers and the teachers were startled at how quickly the gender divide developed, and how deep it was. Indeed, they did not like what they saw. The teachers wanted their classrooms to be much more gender-neutral places. Indeed, many preschool teachers consciously work to make them so. So when we observe children in the usual preschool classroom, we get only a modified reflection of the processes revealed in the stories described above. A much better indication of these processes in children's ordinary lives is found in their free play when they are under only general supervision from adults. Here we see them spontaneously segregating themselves into same-sex clusters, and developing two distinctive "cultures" involving acting out, in play, much the same sex-distinctive themes we have seen in the stories above (Maccoby, 1998). When a same-sex group of children play together over a period of time, they build up a body of shared play themes that are repeatedly elaborated. The manifest content of these themes is of course greatly influenced by the larger culture in which they are growing up, but in their playgroups children utilize cultural themes in the service of their own enterprises. Playmates share memories and understandings of their joint play experiences, as well as mutual expectations and common interests, and they carry some of these things over into new same-sex encounters, where they are replicated. This is the core of what we mean by a group developing a shared "culture."

The sex differences in children's toy choices, in their preferences for stories or TV programs, and in the interaction styles that pervade their play with same-sex peers all appear to be part of the same fabric as the themes that appeared in the narratives children invented for the Nicolopoulou project They all reflect some important differences in what interests and motivates young boys and girls. These differences mean that children typically find others of their own sex to be more compatible as interaction partners, although children differ in the age at which this compatibility begins to matter. There are exceptions, of course: There are some children who find partners of either sex to be compatible, and a few who actively prefer to play with children of the other sex.

To raise again the question that feminists raised in the 1970s: Is gender socially constructed? Absolutely. That is what the children described by Nicolopoulou were busy doing. But of course we must ask: Why do boys and girls socially construct different subcultures? Is there any biological contribution to this difference? I would say, very likely. This duality illustrates the pitfalls in trying to determine whether it is primarily nature or primarily nurture that brings about a gender divergence. Nature and nurture work together, each depending on the other.

A primatologist, Kim Wallen, has made this point strongly in a paper called "Nature Needs Nurture" (1996). He has found that for young rhesus monkeys, the frequency with which they aggressively threaten their peers when placed in a mixed-sex peer group depends on the social conditions of rearing. But these effects are different for male and female animals. When young males are allowed only very limited access to play with peers during the first year of life, remaining almost entirely with their mothers, they are subsequently more aggressive toward other young animals—especially females—and their play is rougher than if they have had opportunities to play freely with peers during their first year. By contrast, limiting the peer-play opportunities of young females during their first year has quite a different effect. When peer-deprived females subsequently find themselves with other young monkeys, they become more submissive than females who have had wider social experience with peers during their first year. Thus the divergence between the two sexes in aggressiveness toward peers can be large or small, depending on their early social experience, but also on their sex, and more specifically (Wallen reports) on the levels of sex hormones present prenatally or natally. Wallen stresses that early exposure to interaction with peers, and probably also the presence of the mother during the first year when aggressive behavior first appears, are *required* conditions for the normal development of aggression in both sexes. The implication obviously is that nature and nurture are not antagonistic forces such that if one is powerful the other must be weak. Whatever different behavioral predispositions the two sexes may be born with, they require being activated or established by certain environmental conditions, a major one being the same-sex playgroup.

## PEER GROUPS AS A SOCIALIZING CONTEXT

Among human children, these playgroups have considerable socializing power. This is well illustrated in some recent work by Martin and Fabes (2001). They have followed three preschool classrooms of 4-year-olds through most of a school year, observing the children every weekday during unstructured playtime. They recorded first of all whether a child was playing with same- or other-sex playmates, or in a mixed group. In addition, they recorded the type of interaction that was occurring. They found that over the course of the year, the more time a boy spent playing with other boys, the greater was the increase in his activity level, amount of rough-and-tumble play, and overt aggression. At the same time, play with other boys was associated with increases in "positive emotionality"— that is, with overt signs of having fun. Also, the more time a boy spent with other boys, the less time he spent close to the available adults. By contrast, the more time girls spent playing with other girls, the more their activity levels and their aggression *decreased*. Girls who often played with other girls spent progressively more time in proximity to adults.

There are many questions about how to interpret these findings. One possibility is that the girls stayed closer to the adults as a way of getting some protection from rough incursions by groups of boys (see Greeno, 1989), but that once they were closer to adults they felt constrained about displaying aggressive behavior toward each other that adults might disapprove. Boys, being farther from adults' watchful eyes, may have felt freer to act on their aggressive impulses. But whatever the reason, it is clear that boys were stimulating one another to increasing levels of rough, active play and aggression, while girls were not. Indeed, the girls were becoming *less* aggressive with continuing playful interaction with one another.[1] More recent analyses (e.g., Fabes, Martin, & Hanish, 2003) reveal that these sex-differentiated patterns seldom occur when children play in mixed-sex groups.

It might appear that there is some inconsistency between what Wallen reported about young rhesus monkeys and what Martin and Fabes report about human children. That is, Wallen found that experience playing with peers appeared to moderate male aggressiveness, while it seemed to have the opposite effect with the 4-year-old boys studied by Martin and Fabes. My guess would be that the dominance hierarchies and cooperative alliances that usually emerge in groups of males who associate with one another frequently do indeed serve to moderate ingroup aggression, but that perhaps these group control processes are not yet fully in place in 4-year-old human children.

## DEVELOPMENTAL TRAJECTORIES
## OF AGGRESSION IN THE TWO SEXES

This Martin and Fabes work appears to fit in nicely with much that we have known for many years about aggression in the two sexes. Simply put, it has been quite clearly established that males are the more confrontational sex. They are more overtly aggressive, and this includes direct verbal as well as physical aggression. That is, even though it has also become clear that the social context has a great deal to do with how and whether aggression is expressed, boys overall have more frequent conflicts among themselves than girls do, and do more hitting, kicking, pushing, teasing, insulting, and attacking the property of others. Much of this work has been done with children between the ages of 3 and about 7, and it is in this age range that rough play and overt physical conflict are at their peak. The frequency of these forms of male interaction decreases through the school years (see summaries in Coie & Dodge, 1998; Ruble & Martin, 1998). The dropoff in physical aggression among boys occurs partly because boys make progress in impulse control, so that they less and less often react to perceived threats or insults from other boys with a quick surge of anger and an immediate hitting-out, as little boys are more likely to do. Also, boys put on muscle as they grow through middle childhood, becoming more and more capable of really hurting one another, so that physical fighting becomes more and more aversive (Coie & Dodge, 1998).

There may be another aspect of male aggression, one that tends to be overlooked. There is evidence that boys make up after a fight more quickly than girls do, so that conflict among them is less disruptive of ongoing group activity than it is among girls (Lagerspetz, Bjorkqvist, & Peltonen, 1988; Lever, 1976). DeWaal (1996) tells us that among chimpanzees:

> Males are the more hierarchical sex and reconcile more readily than females. Females are relatively peaceful, yet if they do engage in open conflict the chances of subsequent repair are low. Unlike males, females avoid confrontation with individuals with whom they enjoy close ties, such as offspring and best friends, whereas they let aggression run its destructive course in case of a fight with a rival. . . . In well-established groups, it is the males who go through frequent cycles of conflict and reconciliation, who test and confirm their hierarchy while at the same time preserving the unity that is required against neighboring communities. (p. 124)

DeWaal's writing alerts us to the fact that we must think of male aggression in the context of male group process. During human childhood and adolescence, coalitions of boys rely on each other for backup in disputes with other boys, and such coalitions become a primary means of maintaining status and avoiding victimhood, just as they are among nonhuman primates. (It is becoming clear that we have greatly exaggerated boys' need for autonomy—they do seek autonomy from adults, but seldom from each other—see Goldstein, 2001). Indeed, at least for some boys, male coalitions might be said to replace individual aggression or dominance strivings as the means to achieve and maintain status as boys grow into adolescence. At the same time, coalitions make aggression by *groups* of boys more possible and more effective.

What about the developmental progression for aggression in girls? We have less evidence about this than we have for boys, but what information we have suggests that for girls, as well as boys, there is a dropoff in direct aggression with age. Indeed, this dropoff begins earlier in girls, reflecting their earlier acquisition of productive language skills and more rapid progress in impulse control during the preschool and early childhood years. Cairns and colleagues (Cairns, Cairns, Neckerman, Ferguson, & Gariepy, 1989) report that, between the fourth and seventh grades, the dropoff in physical aggression for girls occurs primarily in their conflicts with boys; their conflicts with girls remain relatively low through this period.

The new findings from the Duneden longitudinal study (Moffitt, Caspi, Rutter, & Silva, 2002) are giving us some important new insights into the developmental trajectories for aggression and other antisocial behavior in the two sexes. This study is based on approximately 1,000 children growing up in Duneden, New Zealand. The children have been followed from birth to adulthood. The study finds that boys display considerably higher rates of physical aggression and violence at every age studied. Consistent with previous work, a dropoff in physical aggression is shown to occur for both boys and girls during the grade school years. Violent, assaultive acts, though they are rare at all ages, do increase in frequency from early to late adolescence, falling off in young adulthood. In adolescence, such acts tend to co-occur with such other antisocial behaviors as theft and the frequent use of drugs and alcohol.

Moffitt and colleagues are mainly concerned with a cluster of antisocial behavior of which aggression is one element. They make a distinction between children who show a persistent pathway of antisocial behavior from the preschool years into adulthood, and children for whom antisocial behavior emerges during adolescence and has a fairly brief time-course. The life-course-persistent children make up only a small minority of children, but in this group, the boys outnumber the girls by a ratio of 10 to 1. There are many more children who begin to show antisocial tendencies only in adolescence, and among the late-onset group, the sexes are much more similar—boys outnumber the girls by a ratio of only 1.5 to 1.

Among the adolescent girls, there were a few who were arrested or convicted of violent crimes. Moffitt (personal communication) describes three: Several girls whipped another girl with a chain; a group of girls set a Rottweiler to bite another girl; and a group of girls kidnapped a drunk girl from a pub and took her into the country at night and beat her, leaving her in a field. We should note that the victims of this violence were other girls, and the police notes indicate that these appeared to be fights over boyfriends. In case any reader may have doubted it, some girls are capable of real violence that goes far beyond the hair pulling that is our stereotype of female fighting. At the same time, it is demonstrably true that real violence outside the domestic context is far more rare in females than in males.

In our 1974 book *The Psychology of Sex Differences*, Carol Jacklin and I claimed that many of the alleged differences between the sexes had no basis in fact. However, we concluded that aggression was an exception: that there was solid evidence for males being the more aggressive sex. This conclusion was challenged by Tieger in 1980, and we (Maccoby & Jacklin, 1980) replied vigorously with further information and analysis that we believed clearly affirmed a robust sex difference in aggression. The material that I have been reviewing so far would certainly lead us to the same conclusion.

## INDIRECT, "SOCIAL," OR "RELATIONAL" AGGRESSION

In recent years, a different theme has emerged, suggesting that the claim for greater male aggression may have been resting on too narrow a definition of what constitutes aggression—that there are other ways by which individuals can hurt others, including by ignoring them or excluding them from desired social activities, trying to alienate their friends, and engaging in negative gossip about them. There has been increasing research attention to these subtler forms of aggression, variously termed indirect aggression, social aggression, and relational aggression (e.g., Cairns et al., 1989; Crick, 1997; Crick & Grotpeter, 1995; Galen & Underwood, 1997; Lagerspetz et al., 1988). In a number of these studies, girls were found to display subtle aggression at significantly higher levels than boys, with an upsurge in such behavior at the time of transition from childhood to adolescence.[2] Initially, these findings were sometimes interpreted as meaning that girls were fundamentally just as aggressive as boys—they only show it differently.

In fact, a finding that girls utilize indirect forms of aggression more than boys do—if it were reliably documented—would tell us nothing about which sex is more aggressive. So far we simply do not know whether the average frequency with which girls display indirect or "relational" aggression is comparable to the frequency with which boys display the forms of direct aggression more usually associated with males.

If we tried to make this comparison, we would certainly have trouble finding a comparable metric. Or we might consider which sex's aggression is more intense. But perhaps the question of which sex is more aggressive, or the issue of whether relational aggression should be weighed equally with direct overt aggression in some quantitative way, are not the most interesting questions to be asking. The work on the subtler forms of aggression is valuable whether or not it answers these questions. It has called our attention to two main points: Girls are not as unaggressive as we have believed, and there are qualitatively different forms in which aggression is expressed during childhood and youth. Therefore, we need to follow the development of more forms of expressing aggression than the direct forms that have been mainly studied until recently. These are compelling points that require our close attention.

## THE AGENDAS OF THE TWO SEXES

To return to an ethological theme, let me mention something I learned in a course on animal behavior in graduate school many years ago. It seems that in ungulates—deer, elk, wildebeest—adult males and females are alike in the way they attack a predator, such as a snake. They attack it with their hooves, which can be dangerous weapons indeed. When males have competitive fights over territory or females, however, they lower their heads and ram each other with their foreheads—something females are never seen to do—and use their horns, which only males possess. Here it is obvious: The two sexes have the same agendas when it comes to protecting themselves and the young from predators. But the male agenda also includes acquiring and protecting territory, and sequestering a harem—something that is not on the female agenda—and hence there is a whole segment of male aggression that is not found among females at all.

I want to argue that in human children too there are some different elements in the agendas the two sexes have for their interactions with same-sex peers. Each boy understands the importance of letting other boys know that he is willing to protect his own territory—his possessions, his personal space—from uninvited intrusion by other boys. Boys try hard to win in contests with other boys, and want to be seen as "tough"—at least tough enough so that they will not be victimized. Thus, there is more competition, more mock fighting, and occasionally real fighting, in boys' groups than girls' groups. Out of these conflicts a dominance hierarchy typically emerges, which produces some stability in male relationships and moderates fighting.

But there is another equally important element in the male agenda:

It is the establishment of coalitions for the purposes of carrying out group enterprises, sometimes in opposition to other male groups. This kind of cooperation is more common in boys' than in girls' groups, despite the fact that boys are more competitive among themselves. Girls prefer to interact in dyads or trios. Boys also usually have one or two best friends, though these friendships are not as intimate as girls', in the sense that they spend less time exchanging information about each other's lives and tend to know considerably less about their friends' families and histories. But in addition to their "best" friendships, after about age 5, boys typically have a group of more casual friends with whom they carry out joint activities.

This gender divergence is nicely illustrated in some recent work by Benenson and colleagues (Benenson, Apostolaris, & Parnass, 1997) They brought together groups composed of six previously acquainted children. Some groups were composed of six boys, others of six girls, and half the groups were made up of 4-year-olds, the other half of 6-year-olds. Each group was brought into a large playroom equipped with a variety of play materials. Dyadic interaction was common for children of both sexes, though pairs of girls typically sustained episodes of dyadic interaction considerably longer than pairs of boys. More interesting were the findings on coordinated group activity—meaning that several children were engaging in the same activity and integrating their actions with one another. This kind of group activity was relatively rare among 4-year-olds of both sexes. However, by the age of 6, the boys had dramatically increased their level of coordinated group activity, now spending three quarters of their time in such activity, while girls were spending only 16% of their time in this way.

I find these figures quite compelling, and they do point to the emergence of a new element in the agendas of male groups: namely, a growing readiness for collaborative group process. This is especially interesting in view of the well-established fact that discourse among girls is more collaborative (Leaper, 1991) so that girls are more responsive to their conversational (or argumentative) partners than boys are—something that is quite consistent with Benenson's finding that they can sustain dyadic interaction longer. I suspect, too, that girls' mutual responsiveness, and their greater understanding of each other's points of view, help them not to misattribute hostile intent to one another, as boys often do. But somehow girls' interpersonal sensitivity seldom seems to translate into groups of four or five girls getting together to accomplish something jointly, unless an outside structure, such as a school athletic program or a shared school assignment, puts them into a team situation.

I want to suggest that boys' groups empower them, through their joint endeavors, in ways that girls' responsiveness to each other does not

(Maccoby, 2002). When it comes to aggression, the implication is that boys have something to gain by mutually controlling aggression within the in-group, so as to be more effective in their joint activities and in their efforts to compete with or confront an out-group.

My main point here is that we have spent a great deal of time and effort examining sex differences. Now I think we would benefit by focusing more on each sex in its own terms. That is, we need to think about the topography of aggressive behavior in each sex, the specific contexts in which it occurs, and the purposes it appears to serve.

## THE MEANING AND CONTEXTS OF INDIRECT ("RELATIONAL") AGGRESSION

Let us, then, consider the subtler forms of aggression in these terms. It is difficult to find an apt word or phrase for the kind of aggression we want to talk about. All aggression, including physical fighting, is social. But in the currently accepted usage, the term *social aggression* has come to mean acts intended to inflict damage on a victim's social relationships or social status. But within this general category, some distinctions may be helpful. Xie, Cairns, and Cairns (2004) make a useful distinction between attacks on another's social relationships that are confrontational and those that are not. To say to another "I don't like you any more" or "I won't be your friend unless you . . . " are confrontational forms of social aggression, while gossiping behind the victim's back or alienating a third party from the victim are nonconfrontational (henceforth abbreviated as NC). The latter has been called "indirect aggression" by Lagerspetz and colleagues (1988) and "social aggression" in the Cairns project (Cairns & Cairns, 1994). Direct social aggression and NC social aggression have been combined under the heading "relational aggression" by Crick and Grotpeter (1995). Xie and colleagues make a case for distinguishing them. On the basis of their own work and that of others, they report that young people who are physically aggressive in childhood and early adolescence tend to do poorly in school, be unpopular with their peers, and subsequently engage in a variety of antisocial behaviors that get them into trouble with the law. None of these maladaptations are found in children and adolescents who frequently use NC social aggression in peer conflicts. Indeed, the NC socially aggressive children and adolescents (especially girls) tend to play a central role in their social networks.

Xie and colleagues (2004) point out that in confrontational aggression of any kind—including attacks on a victim's social relationships—the perpetrator's identity must be known, with the attendant risks of blame, revenge, or loss of status. In NC social aggression, not only can the perpetrator remain anonymous, but a connection to social networks is necessary. As Xie and colleagues say, it takes two to fight—confrontationally—but it takes at least three to gossip. They say it is no surprise, then, that reports of NC social aggression increase strongly in early adolescence[3] (Cairns et al., 1989), for it is at this time that children become more sophisticated in understanding the dynamics of social networks and more motivated to achieve status within them. Perhaps it is no surprise as well that the increase is typically especially strong among girls (see summary of evidence in Xie et al., 2004). Girls, after all, are typically more concerned about relationships—their own and others'—and are generally more sophisticated than boys in terms of their knowledge of other people's social ties. Thus, they are in a better position to manipulate these ties if they find it in their interests to do so. But they are also more vulnerable to being hurt when they are targeted. There is good evidence now that girls are considerably more upset when they are the victims of slights or put-downs from other girls; boys who are slighted by other boys tend to shrug off such treatment (Galen & Underwood, 1997)—or at least say that they do. In the usual case, the greater intimacy of girls' friendships makes them more vulnerable to betrayal when friendships break up and social networks shift.

It is an open question how useful the distinction between confrontational and NC social aggression will continue to be as new evidence comes in. In a recent paper (Xie, Swift, Cairns, & Cairns, 2002), we learn that these two kinds of social aggression are similar in some respects: for example, neither predicts high levels of subsequent antisocial behavior, as physical aggression does. But NC social aggression is associated with network centrality, and tends to be nonreactive and nonreciprocal, whereas confrontational social aggression is both.


## "GIRL TALK"

Girls' gossip has a different contextual meaning than gossip has among boys at this age. It occurs in the context of "girl talk." Girls spend considerably more time talking with their friends than boys do—indeed, girl talk rather mystifies boys. Penelope Eckert (1990) quotes a high school boy as saying:

> "I think girls just talk too much, you know, they—they talk constantly between themselves and—about every little thing. Guys, I don't think we talk about that much. (*What kinds of things do you talk about?*) Not much. Girls .. cars, parties, you know. I think girls talk about, you

know, every little relationship, every little thing that's ever happened, you know. (p. 91)

Yes, girls do talk more, and this starts early. Speaking now about what we know about girls in the United States and Britain, the hallmark of girls' friendships is talk—face-to-face and over the telephone—involving the sharing of confidences, as we all know, but much more. While it is true that much of girls' social time is spent with one or two best friends, girls do cluster together in larger groups as well, such as for slumber parties or as groups of young teens who go to the shopping malls together. What are pairs or groups of girls up to? What do they talk about? What is their agenda? Under what circumstances does talk turn into hurtful gossip or shunning of certain girls? We know woefully little about these things. But this form of aggression needs to be seen in the larger context of the processes going on in the social situations where they occur.

Xie and colleagues (2004) help us to uncover some of the dynamics of these processes. Their work suggests that the breakup of a dyadic friendship often involves a larger social network, and that instances of NC social aggression are embedded in the changing interpersonal relationships within this larger network. They give an example:

> Ellen, a fourth-grade participant, found herself being refused by a group of girls to play jump rope. She also noticed that her best friend—Katherine—tried to avoid her. It turned out that the group had just lost or ostracized two girls, and Katherine was made a member. The girls in that group did not approve of Katherine and Ellen being together any more. In the end, Katherine told Ellen that she would start sitting with that group of girls for lunch and she did not like Ellen any more. (p. 121)

In this instance, it appears that the group that was losing and acquiring members acted jointly, as a group, and we do not get a picture of leadership or dominance by any particular girl. However, as we have seen, there are certain girls who are centrally "embedded" in a girls' group (as reported by peers, and in terms of their self-reports), and these girls are more likely than others to be involved in NC social aggression Why? Xie and colleagues note that central girls are in a better position than others to recruit allies for the transmission of gossip. And their connections to each of the group members mean that they are more involved in conflicts among them—perhaps as mediator?—and play a larger role than other girls in influencing who shall be included in, or excluded from, the group. They speculate that central girls control and manipulate the social alignments within their group.

Core members of a dominant group may also be protected from social attacks. An example given by a fourth-grade girl:

> When Cindy started telling all these things about Stella, I told her not to
> do it, . . . cause if you're going to go ahead and talk about somebody,
> you know you're not gonna have any friends, cause you know many
> people like that friend and you don't, so who's going to like you if you
> don't like her. So I told her to stop and I just ignore her most of the time.
> (in Xie et al., 2004, p. 120)

Instances of protecting a core group member are rare among the reports
that Cairns and colleagues obtained from fourth- and seventh-grade girls,
but they do illustrate the impressive level of social sophistication that can
be reached by girls as they manage social aggression among themselves.

An especially insightful analysis of what is going on in girls' discourse comes from the work of Penelope Eckert (1996), an anthropolog-
ical linguist. Eckert spent two years closely sharing the school-day lives
of the older girls in a multiethnic elementary school, as they moved
through the fifth and sixth grades. She was with them in the classrooms,
in the corridors, in the girls' bathrooms, on the school buses, at sporting
events, at school social events. She became an accepted part of the scen-
ery, so that her note taking and tape recording came to be largely ignored. She "listened in" on girls' conversations in all these settings.

Eckert sees gender as something that is co-constructed along with
other aspects of identity in what she calls a "community of practice," in
which a group of people develop shared ways of doing things, shared
ways of talking, and shared beliefs and values. In the age period from
about 11 through 13, children are engaged in a transition from a mainly
same-sex social order to a heterosexual one involving what Eckert calls
*mutual and conscious gender differentiation*, when "boys appropriate
arenas for the production of accomplishment, and girls move into the
elaboration of stylized selves" (p. 184). Girls stop running, she says, and
become engaged in the technology of beauty and personality, involving
new attention to hairstyles and makeup, clothes, and new ways of walk-
ing. What Eckert saw was the formation of a loose, amorphous heterosexual grouping of children in a central area of the playground. The
membership shifted from day to day, and there were some children who
never joined it at all. From time to time girls who were members of this
group would split off into pairs or into larger groups of girls who would
conspicuously walk around talking, and what they talked about had to
do with who was in and who was out, or which boys "liked" which girls
and vice versa. Anything having to do with heterosexuality was seen by
both boys and girls as a girls' pastime—girls are the experts, the arrang-

ers, and boys are passive participants at best. As an example: One boy broke up with his girlfriend of 6 months because her friends asked him to—they wanted to punish her for being a "bitch." Eckert says: "Girls become heighteners of the social, breathing excitement into heretofore normal everyday people and situations . . . and propelling themselves into the public arena" (p. 185). In other words, a whole arena of personal feelings and affiliations that were private now become public.

To me, Eckert's account rings true. If she is right, it becomes clear why many girls are more upset than boys over slights and exclusions. We have to be aware, of course, that this account is based on participant observation in a single school at a single 2-year period of time. But its great virtue is that it alerts us to the importance of trying to understand what the enterprise is that girls are engaged in when NC social aggression occurs. It would be very profitable, I believe, if we were to take this question as a major item on our research agenda.

Equally interesting, I think is the question of why some girls stay out of this arena of female excitement and tension. What are the consequences of steering clear of it, or becoming involved only much later in adolescence? And, for those who are involved at the usual time (early adolescence), why do some girls, but not others, use NC social aggression as a means of attaining their social objectives? The recent spurt of media attention to "mean girls" has seemed to imply that girls' attacking and undermining other girls is very widespread—that many or even most girls engage in it fairly often. I suspect this is a considerable exaggeration. Also, the media hype about "alpha" girls puts a male template on female group behavior that probably does not fit—what girls are doing when they are being mean probably is not a matter of an alpha girl seeking to maintain dominance in a same-sex hierarchy, the way it would be for an alpha male. Yes, girls are concerned about their status, but status for girls may be more a matter of popularity or some degree of celebrity in the eyes of peers of both sexes. But this is speculation—we simply have not studied things from this point of view.

I have been insisting that males are the more aggressive sex when it comes to direct physical or verbal confrontations. It is time for us to pay close attention to a very robust exception: Things are different when it comes to domestic violence. The comprehensive review by Moffit and colleagues (2002) indicates that women are at least as involved as men in initiating or sustaining fights with domestic partners. Their domestic aggression includes verbal abuse, threatening, hitting, pushing, and throwing objects, and women are not always—or even usually—doing this in self-defense. Recent data indicate that all this is presaged by what happens between dating couples (see Capaldi, Kim, & Shortt, Chapter 11, this volume).

## OVERVIEW

In this chapter I have argued that gender is indeed socially constructed, and that much of the construction goes on in sex-segregated play groups that are relatively unconstrained by adult influence. I have also argued that the twin processes of social construction and biological influences are not in any way incompatible; rather, that they coexist and interact as development proceeds. One fascinating question is whether and how biological factors can be implicated in the way individuals select, and are influenced by, certain categories of others.

Same-sex playmates amplify in one another certain behaviors that may be quite subdued in other contexts. We know much more about these processes among boys than among girls. But it is safe to say that in their same-sex groups, both boys and girls appear to be enacting some gender-specific agendas—agendas that change markedly with age. Let me stress that during many of their daily activities, children are usually *not* engaged in enacting these sex-differentiated themes, so that much of the time gender differences may fade to insignificance. Until recently, much of the research on childhood aggression in the two sexes has simply compared boys and girls in terms of how they differ on a broad personality trait of aggressiveness or, more broadly, antisocial tendencies. I believe this kind of work aggregates too broadly. I want to urge that we now concentrate on studying each sex individually in its own terms, trying to identify a set of sex-distinctive agendas and the social contexts in which they are most likely to be enacted. Once we understand these things more fully, we should have better insights into the role aggression plays in the social development of the two sexes.

### NOTES

1. "Social" or "relational" aggression was not coded in the Martin and Fabes work. It would be interesting to know whether, when girls play with other girls, these forms of aggression increase or decrease.
2. There are a number of studies in which a sex difference in social or relational aggression has not been found; indeed, in some studies boys have been found to display this behavior at higher rates than girls. Much depends on what behaviors are included in the category, and how they are assessed. See Underwood (2003) and Crick, Casas, and Nelson (2002) for summaries of studies.
3. Cairns and colleagues assessed social aggression by asking preteens and adolescents to describe two recent conflicts with peers: one with a same-sex peer, one with an other-sex peer. The descriptions were coded for themes of physical aggression and social aggression (rejection from a clique, negative gossip, and alienation of affection). This method does not, of course, permit estimating the frequency with which these different kinds of aggression occur, but it does permit tracing changes with time in the predomin-

ance of a given aggressive theme for the recent conflicts that were salient enough for subjects to choose to describe them.

# REFERENCES

Benenson J. F., Apostolaris, N. H., & Parnass, J. (1997). Age and sex differences in dyadic and group inter-action. *Developmental Psychology, 33,* 538–543.

Cairns, R. B., & Cairns, B. D. (1994). *Lifelines and risks: Passages of youth in our time.* New York: Cambridge University Press

Cairns, R. B., Cairns, B. D., Neckerman, H. J., Ferguson, L. I., & Gariepy, J. L. (1989). Growth and aggression: 1. Childhood to early adolescence. *Developmental Psychology, 25,* 320–330.

Coie, J. D., & Dodge, K. A. (1998). Aggression and anti-social behavior. In W. Damon & N. Eisenberg (Eds.), *Handbook of child psychology: Vol. 3. Social, emotional, and personality development* (5th ed., pp. 779–862). New York: Wiley.

Crick, N. R. (1997). Relational and overt aggression in preschool. *Developmental Psychology, 33,* 579–588.

Crick, N. R., Casas, J. F., & Nelson, D. A. (2002) Toward a more comprehensive understanding of peer maltreatment: Studies of relational victimization. *Current Directions in Psychological Science, 11,* 98–101.

Crick, N. R., & Grotpeter, J. K. (1995). Relational aggression, gender, and social-psychological adjustment. *Child Development, 66,* 710–722.

DeWaal, F. (1996). *Good natured: The origins of right and wrong in humans and other animals.* Cambridge, MA: Harvard University Press

Eckert, P. (1990). Cooperative competition in adolescent "girl talk." *Discourse Processes, 13,* 91–122.

Eckert, P. (1996). Vowels and nail polish: The emergence of linguistic style in the preadolescent heterosexual marketplace. In J. Ahlers, L. Bilmes, M. Chen, M. Oliver, H. Warner, & S. Wertheim (Eds.), *Gender and belief systems* (pp. 183–190). Berkeley, CA: Berkeley Women and Language Group.

Fabes, R. A., Martin, C. L., & Hanish, L. D. (2003). Young children's play qualities in same-, other-, and mixed-sex peer groups. *Child Development, 74,* 921–932.

Galen, B. R., & Underwood, M. K. (1997). A developmental investigation of social aggression among children. *Developmental Psychology, 33,* 589–600.

Goldstein, J. (2001). *War and gender.* Cambridge, UK: Cambridge University Press.

Greeno, K. (1989). *Gender differences in children's proximity to adults.* Unpublished doctoral dissertation, Department of Psychology, Stanford University.

Lagerspetz, K. M. J., Bjorkqvist, K., & Peltonen, T. (1988). Is indirect aggression typical of females? Gender differences in aggressiveness in 11–12-year-old children. *Aggressive Behavior, 14,* 303–315.

Leaper, C. (1991). Influence and involvement in children's discourse: Age, gender and partner effects. *Child Development, 62,* 797–811.

Lever, J. (1976). Sex differences in the games children play. *Social Problems, 23,* 478–487.

Maccoby, E. E. (1998). *The two sexes: Growing up apart, coming together.* Cambridge, MA: Harvard University Press.

Maccoby, E. E. (2002). Gender and group process: A developmental perspective. *Current Directions in Psychological Science, 11,* 54–58.

Maccoby, E. E., & Jacklin, C. N. (1980). Sex differences in aggression: A rejoinder and reprise. *Child Development, 51,* 964–980.

Maccoby, E. E., & Jacklin, C. N. (1974). *The psychology of sex differences.* Stanford, CA: Stanford University Press.

Martin, C. L., & Fabes, R. A. (2001). The stability and consequences of young children's same-sex peer interactions. *Developmental Psychology, 37,* 431–446.

Moffitt, T. E., Caspi, A., Ruttter, M., & Silva, P. A. (2002). *Sex differences in antisocial behaviour, conduct disorder, and violence in the Duneden Longitudinal Study.* Cambridge, UK: Cambridge University Press

Nicolopoulou, A. (1997). Worldmaking and identity formation in children's narrative play-acting. In B. Cox & C. Lightfoot (Eds.), *Sociogenic perspectives in internalization* (pp. 157–187). Hillsdale, NJ: Erlbaum.

Ruble, D. N., & Martin, C. L. (1998). Gender development. In W. Damon & N. Eisenberg (Eds.), *Handbook of child psychology: Vol. 3. Social, emotional and personality development* (5th ed., pp. 933–1016). New York: Wiley.

Tieger, T. (1980). On the biological basis of sex differences in aggression. *Child Development, 51,* 943–963.

Underwood, M. K. (2003). *Social aggression among girls.* New York: Guilford Press.

Wallen, K. (1996). Nature needs nurture: The interaction of hormonal and social influences on the development of behavioral sex differences in rhesus monkeys. *Hormones and Behavior, 30,* 364–378.

Weizmann, T. M., & Pardue, M. (Eds.). (2001). *Exploring the biological contributions to human health: Does sex matter?* Washington, DC: Board on Health Sciences Policy, Institute of Medicine, National Academy Press.

Xie, H., Cairns, B. D., & Cairns, R. B. (2004). The development of aggressive behaviors among girls: Measurement issues, social functions and differential trajectories. In D. J. Pepler, K. Madsen, C. Webster, & K. Levene (Eds.), *The development and treatment of girlhood aggression* (pp. 103–134). Mahwah, NJ: Erlbaum.

Xie, H., Swift, D. J., Cairns, B. D., & Cairns, R. B. (2002). Aggressive behavior in social interaction: A narrative analysis of interpersonal conflicts during early adolescence. *Social Development, 11,* 205–224.

# CHAPTER 2

# Biology–Behavior Integration and Antisocial Behavior in Girls

Elizabeth J. Susman *and* Kathleen Pajer

The biological factors involved in research on female violence and aggressive behavior have largely been ignored until recently. Past research rarely examined biological issues as influences on and consequences of the most hurtful of human behavior. When biological issues were the focus of inquiry, the inclusion of women in these studies was a rarity. The marked absence of such research is due to a combination of theoretical, methodological, and sociopolitical issues.

The purpose herein is to present a developmental perspective on the relationship between biological substances and processes and aggressive and antisocial behavior in girls. The term "antisocial behavior" refers to externalizing behavior problems, conduct disorder symptoms, delinquency, and violence. We propose that the best way to understand female antisocial behavior is to understand the dialectical nature of the interactions between biological, psychological, and contextual processes. The chapter presents a brief history of the research on biological processes and aggressive and antisocial behavior, discusses basic theoretical and physiological principles related to biobehavioral development and antisocial behavior, presents findings on endocrine parameters of antisocial behavior, and suggests future directions that will inform research, prevention, and clinical practice.

## HISTORY OF BIOLOGICAL ISSUES
## AND ANTISOCIAL BEHAVIOR

Despite the voluminous literature on aggressive and antisocial behavior, there was a paucity of biological research on the topic until two decades ago. Innovative studies now focus on complex biological parameters, but the number of these studies remains relatively low and the number that includes females is even lower. Moreover, one of the limitations of the current body of work is that many of the studies examine various types of aggression rather than the complex set of behaviors used to designate individuals as antisocial. Because there is little research specifically on biological factors in antisocial behavior and because many antisocial individuals also demonstrate destructive aggression, both types of studies are reviewed in this chapter.

The first studies of biological factors in aggressive behavior were conducted in adult human males. Hypotheses derived from male rat model studies showed a positive correlation between aggressive behavior and testosterone levels. Studies of cortisol, corticotropin-releasing hormone (CRH), serotonin, and autonomic nervous system (ANS) functioning (heart rate and heart rate variability) followed shortly thereafter. Simultaneous with studies of adult males, male and female adolescents became the focus of studies that assessed hormones and aggressive behavior, hostile emotions, and sexual activity (Susman & Petersen, 1992). The models tended to be correlational, cross sectional, and relatively atheoretical, but the inclusion of females was noteworthy. Recent reviews tally the findings and rapid progress in the biosocial aspects of antisocial behavior (Archer, 1991; Mazur & Booth, 1998; Raine, 2002; Raine, Brennan, Farrington, & Mednick, 1997; Stoff, Breiling, & Mazur, 1997; Susman & Finkelstein, 2001). Currently, studies continue to link genetic, endocrine, neurotransmitter, neural structures, and ANS functioning with antisocial behavior. Females are included in some but not all of these studies. The inclusion of contextual factors, like neighborhoods, as moderators or mediators of biological processes and antisocial behavior add an important new dimension to the history of biosocial research on antisocial behavior.

### Why Do We Know So Little about the Biology of Antisocial Behavior in Girls?

A metatheoretical issue imposing on the entire area of biosocial issues and antisocial behavior is that biology was considered to be irrelevant to the development and progression of antisocial behavior. Under the predominance of the psychology of the individual and contextualism in the last few decades, antisocial behavior was considered to result from endogenous psychological or exogenous environmental factors. Endogenous factors included hostility and mental health disorders, and exogenous factors included parental attitudes and practices, deviant peer influences, and dangerous and impoverished neighborhoods. Inherent in psychological and contextual metamodels was the belief that biological factors are deterministic. Recent perspectives on the biology of aggression include the concept of reciprocal determinism, which is the notion that biological, psychological, and contextual factors are mutually interactive and causal.

However, beyond the fact that biological processes were not considered important in the genesis or treatment of antisocial behavior, there are two reasons that antisocial females were barely studied at all. First, there was an assumption that girls were not aggressive. This assumption was based on the fact that girls are rarely arrested for aggressive or violent crimes. Physical aggression, delinquency, and criminal acts are much more prevalent in males that in females. Therefore, the justice system and research emphasis was on physical aggression and violent behavior in males, which led to the systematic exclusion of females, as their low levels of antisocial behavior posed less threat to society (Ahnsjo, 1941; Baker, Mack, Moffitt, & Mednick, 1989; Cowie, Cowie, & Slater, 1968a, 1968b; Gibbens & Prince, 1967; Glueck & Glueck, 1934).

However, it is now clear that the rate of physical aggression in girls is rising and that even when girls do not directly commit aggressive acts, they may use others to do so (Campbell, 1986; Litt, 1995; Loper & Cornell, 1996; Molidor, 1996; Office of Juvenile Justice and Delinquency Prevention, 1996; Poe-Yamasata & Butts, 1996; Russell, 1985). Beginning in the 1980s, Langerspetz (Langerspetz, Bjorkqvist, & Peltonen, 1988) and then others (Bjorkqvist, 1994; Crick, 1996; Goodman & Kohlsdorf, 1994; Zoccolillo, 1993) increasingly recognized relational aggression as a predominant phenotype in girls, especially in adolescents. Relational aggression includes threatening to withdraw friendship, using social exclusion and hostile accusations, and backbiting verbal abuse (Crick, 1996; Crick & Grotpeter, 1995). Ignored also was how male- and female-typical antisocial behavior may have similar biological correlates. The second reason females have been omitted from research on biological factors in antisocial behavior is that scientists assumed that menstrual cycle variations in hormones would hopelessly confound the relationship between biological parameters and antisocial behavior. This conclusion likely was derived from the fact that sex steroids (estradiol and testosterone) vary systematically with the phase of the menstrual cycle. Typical of the change in hormone concentrations is a rise in estrogen that begins around day 6 to 7 of the menstrual cycle, a peak at midcycle, and then a gradual decline until the onset of menstruation. These variations are known to be related to changes in cognition and moods and are similarly expected to either accentuate or decrease the probability of antisocial behavior. However, the effect of the menstrual cycle on hormone levels is quite predictable (indeed the absence of this relationship may be significant), and we now know that the effect of the menstrual cycle can be controlled in either the design or in post hoc analyses.

## THEORETICAL PRINCIPLES: MODELS OF BIOBEHAVIORAL DEVELOPMENT

### Contextualism

The interest in contextual influences on development (peer, family, and neighborhood), developmental contextualism (Lerner, 1998), parallels lifespan developmental theory. The lifespan perspective is concerned with the embeddedness of evolution and ontogeny, consistency and change, human plasticity, and the role a developing person plays in his or her own development (Lerner, 1987). Thus, a lifespan perspective played a formative role in the genesis of contextualism, a concept that integrates biological and psychological levels with the contextual levels of analysis. The influence of contextual factors on antisocial behavior considers both structural and functional aspects of the environment (Sampson, Raudenbush, & Earls, 1997) but does not integrate the biological level of functioning.

### Reciprocal Interaction and Bidirectionality

The configural, or systems, and bidirectional perspectives view processes from different levels as having equal potencies in development (Cairns, 1997; Lerner, 1998; Magnusson & Stattin, 1998; Susman, 1997, 1998). The biological changes that transpire in development both influence and reciprocally are influenced by psychological, behavioral, and social processes (Lerner, 1987; Lerner & Foch, 1987). A more descriptive term for bidirectionality is dynamic integration, as the latter refers to the constantly changing relations among the levels of analysis. For instance, genes no longer are considered static deterministic influences on development. Rather, genes require a specific environment in which to be expressed.

Magnusson (1999) brings together the concepts of contextualism, reciprocal interaction, and bidirectionality in his metamodel of holistic interactionism. A basic proposition of an interactionism framework is that the individual is an active, intentional part of an integrated complex, continuous, dynamic, and reciprocal and adaptive person–environment system from the fetal period until death (Magnusson, 1999; Magnusson & Cairns, 1996). Novel patterns of functioning arise during ontogeny, and differences in the rates of development, like differences in the nature of aggressive or delinquent episodes, may produce differences in the organization and configuration of psychological functions that are extremely sensitive to the environmental circumstances in which they are formed (Magnusson & Cairns, 1996). It follows that biological development will be sensitive to experiences and proximal environments.

Consistent with the holistic interactionism perspective, the developmental *integration* model views antisocial development as a product of a complex genotype, brain–behavior–biology and contextual integration that varies between males and females. Nonetheless, in both males and females, processes at different levels of functioning are not independent but are merged in a holistic manner. A developmental integration model does not imply that all aspects of antisocial behavior need to be considered simultaneously. Rather, the developmental integration model, like the developmental contextual and holistic interactionism models, acts as a guide for selecting constructs and measures at different levels of analysis. Within these perspectives, developmental processes are accessible to systematic, scientific inquiry since they occur in a specific way within organized structures and are guided by specific principles that are finite (Magnusson & Stattin, 1998). Critical to integration models is the interpretation of findings at one level of functioning in relation to levels above and below the level of empirical verification. For instance, in the case of examining complex antisocial behaviors, biological or psychological levels of empirical verification can only be meaningfully interpreted in relation to contextual processes.

The functioning of a person, then, can be viewed as a product of phenomena of life existing at numerous levels: inner-biological, individual-psychological, peer network, community, societal, cultural, and the larger physical ecology and historical context. A dynamic integration perspective focuses on the simultaneous fusion among these levels of analysis, such as the integration of hypothalamic, pituitary, and gonadal hormones and physical and psychological changes. Unfortunately, when biological processes are included in research, measures representing only one biological system tend to be considered—that is, hormones, neurotransmitters, or psychophysiological measures—a strategy that fails to consider the dynamic, systemic, and holistic nature of human functioning. Thus, conclusions regarding the interconnections between biological processes and aggressive and antisocial behavior are relatively simplistic, even though multidimensional behaviors, attitudes, and various forms of violent behavior are immeasurably complex.

## BIOLOGICAL BASIS FOR
## HYPOTHESIZED SEX DIFFERENCES

Biological sex differences can originate from initial chromosomal differences at fertilization, are followed by development of gonadal sex, and culminate in the emergence of secondary sexual characteristics (George, 1996). Chromosomal sex refers to the genotype for males (46 XY) and females (46 XX). Gonadal sex refers to the structures that comprise the internal structures of the reproductive system that are apparent at week 4 of human embryogenesis. Secondary sexual characteristics refer to development of pubic hair in boys and girls and breast and genital development in females and males, respectively, that emerge at puberty. These differences collectively constitute male and female phenotypes.

Sexual differentiation of the brain relevant to antisocial behavior is not well understood compared to differentiation of the reproductive system; thus, it is difficult to link brain structures and functioning with antisocial behavior. Nonetheless, advances in the science of brain development have identified sex differences in brain areas that may be involved in antisocial behavior: prefrontal cortex (Duff & Hampson, 2001), limbic nucleus (Kruijver et al., 2000), caudate and amygdala (Durston et al., 2001), and other area brain regions, as well as brain functioning (Segovia et al., 1999).

The systems implicated in antisocial behavior include the ANS, the endocrine system, neurotransmitter systems, and other lesser examined systems (for reviews, see Brain & Susman [1997]; Raine, [2002]; Susman & Finkelstein [2001]). The focus herein primarily is on the endocrine system and antisocial behavior, as the few studies in females that integrate the biology of antisocial behavior examined hormones of gonadal or adrenal origin. New evidence implicates neurohormones, hormones synthesized in the brain rather than in peripheral sites, as influences on sexually dimorphic antisocial behavior. It is currently not feasible to examine the contribution of neurally derived hormones to antisocial behavior; however, future research will undoubtedly reveal a significant function for neurosteroids in sexual differentiation of the brain–behavior relationship.

### The Endocrine System and Antisocial Behavior

The primary function of the endocrine system is to regulate metabolic processes by means of a group of chemical messengers called hormones. A second regulatory system, the neural system, regulates metabolic processes through electrochemical systems. The endocrine and neural systems interact by neural substances (e.g., locus ceruleus) that control secretion of hormones. For instance, hypothalamic releasing factors regulate the secretion of epinephrine of adrenomedullary origin and cortisol from adrenocortical origin under stressful conditions. The two endocrine systems most frequently linked to antisocial behavior are the hypothalamic–pituitary–gonadal (HPG) (testosterone and estrogen) and hypothalamic–pituitary–adrenal (HPA) (cortisol) systems.

## Testosterone and Estrogen

The steroid hormone testosterone is implicated in physical aggression in animals and antisocial behavior in humans (for reviews, see Archer [1991]; Brain [1994]; Brain & Susman [1997]; Mazur & Booth [1998]; Susman & Finkelstein [2001]). The positive relationship between testosterone and aggressive behavior is hypothesized to be derived from pre- and early postnatal organizational effects of hormones on brain development, although recent speculation is that hormones can affect brain functioning at any period of development. The argument for the relationship between testosterone and aggressive behavior is that since males are exposed to higher concentrations of androgens than females during pre- and postnatal development and onward, and males express more physical aggression and violence than females, androgens are implicated in the higher levels of aggressive behavior and dominance in males than in females (Brain, 1994; Mazur & Booth, 1998). Since testosterone levels rise at puberty and externalizing behavior problems concurrently rise in boys, it follows that testosterone is hypothesized to influence aggressive behavior in boys at puberty.

The empirical evidence linking testosterone and aggressive and dominant behavior in males is somewhat consistent across studies. In females, testosterone is too infrequently examined to unequivocally evaluate its relationship to antisocial behavior. In those instances when testosterone was considered in females, higher levels of testosterone were positively related to current smoking and intensity of smoking (Martin et al., 2001), coitus (Halpern, Udry, & Suchindran, 1997), and aggressive dominance in incarcerated women (Dabbs & Hargrove, 1997). Testosterone also was higher among delinquent young women than in college students (Banks & Dabbs, 1996). In early adolescent girls, testosterone was not related to aggressive problem behaviors (Susman et al., 1987), negative affect (Brooks-Gunn & Warren, 1989), dominance and conflict in interactions with parents (Inoff-Germain et al., 1988), or free play aggressive behavior (Sanchez-Martin et al., 2000). The lack of relationships between testosterone and the various forms of antisocial behavior to some extent likely reflects the measurement of male rather than female phenotypic antisocial behavior. Alternatively, testosterone

levels are low in young adolescent girls compared to boys, thereby re-
stricting variability and reducing the power of correlations to capture
significant relationships.

Estrogens are less frequently examined in relation to antisocial
behavior compared to testosterone. Of note is that girls with higher concentrations of estradiol ($E_2$) were likely to show greater dominance while
interacting with their parents than girls with lower levels (Inoff-Germain
et al., 1988). Estrogen is likely to have indirect effects on antisocial
behavior in girls. Estrogen is involved in breast development and onset
of menarche at puberty. Increases in estrogen and related menarche occur earlier in some girls than in others. The *early maturational or early
timing hypothesis* (e.g., Brooks-Gunn, Peterson, & Eichorn, 1985; Caspi
& Moffit, 1991; Petersen & Taylor, 1980; Tschann et al., 1994) posits
that being an early developer is especially disadvantageous for girls
(Stattin & Magnusson, 1990). Girls who have early breast development
and menarche, that is, early timing of puberty relative to same-age peers,
are prone to exhibit behavior problems (Caspi & Moffitt, 1991) and affiliation with older (Stattin & Magnusson, 1990) and deviant peers (Ge,
Brody, Conger, Simmons, & Murry, 2002; Ge, Conger, & Elder, 1996).
One explanation for antisocial behavior in early timing girls is that these
girls interact with older and more deviant peers. Alternatively, estrogen
may have direct effects on the brain that influence impulsive or non-
reflective behavior. The extensive distribution of estrogen receptors in
the brain suggests that estrogens can influence a variety of behaviors.

Although sex steroids are inconsistently linked to antisocial behavior in correlational observational studies, the causal influence of sex steroid levels on antisocial behavior cannot be inferred. An experimental
design is the preferred method for establishing a cause–effect relationship between hormones and antisocial behavior. To examine the causal
influence of sex steroids on behavior, physiological doses of testosterone
(boys) or estrogen (Premarin) (girls) were administered to delayed puberty boys and girls, respectively, in a placebo-controlled, randomized,
double-blind, crossover design study (Finkelstein et al., 1997, 1998;
Kulin et al., 1997; Liben et al., 2002; Schwab et al., 2001; Susman et al.,
1998). Each 3-month treatment period was preceded and followed by a
3-month placebo period. The doses of gonadal steroids were calculated
to simulate concentrations in blood in healthy early (low dose), middle
(middle dose) and late (high dose) pubertal adolescents. Aggressive
behavior was assessed by self-reports about physical and verbal aggression, aggression against peers and adults, aggressive impulses and
aggressive inhibitory behaviors. Significant increases in self-reported aggressive impulses and in physical aggression against both peers and
adults were seen in girls at the low and middle dose but not at the high

dose of estrogen (Finkelstein et al., 1997). In contrast, in boys, significant increases in aggressive impulses and physical aggression against peers and adults were reported, but only at the middle dose of testosterone. Administering midpubertal levels of testosterone to hypogonadal boys, but not girls, resulted in significantly increased self-reports of nocturnal emissions, touching girls, and being touched by girls (Finkelstein et al., 1998). There were no effects for testosterone treatment on behavior problems in boys, but increases in estrogen were paralleled by increases in withdrawal behavior in girls (Susman et al., 1998). Significant is that experimental treatment with estrogen resulted in increases in aggressive behavior in girls at lower doses than was required for testosterone doses in boys. This dose response pattern suggests that girls are more sensitive to the rise in estrogen than boys are to the rise in testosterone during puberty.

## Adrenal Androgens

The adrenal glands are the major source of androgens in girls during early adolescence. Adrenal androgens begin to rise at adrenarche, which refers to the activation of adrenal androgen production from the zona reticularis between ages 6 and 9 (Ibáñez, Dimartino-Nardi, Potau, & Saenger, 2000). Continuing into gonadarche, the adrenal androgens rise before declining with advancing age. The adrenal androgens are dehydroepiandrosterone (DHEA) and its sulfated form (DHEAS) and androstenedione ($\Delta$4A). In healthy pubertal-age girls (Brooks-Gunn & Warren, 1989), higher DHEAS correlated negatively with aggressive affect. The interaction between negative life events and DHEAS and aggressive affect also was significant. Girls with lower concentrations of DHEAS who experienced negative life events had more aggressive affect than girls with fewer negative life events. In a parallel study of 9- to 14-year-old healthy boys and girls, there was a relatively consistent pattern of higher DHEA and ($\Delta$4A and lower DHEAS and problem behaviors (Nottelmann et al., 1987; Nottelmann, Inoff-Germain, Susman, & Chrousos, 1990; Susman et al., 1987; Susman, Dorn, & Chrousos, 1991). Adrenal androgens also were correlated in girls with dominance while interacting with their parents (Inoff-Germain et al., 1988). The links between adrenal androgens and problem behavior extended to sexual behavior as well. Higher levels of adrenal androgens were related to girls' sexual behavior and activities during adolescence (Udry & Talbert, 1988). Additional support for the relationship between adrenal androgens and behavior problems was reported in girls with early adrenarche. These girls had higher levels of adrenal androgens and more behavior problems than the on-time adrenarche girls (Dorn, Hitt, & Rotenstein,

1999). Although adrenal androgens have a weaker binding affinity compared to testosterone, the relationship between adrenal androgens and antisocial behavior in girls appears to parallel the relationships between testosterone and aggressive behavior in males.

Overall, the findings demonstrate the associations between sex steroids, adrenal androgens, and aggressive and antisocial behavior. There remain few studies of the biology of antisocial behavior in girls. In studies that have included girls there are null findings in some and inconsistent findings across other studies. For instance, testosterone was related to antisocial and violent behavior but not to lesser forms of antisocial behavior, like aggressive behavior, in children and adolescents. Carefully selected gender-typical measures of antisocial behavior in future observational and clinical trial studies undoubtedly will uncover unique relationships between testosterone, estrogen, and adrenal androgens and antisocial behavior in girls. The current interest in gender-typical phenotypic types of antisocial behavior, such as relational aggression, is likely to lead to greater specification of the integration of hormones and behavior in girls.

## The Role of Serotonin in Antisocial Behavior

It is becoming apparent that the neurotransmitter serotonin (5-HT) also has an important role in the relationships between the HPA and HPG axes and behavior problems (Coccaro, Kavoussi, & Hauger, 1995; Higley et al., 1996; Hoi-Por, Olsson, Westberg, Melke, & Eriksson, 2001; Matykiewicz, Grange, Vance, Wang, & Reyes, 1997; Modai et al., 1989; Moffitt et al., 1998; Rubinow, Schmidt, & Roca, 1998; Virkkunen, Nuutila, Goodwin, & Linnoila, 1987). Some data on women do exist. Constantino, Morris, and Murphy (1997) reported that the levels of 5-hydroxyindoleacetic acid (5-HIAA, the primary metabolite of 5-HT) in cerebrospinal fluid were significantly lower in the offspring of mothers who were categorized as antisocial than in nonantisocial mothers. Tryptophan (the dietary precursor for serotonin) depletion during the luteal phase of the menstrual cycle increases premenstrual aggression in women (Bond, Wingrove, & Critchlow, 2001). Buspirone, a $5\text{-HT}_{1a}$ agonist, produced a blunted prolactin response in violent (including females) compared to nonviolent parolees (Cherek, Moeller, Kahn-Dawood, Swann, & Lane, 1999), indicating lower 5-HT levels in the violent parolees. Coccarro and colleagues have demonstrated that men and women with aggressive character disorders (including antisocial personality disorder) have lower 5-HT (Coccaro, Kavoussi, Sheline, Berman, & Csernansky, 1997; New et al., 1997).

Similarly, data derived from animal model studies suggest the existence of a complex relationship between 5-HT, the neuroendocrine system, and aggression in females. Reduced extracellular levels of 5-HT were found in the amygdala of aggressive female rats, but *only* in those who had been exposed to elevated levels of androgens in the neonatal period (Sunblad & Eriksson, 1997). Intruder aggression in female rats is abolished by ovariectomy, but is diminished by fluoxetine, a selective serotonin reuptake inhibitor that raises serotonin levels. As discussed earlier, the social context may be a particularly important moderator of neuroendocrine–behavioral processes in females. Female macaque monkeys who were socially subordinate to other females and males were more likely to have low cerebrospinal fluid 5-HIAA levels. These monkeys were significantly more likely to engage in spontaneous, aggressive wounding inappropriate to the social context, whereas the dominant females who engaged in higher rates of competitive aggression (for food or males) were more likely to have high cerebrospinal fluid 5-HIAA levels. Overall, these revealing new findings suggest that at the neurotransmitter level, the biology of males and females is remarkably similar.

## The Physiology of Stress and Antisocial Behavior

Recent reports reveal that attenuation of basal cortisol levels is related to antisocial behavior in children, adolescents, and adults. Attenuation of cortisol levels is indicative of low ANS arousal. The majority of these studies included only males. Cortisol levels are lower in aggressive and antisocial males (Bergman & Brismar, 1994; Vanyukov et al., 1993; Virkunnen, 1985), prepubertal boys of parents with a substance use disorder (Moss, Vanyukov, & Martin, 1995), and in boys with disruptive behavior disorder (McBurnett et al., 1991; McBurnett, Lahey, Rathouz, & Loeber, 2000). In a few studies, hyperresponsivity of the HPA axis is related positively to antisocial behavior (e.g., Fishbein, Dax, Lozovsky, & Saffe, 1992). In a study that compared boys and girls, anticipating and then experiencing a stressful event (Susman, Dorn, Inoff-Germain, Nottelmann, & Chrousos, 1997), low basal cortisol levels predicted antisocial behavior 1 year later in girls as well as in boys.

The paradigm shift toward interest in antisocial behavior in girls has led to a serious examination of attenuation of basal cortisol levels in antisocial girls. Pajer, Gardner, Kirillova, and Vanyukov (2001) report that girls with conduct disorder diagnoses had significantly lower cortisol levels than girls in the comparison group across three early morning plasma samples. The differences were not due to methodological factors such as demographic characteristics, use of oral contraceptives, antidepressants, or season. A second study included girls with varying rates of neurobehavioral disinhibition (Pajer et al., 2001). This construct of neurobehavioral disinhibition includes neuropsychological, psychological, and behavioral features of antisocial behavior, with a high score indicating poor functioning. Saliva cortisol levels were significantly negatively correlated with neurobehavioral disinhibition in girls. Girls with low cortisol were characterized by poor executive cognitive function, lack of empathy, impulsivity, and aggression. Pajer and colleagues suggest that adolescent girls with conduct disorder appear to experience stress system dysregulation similar to or even greater than that reported in males.

The mechanism responsible for the relationship between attenuation of cortisol levels and antisocial behavior is not yet determined. Three theories are proposed as explanations for attenuation of cortisol in antisocial individuals.

### Genetic Vulnerability

The genetic theory is that attenuation of cortisol in antisocial individuals is the result of intergenerational transmission, from parent to child, of genes that predispose toward both aggressive behavior and low cortisol levels. To date no studies have examined the genomic characteristics of parent–child antisocial behavior and components of the stress axis. The likelihood is low that any single gene will account for both low cortisol level and a polygenetic trait like antisocial behavior.

### Dysfunctions of the Stress System

The stress response arousal system in antisocial individuals does not appear to respond in the normal way to novelty and challenges. Dysfunctions may exist at multiple levels of the stress system: hypothalamic, pituitary or adrenal glands, or sympathetic nervous system. At the hypothalamic level, Virkunnen and colleagues (1994) showed that cerebrospinal fluid, corticotropin-releasing hormone (CRH) was low in a population of substance abusers and offenders. In pregnant adolescents, lower levels of CRH were related to a higher number of conduct disorder symptoms at early pregnancy and were predictive of conduct disorder symptoms in the postpartum period. Lower production rates or higher clearance rates of CRH may indicate the dynamic bidirectional effects of pregnancy-related changes in CRH on antisocial behavior and the effects of the girls' antisocial behavior on CRH. Alternatively, attenuation of CRH may be an aspect of the pathophysiology of antisocial behavior that is independent of pregnancy but is a common and yet unidentified third factor influencing the relationship between CRH and conduct disorder symptoms. Progesterone, for instance, may be a mediator of CRH and antisocial behavior. The addition of progesterone to *in vitro* placental, amnion, chorion, and decidua tissues resulted in decreased CRH production at term (Jones, Brooks, & Challis, 1989).

Abnormalities also can occur at the pituitary and adrenal levels (Pajer et al., 2001). Deceased sensitivity may exist at the pituitary level to CRH or deceased sensitivity at the adrenal cortex level to adrenocorticotropic hormone (ACTH). At the adrenal level, dysfunctions of glucocorticoid receptors may exist as well. There is also evidence for stability of low cortisol secretion. Subjects with attention-deficit/hyperactivity disorder (ADHD) who maintained their diagnosis across 1 year had a blunted response to the stressor in comparison to those subjects with ADHD who no longer retained the disorder 1 year later (King, Barkley, & Barrett, 1998). The evidence for a centrally mediated process regulating the relationship between CRH, ACTH, and cortisol secretion and antisocial behavior is based on findings showing that sympathetic nervous sytem activity (SNS) is attenuated in antisocial males. Aggressive children had lower heart rates than nonaggressive children (Raine, Venables, & Mednick, 1997). Low resting heart rate or low heart rate variability may have its origin in the fetal period (Ponirakis, Susman, & Stifter, 1998) and is a predictable biological correlate of antisocial and aggressive behavior in children, adolescents, and adults, reflecting reduced noradrenergic functioning and a fearless, stimulation-seeking temperament (Raine, 2002). The generalizability of the findings for low resting heart rate and antisocial behavior generated in males has not yet been established in women.

The biobehavioral integration model proposed earlier suggests that contextual factors, such as family or neighborhood influences, will influence components of both the stress system and antisocial behavior. It is most likely the case that a nasty cycle exists, with abnormalities of the central neuroendocrine and/or autonomic nervous system predisposing to antisocial behavior and vice versa.

### Hypoarousal/Sensation Seeking

The link between attenuation of cortisol, hypoarousal, and antisocial behavior can also be attributed to the need for stimulation in low-arousal individuals. These individuals seek sensation stimuli that will increase arousal and thus, cortisol levels. Indeed, there was a significant inverse relationship between cortisol and sensation seeking with high-sensation men having lower cortisol levels (Rosenblitt, Soler, Johnson, & Quadagno, 2001). There was no relationship between sensation seeking and cortisol for women. The context of being a woman in contemporary cultures, and the related socialization of gender roles, mitigates sensation-seeking experiences (e.g., auto racing, gambling) in women. It is usually not considered that the context of committing a crime, being a successful criminal, or otherwise being chronically antisocial may constitute experiences that demand lower levels of cortisol. To continuously engage in antisocial acts requires a suppression of emotions, like shame and guilt, and high levels of emotional arousal. Thus, it may be the case that success in chronic antisocial acts leads to attenuation of emotions and cortisol and other products of the stress system and results in magnified fearlessness and stimulus seeking.

### Adaptation to an Adverse Environment

The person is an active, self-organizing organism who is purposeful in adapting to dynamic person–environment systems (Cicchetti, 1994). Neonatal acquisition of the connection between fear and specific environmental contexts is essential for adaptation and survival. Adaptation is influenced by prenatal regulatory systems, but from the neonatal period onward, adaptation to a dangerous physical and social environment is essential for survival and is the major developmental task for the neonate. In the process of adaptation, the infant must distinguish dangerous from nondangerous cues and respond accordingly in order to survive. Initially, reflex actions (e.g., pulling away from heat) are responsible for the neonate's adaptation to the harsh environment. With advancing development, Crittenden (1999) proposes that meanings and perceptions of danger elicit mental and behavioral organization into protective strategies that are innate and have evolutionary adaptive value.

The efficacy of adaptation strategies varies across individuals. An optimal pattern of physiological and psychological adaptive responses to perceived threat-inducing situations is characterized by activation of the amygdala and CRH and locus ceruleus–norepinephrine stress system consisting of increases in heart rate, CRH, ACTH and cortisol, adrenaline, and the emotions of fear and anxiety. These physiological and emotional linkages form the basic physiological conditions for the individual to be prepared to act effectively in dangerous and demanding situations, to avoid some situations, or to flee still other situations.

If the childhood environment is noncontingently responsive, if pain or distress is an unpredictable or frequent occurrence, and if the environment is dangerous and unpredictable, the amygdala, emotional, cognitive, and stress systems may adapt in a manner that is inconsistent with the demands of the environment (Susman & Magnusson, 2003). Specifically, under these chronically fearful and challenging conditions, individuals adapt by attenuation or down regulation of arousal so as to avoid chronic arousal and excessive energy expenditure. Such energy expenditure related to chronic arousal would otherwise lead to eventual traumatic stress disorder and cardiovascular and immune system pathophysiology. Thus, as an adaptive strategy in early development, the stress response system/arousal system does not respond in a typical way to novelty and challenges.

A seemingly valid conclusion is that cortisol levels are attenuated in antisocial girls as well as in boys. Dysfunctions in the stress system may be a marker for the more developmentally persistent form of antisocial behavior. Methodological issues may affect the pattern of association between cortisol and aggressive and antisocial behavior as well. A developmental integration perspective suggests that attenuation of basal cortisol level will be influenced by the context in which cortisol is assessed (home, laboratory, or school). However, the context within which blood or saliva is collected is rarely considered. Similarly, hypo- or hyperresponsivity of the HPA axis in antisocial individuals may depend on whether a social interaction or physiological challenge test artificially stimulated the HPA axis and the substances assayed for cortisol level (i.e., urine, plasma, or saliva). Replication across studies using identical environmental conditions will establish the validity of patterns of cortisol secretion in males and females and antisocial behavior.

## IMPLICATIONS FOR RESEARCH, PREVENTION, AND CLINICAL PRACTICE

### Implications for Research

Advances in understanding the origins and pathways of antisocial behavior in girls will profit from continuing examination of biological systems and substances—hormones, SNS, genes, and neurotransmitters—that are integrated with behavioral aspects of antisocial behavior. For instance, other hormone systems may be identified that enhance or reduce the probability of aggression. Specifically, oxytocin and vasopressin (AVP) are linked to aggression and support seeking in animal studies of both sexes (Delville & Ferris, 1995; Delville, Mansour, & Ferris, 1996; Delville, Melloni, & Ferris, 1998; Ferris, 1996; Ferris et al., 1997; Potegal, Ferris, Hebert, Meyerhoff, & Skaredoff, 1996), but there are very few studies on humans (Coccaro, Kavoussi, Hauger, Cooper, & Ferris, 1998; Erkut, Pool, & Swaab, 1998). Oxytocin and AVP are released under stressful conditions from the hypothalamo-neurohypophyseal system. AVP has a stimulatory effect on the HPA axis, whereas oxytocin has a suppressive effect on the stress system (Gibbs, 1986). Oxytocin is higher in females than in males, whereas AVP is higher in males than in females. Therefore, oxytocin may reduce stress-related aggressive behavior in females and AVP may exaggerate antisocial behavior in males.

## Implications for Prevention

Interventions to prevent antisocial behavior must embody the accepted hallmarks of a properly designed and successful prevention intervention program, which include developmental theory, epidemiologically sound sampling, and inclusion of empirically derived risk factors (American Psychological Association, 1996; Coie, 1996; Costello & Angold, 1993). The National Institute of Mental Health (NIMH) Committee on Prevention Research (1995) gave considerable emphasis to the importance of biological risk factors in the design of prevention research.

The content of interventions may not change based on the presence of a biological marker of risk, but the scope of identifying girls at risk will be more comprehensive. There is not necessarily an isomorphism between the structure of risk and the structure of prevention programs, although the former informs the latter. Additionally, singling out a single variable, like hormones, as targets for intervention is consistent neither with current approaches to prevention (e.g., Coie, 1996) nor with models of development. The inclusion of biological parameters adds a dimension that is inherently integrated with behavior throughout the lifespan. Inclusion of biological parameters also will yield information regarding when preventive interventions may have the best chance of success.

Consider the case of early timing of puberty and the established rise in antisocial behavior. At puberty, the direct effects of hormone changes can occur prior to the external manifestations of puberty, that is, the appearance of secondary sexual characteristics. In early-maturing adolescents, the effects of hormone changes can occur 2–3 years before they are anticipated by parents and teachers. The earlier timing of puberty (Herman-Giddens et al., 1997) adds to the problem of the mismatch between the age of instigation of previous prevention programs and the biological changes of puberty. Parents and others are unaware of the early onset of puberty, the early manifestations of secondary sexual characteristics, and the early hormone changes. Body self-awareness, parental monitoring, and emotion recognition programs are especially important to implement early in puberty, prior to when girls may begin to exhibit externalizing behavior problems. Early parent-monitoring interventions are especially important for early-maturing adolescents, as early puberty is associated with an increase in antisocial behavior in girls. Prevention programs tend not to include biological developmental issues that are related to antisocial behavior. Parents will benefit from instruction on the manifestations of puberty in girls (e.g., changes in body size and proportion, pubic hair, and breast and genital development). Programs to increase parental monitoring to avoid long periods of unsupervised time, to introduce strict rules about solitary behavior, to structure the adolescents' free time, and to encourage affiliation with same-age peers may be effective in reducing antisocial behavior in early-maturing girls. Since aggressive girls act out sexually and become pregnant early (Huizinga, Loeber, & Thornberry, 1993), successful programs to reduce aggressive behavior could profitably be combined with programs to prevent teenage pregnancy and other health-compromising behaviors (e.g., alcohol and drug use).

## Implications for Practice

At the outset, it is acknowledged that it is medically contraindicated to use pharmacological interventions to change hormone levels in healthy children. Nonetheless, hormone effects are modifiable through psychosocial intervention. Emotion management techniques and more active types of psychotherapy such as role playing and computer games about interpersonal skills may be useful in girls who tend to be hypoaroused. Interdisciplinary teams will be required to implement the clinical strategies designed to reduce antisocial behavior. The inclusion of pediatricians, family practitioners, and nurses in prevention efforts will broaden the scope of assessment of children at risk. These health professionals will carry out biological and physical assessments that complement psychological and family assessments.

Biological research in antisocial behavior may also be useful in the development of pharmacological interventions. For example, the use of serotonin-enhancing antidepressants to treat female conduct disorder is a common practice, based on the long-standing psychoanalytic perspective that these "girls are not really bad, they are just depressed." However, most of these agents decrease cortisol levels (citalopram is an exception). If at least a subgroup of antisocial girls has low cortisol already, then such an intervention may not be useful and may actually exacerbate the situation. Alternatively, girls who are very aggressive in their antisocial behavior may do better on a medication such as buspirone, which increases serotonin levels but does not affect cortisol.

## SUMMARY AND CONCLUSIONS

The history of the biology of antisocial behavior is relatively short. Nonetheless, findings on the psychobiology of antisocial and aggressive behavior in girls are accumulating at a modest pace. Recent trends in developmental theory will facilitate additional research on biological issues in the future, as theories now consider a nondeterministic role for biological processes in development. The emphasis on contextual issues in development further illuminates differences in males and females and the biology of aggressive and antisocial behavior. The existing findings on sex differences are rich with implications for future hypothesis testing that will inform research, prevention, and practice.

## REFERENCES

Ahnsjo, S. (1941). Delinquency in girls and its prognosis. *Acta Paediatrica*, 28(Suppl. 3), 107–326.

American Psychological Association. (1996, December). *Reducing violence: A research agenda*. Washington, DC: Author.

Archer, J. (1991). The influence of testosterone on human aggression. *British Journal of Psychology*, 82, 1–28.

Baker, L., Mack, W., Moffitt, T., & Mednick, S. (1989). Sex differences in property crime in a Danish adoption cohort. *Behavior Genetics*, 19(3), 355–370.

Banks, T., & Dabbs, J. M. (1996). Salivary testostorone and cortisol in a delinquent and violent urban subculture. *Journal of Social Psychology*, 136, 49–56.

Bergman, B., & Brismar, B. (1994). Hormone levels and personality traits in abusive and suicidal male alcoholics. *Alcohol, Clinical, and Experimental Research*, 18, 311–316.

Bjorkqvist, K. (1994). Sex differences in physical, verbal, and indirect aggression: A review of recent research. *Sex Roles*, 30, 177–188.

Bond, A., Wingrove, J., & Critchlow, D. (2001). Tryptophan depletion increases aggression in women during the premenstrual phase. *Psychopharmacology*, 156, 477–480.

Brain, P. (1994). Hormonal aspects of aggression and violence. In A. J. Reiss Jr., K. A. Miczek, & J. I. Roth (Eds.), *Understanding and preventing violence: Vol. 2. Behavioral influences* (pp. 173–244). Washington, DC: National Academy Press.

Brain, P., & Susman, E. J. (1997). Hormonal aspects of antisocial behavior and violence. In D. M. Stoff, J. Breiling, & J. Maser (Eds.), *Handbook of antisocial behavior* (pp. 314–323). New York: Wiley.

Brooks-Gunn, J., Petersen, A. C., & Eichorn, D. (1985). The study of maturational timing effects in adolescence. *Journal of Youth and Adolescence*, 14, 149–161.

Brooks-Gunn, J., & Warren, M. P. (1989). Biological and social contributions to negative affect in young adolescent girls. *Child Development*, 60, 40–55.

Cairns, R. (1997). Socialization and sociogenesis. In D. Magnusson (Ed.), *The lifespan development of individuals: Behavioral, neurobiological and psychosocial perspectives: A synthesis* (pp. 277–295). New York: Cambridge University Press.

Campbell, A. (1986). Self-report of fighting by females: A preliminary study. *British Journal of Criminology, 26*(1), 28–46.

Caspi, A., & Moffitt, T. E. (1991). Individual differences are accentuated during periods of social change: The sample case of girls at puberty. *Journal of Personality and Social Psychology, 61,* 157–168.

Cherek, D., Moeller, F., Kahn-Dawood, F., Swann, A., & Lane, S. (1999). Prolactin response to buspirone was reduced in violent compared to nonviolent parolees. *Psychopharmacology, 142,* 144–148.

Cicchetti, D. (1994). Development and self-regulatory structures of the mind. *Development and Psychopathology, 6,* 533–549.

Coccaro, E. F., Kavoussi, R. J., & Hauger, R. L. (1995). Physiological responses to *d*-fenfluramine and ipsapirone challenge correlate with indices of aggression in males with personality disorder. *International Clinical Psychopharmacology, 10,* 177–179.

Coccaro, E. F., Kavoussi, R. J., Hauger, R. L., Cooper, T. B., & Ferris, C. F. (1998). Cerebrospinal fluid vasopressin levels. Correlates with aggression and serotonin function in personality-disordered subjects. *Archives of General Psychiatry, 55,* 708–714.

Coccaro, E. F., Kavoussi, R. J., Sheline, Y. I., Berman, M. E., & Csernansky, J. G. (1997). Impulsive aggression in personality disorder correlates with platelet 5-HT 2A receptor binding. *Neuropsychopharmacology, 16*(3), 211–216.

Coie, J. D. (1996). Prevention of violence and antisocial behavior. In R. S. Peters & R. J. McMahon (Eds.), *Preventing childhood disorders, substance abuse, and delinquency* (pp. 1–18). Thousand Oaks, CA: Sage.

Constantino, J. N., Morris, J. A., & Murphy, D. L. (1997). CSF 5-HIAA and family history of antisocial personality disorder in newborns. *American Journal of Psychiatry, 154*(12), 1771–1773.

Costello, E. J., & Angold, A. (1993). Toward a developmental epidemiology of the disruptive behavior disorders. *Development and Psychopathology, 5,* 91–101.

Cowie, J., Cowie, V., & Slater, E. (1968a). *Delinquency in girls.* London: Macmillan.

Cowie, J., Cowie, V., & Slater, E. (1968b). Early studies of delinquency in girls. In J. Cowie, V. Cowie, & E. Slater, *Delinquency in girls* (pp. 1–24). London: MacMillan.

Crick, N. (1996). The role of overt aggression, relational aggression, and prosocial behavior in the prediction of children's future social adjustment. *Child Development, 67,* 2317–2327.

Crick, N., & Grotpeter, J. K. (1995). Relational aggression, gender, and social-psychological adjustment. *Child Development, 66,* 710–722.

Crittenden, P. M. (1999). Danger and development: The organization of self-protective strategies. In J. I. Vondra & D. Barnett (Eds.), Atypical attachment in infancy and early childhood among children at developmental risk. *Monographs of the Society for Research in Child Development 49,* 145–171.

Dabbs, J., & Hargrove, M. F. (1997). Age, testosterone, and behavior among female prison inmates. *Psychosomatic Medicine, 59,* 477–480.

Delville, Y., & Ferris, C. F. (1995). Sexual differences in vasopressin receptor binding within the ventrolateral hypothalamus in golden hamsters. *Brain Research, 681,* 91–96.

Delville, Y., Mansour, K. M., & Ferris, C. F. (1996). Testosterone facilitates aggression by modulating vasopressin receptors in the hypothalamus. *Physiology and Behavior, 60*(1), 25–29.

Delville, Y., Melloni, R. J., & Ferris, C. (1998). Behavioral and neurobiological consequences of social subjugation during puberty in golden hamsters. *Journal of Neuroscience, 18*, 2667–2672.

Dorn, L. D., Hitt, S., & Rotenstein, D. (1999). Biopsychological and cognitive differences in children with premature vs. on-time adrenarche. *Archives of Pediatrics and Adolescent Medicine, 153*, 137–146.

Duff, S. J., & Hampson, E. (2001). A sex difference on a novel spatial working memory task in humans. *Brain and Cognition, 47*, 470–493.

Durston, S., Hulshoff Pol, H. E., Casey, B. J., Giedd, J. N., Buitelaar, J. K., & van Engeland, H. (2001). Anatomical MRI of the developing human brain: What have we learned? *Journal of the American Academy of Child and Adolescent Psychiatry, 40*, 1012–1020.

Erkut, Z. A., Pool, C., & Swaab, D. F. (1998). Glucocorticoids suppress corticotropin-releasing hormone and vasopressin expression in human hypothalamic neurons. *Journal of Clinical Endocrinology and Metabolism, 83*, 2066–2073.

Ferris, C. (1996). Serotonin diminishes aggression by suppressing the activity of the vasopressin system. *Annals of the New York Academy of Sciences, 794*, 98–103.

Ferris, C. F., Melloni, R. H., Koppel, G., Perry, K. W., Fuller, R. W., & Delville, Y. (1997). Vasopressin/serotonin interactions in the anterior hypothalamas control aggressive behavior in golden hamsters. *Journal of Neuroscience, 17*, 4331–4340.

Finkelstein, J. W., Susman, E. J., Chinchilli, V. M., D'Arcangelo, M. R., Kunselman, S. J., Schwab, J., Demers, L. M., Liben, L. S., & Kulin, H. E. (1998). Effects of estrogen or testosterone on self-reported sexual responses and behaviors in hypogonadal adolescents. *Journal of Clinical Endocrinology and Metabolism, 83*(7), 2281–2285.

Finkelstein, J. W., Susman, E. J., Chinchilli, V. M., Kunselman, S. J., D'Arcangelo, M. R., Schwab, J., Demers, L. M., Liben, L., Lookingbill, M. S., & Kulin, H. E. (1997). Estrogen or testosterone increases self-reported aggressive behavior in hypogonadal adolescents. *Journal of Clincial Endocrinology and Metabolism, 82*, 2433–2438.

Fishbein, D. H., Dax, E., Lozovsky, D. B., & Jaffe, J. H. (1992). Neuroendocrine responses to a glucose challenge in substance users with high and low levels of aggression, impulsivity, and antisocial personality. *Neuropsychobiology, 25*, 106–114.

Ge, X., Brody, G. H., Conger, R. D., Simmons, R. L., & Murry, V. (2002). Contextual amplification of pubertal transitional effect on African American children's problem behaviors. *Developmental Psychology, 38*, 42–54.

Ge, X., Conger, R. D., & Elder, G. H., Jr. (1996). Coming of age too early: Pubertal influences on girls' vulnerability to psychological distress. *Child Development, 67*, 3386–3400.

George, F. W. (1996). Sexual differentiation. In J. E. Griffin & S. R Ojeda (Eds.), *Textbook of endocrine physiology* (pp. 147–163). New York: Oxford University Press.

Gibbens, T. C., & Prince, J. (1967). Studies of female offenders. In N. Goodman & J. Price (Eds.), *Studies of female offenders* (pp. 1–27). London: HMSO.

Gibbs, D. M. (1986). Vasopressin and oxytocin: Hypothalamic modulators of the stress response: Review. *Psychoneuroendocrinology, 11*, 131–140.

Glueck, S., & Glueck, E. T. (1934). *Five hundred delinquent women.* New York: Knopf.

Goodman, S. H., & Kohlsdorf, B. (1994). The developmental psychopathology of conduct problems: Gender issues. In D. C. Fowles, P. Sutker, & S. H. Goodman (Eds.), *Progress in experimental personality and psychopathology research* (pp. 121–161). New York: Springer.

Halpern, C. T., Udry, J. R., & Suchindran, C. (1997). Testosterone predicts initiation of coitus in adolescent females. *Psychosomatic Medicine, 59*, 161–171.

Herman-Giddens, M. E., Slora, E. J., Wasserman, R. C., Bourdony, C. J., Bhapkar, M. V., Koch G. G., & Hasemier, C. M. (1997). Secondary sexual characteristics and menses in young girls seen in office practice: A study from the pediatric research in office settings network, *Pediatrics, 99*, 506–512.

Higley, J. D., King, S. T., Jr., Hasert, M. F., Champoux, M., Suomi, S. J., & Linnoila, M. (1996). Stability of interindividual differences in serotonin function and its relationship to severe aggression and competent social behavior in rhesus macaque females. *Neuropsychopharmacology, 14*(1), 67–76.

Hoi-Por, H., Olsson, M., Westberg, L., Melke, J., & Eriksson, E. (2001). The serotonin reuptake inhibitor fluoxetine reduces sex steroid-related aggression in female rats: An animal model of premenstraul irritiability? *Neuropsychopharmacology, 24*, 502–510.

Huizinga, D., Loeber, R., & Thornberry, T. P. (1993). Longitudinal study of delinquency, drug use, sexual activity, and pregnancy among children and youth in three cities. *Public Health Reports, 108*, 90–96.

Ibáñez, L., Dimartino-Nardi, J., Potau, N., & Saenger, P. (2000). Premature adrenarche—normal variant or forerunner of adult disease? *Endocrine Reviews, 21*, 671–696.

Inoff-Germain, G. E., Arnold, G. S., Nottelmann, E. D., Susman, E. J., Cutler, G. B., Jr., & Chrousos, G. P. (1988). Relations between hormone levels and observational measures of aggressive behavior of early adolescents in family interactions. *Developmental Psychology, 24*, 129–139.

Jones, S. A., Brooks, A. N., & Challis, J. R. G. (1989). Steroids modulate corticotropin-releasing hormone production in human fetal membranes and placenta. *Journal of Clinical Endocrinology and Metabolism, 64*, 825–830.

King, J. A., Barkley, R. A., & Barrett, S. (1998). Attention-deficit hyperactivity disorder and the stress response. *Biological Psychiatry, 44*, 72–74.

Kruijver, F. P., Zhou, J. N., Pool, C. W., Hofman, M. A., Gooren, L. J., & Swaab, D. F. (2000). Male-to-female transsexuals have female neuron numbers in a limbic nucleus. *Journal of Clinical Endocrinology and Metabolism, 85*, 2034–2041.

Kulin, H. E., Finkelstein, J. W., D'Arcangelo, R. , Susman, E. J., Chinchilli, V., Kunselman, S., Schwab, J., Demers, L., & Lookingbill, G. (1997). Diversity of pubertal testosterone changes in boys with constitutional delay in growth and/or adolescence. *Journal of Child Clinical Endocrinology, 10*, 1–6.

Langerspetz, K. M. J., Bjorkqvist, K., & Peltonen, T. (1988). Is indirect aggression typical of females? *Aggressive Behavior, 14,* 403–414.

Lerner, R. (1987). A life-span perspective for early adolescence. In R. M. Lerner & T. T. Foch (Eds.), *Biological–psychological interactions in early adolescence* (pp. 1–34). Hillsdale, NJ: Erlbaum.

Lerner, R. (1998). Theories of human development: Contemporary perspectives. In W. Damon & N. Eisenberg (Eds.), *Handbook of child psychology* (pp. 1–24). New York: Wiley.

Lerner, R. M., & Foch, T. T. (Eds.). (1987). *Biological–psychological interactions in early adolescence.* Hillsdale, NJ: Erlbaum.

Liben, L. S., Susman, E. J., Finkelstein, J. W., Chinchilli, V. M., Kunselman, S., Schwab, J., Dubas, J. S., Demers, L. M., Lookingfill, G., Dariangelo, M. R., Krogh, H. R., & Kulin, H. E. (2002). The effects of sex steroids on spatial performance: A review and an experimental clinical investigation. *Developmental Psychology, 38,* 236–256.

Litt, I. F. (1995). Violence among adolescents: Don't overlook the girls. *Journal of Adolescent Health, 17,* 333.

Loper, A., & Cornell, D. (1996). Homicide by juvenile girls. *Journal of Child and Family Studies, 5,* 323–336.

Magnusson, D. (1999). Holistic interactionism: A perspective for research on personality development. In L. A. Pervin & O. P. John (Eds.), *Handbook of personality: Theory and research* (2nd ed., pp. 219–247). New York: Guilford Press.

Magnusson, D., & Cairns, R. B. (1996). Developmental science: Principles and illustrations. In R. B. Cairns, G. H. Elder, Jr., & E. J. Costello (Eds.), *Developmental science* (pp. 7–30). New York: Cambridge University Press.

Magnusson, D., & Stattin, H. (1998). Person–context interaction theories. In W. Damon & R. M. Lerner (Eds.), *Handbook of child psychology: Vol. 1. Theoretical models of human development* (pp. 68–75). New York: Wiley.

Martin, C. A., Logan, T. K., Portis, C., Leukefeld, C. G., Lynam, D., Staton, M., Brogli, B., Flory, K., & Clayton, R. (2001). The association of testosterone with nicotine use in young adult females. *Addictive Behaviors, 26,* 279–283.

Matykiewicz, L., Grange, L. L., Vance, P., Wang, M., & Reyes, E. (1997). Adjudicated adolescent males: Measures of urinary 5-hydroxyindoleacetic acid and reactive hypoglycemia. *Personality and Individual Differences, 22*(3), 327–332.

Mazur, A., & Booth, A. (1998). Testosterone and dominance in men. *Behavioral and Brain Sciences, 21,* 353–397.

McBurnett, K., Lahey, B. B., Frick, P. J., Risch, C., Loeber R., Hart, E. L., Christ, M. A., & Hanson, K. A. (1991). Anxiety, inhibition, and conduct disorder in children: II. Relation to salivary cortisol. *Journal of the American Academy of Child and Adolescent Psychiatry, 30,* 192–196.

McBurnett, K., Lahey, B. B., Rathouz, P. J., & Loeber, R. (2000). Low salivary control and persistent aggression in boys referred for disruptive behavior. *Archives of General Psychiatry, 57,* 38–43.

Modai, I., Apter, A., Meltzer, M., Tyano, S., Walevski, A., & Jerushalmy, Z.

(1989). Serotonin uptake by platelets of suicidal and aggressive adolescent psychiatric inpatients. *Neuropsychobiology, 21*(1), 9–13.

Moffitt, T., Brammer, G., Caspi, A., Fawcett, J., Raleigh, M., Yuwiler, A., & Silva, P. (1998). Whole blood serotonin relates to violence in an epidemiological sample. *Biological Psychiatry, 43*, 446–457.

Molidor, C. (1996). Female gang members: A profile of aggression and victimization. *Social Work, 41*, 251–257.

Moss, H. B., Vanyukov. M. M., & Martin, C. S. (1995). Salivary cortisol responses and the risk for substance abuse in prepubertal boys. *Biological Psychiatry, 38*, 547–555.

National Institute on Mental Health, Committee on Prevention Research. (1995). *A plan for prevention research for the National Institute of Mental Health.* Washington, DC: Author.

New, A. S., Trestman, R. L., Mitropoulou, V., Benishay, D. S., Coccaro, E., Silverman, J., & Siever, L. J. (1997). Serotonergic function and self-injurious behavior in personality disorder patients. *Psychiatry Research, 69*, 17–26.

Nottelmann, E. D., Inoff-Germain, G., Susman, E. J., & Chrousos, G. P. (1990). Hormones and behavior at puberty. In J. Bancroft & J. M. Reinisch (Eds.), *Adolescence and puberty* (pp. 88–123). New York: Oxford University Press.

Nottelmann, E. D., Susman, E. J., Dorn, L. D., Inoff-Germain, G. E., Loriaux, D. L., Cutler, G. B., Jr., & Chrousos, G. P. (1987). Developmental processes in early adolescence: Relations among chronological age, pubertal stage, height, weight, and serum levels of gonadotropins, sex steroids, and adrenal androgens. *Journal of Adolescent Health Care, 8*, 246–260.

Office of Juvenile Justice and Delinquency Prevention. (1996). *Female offenders in the juvenile justice system.* Washington, DC: National Center for Juvenile Justice.

Pajer, K., Gardner, W., Kirillova, G., & Vanyukov, M. (2001). Sex differences in cortisol level and neurobehavioral disinhibition in children of substance abusers. *Journal of Child and Adolescent Substance Abuse, 10*, 65–72.

Petersen, A. C., & Taylor, B. (1980). The biological approach to adolescence: Biological change and psychosocial adaptation. In J. Adelson (Ed.), *Handbook of the psychology of adolescence* (pp. 115–155). New York: Wiley.

Poe-Yamasata, E., & Butts, J. (1996). *Female offenders in the juvenile justice system: Statistics summary.* Washington, DC: Office of Juvenile Justice and Delinquency Prevention, USA Department of Justice.

Ponirakis, A., Susman, E. J., & Stifter, C. (1998). Negative emotionality and cortisol during adolescent pregnancy and its effects on infant health and autonomic nervous system reactivity. *Developmental Psychobiology, 33*, 163–174.

Potegal, M., Ferris, C. F., Hebert, M., Meyerhoff, J., & Skaredoff, L. (1996). Attack priming in female syrian golden hamsters is associated with a c-fos-coupled process within the corticomedial amygdala. *Neuroscience, 75*(3), 869–880.

Raine, A. (2002). Biosocial studies of antisocial and violent behavior in children and adults: A review. *Journal of Abnormal Child Psychology, 30*, 311–326.

Raine, A., Brennan, P. J., Farrington, D. P., & Mednick, S. A. (1997). Biosocial bases of violence. In A. Raine, D. Farrington, P. Brennan, & S. A. Mednick (Eds.), *Unlocking crime: The biosocial key* (pp. 1–20). New York: Plenum Press.

Raine, A., Venables, P. H., & Mednick, S. A. (1997). Low resting heart rate at age 3 years predisposes to aggression at age 11 years: Evidence from the Mauritius child health project. *Journal of the American Academy of Child and Adolescent Psychiatry, 36,* 1457–1464.

Rosenblitt J. C., Soler, H., Johnson, S. E., & Quadagno, D. M. (2001). Sensation seeking and hormones in men and women: Exploring the link. *Hormones and Behavior, 40,* 396–402.

Rubinow, D., Schmidt, P., & Roca, C. (1998). Estrogen–serotonin interactions: Implications for affect regulation. *Biological Psychiatry, 44,* 839–850.

Russell, D. H. (1985). Girls who kill. *International Journal of Offender Therapy and Comparative Criminology, 29,* 171–176.

Sampson, R. J., Raudenbush, S. W., & Earls, F. (1997). Neighborhoods and violent crime: A multilevel study of collective efficacy. *Science, 277,* 918–924.

Sanchez-Martin, J. R., Fano, E., Ahedo, L., Cardas, J., Brain, P. F., & Azpiroz, R. (2000). A. Relating testosterone levels and free play social behavior in male and female preschool children. *Psychoneuroendocrinology, 25,* 773–783.

Schwab, J., Susman, E. J., Finkelstein, J. W., Chinchilli, V. M., Kunselman, S. J., D'Arcangelo, R. M., Demers, L. M., Lookingbill, G., & Kulin, H. E. (2001). The role of sex hormone replacement therapy on self-perceived competence in adolescents with delayed puberty. *Child Development, 72,* 1439–1450.

Segovia, S, Guillamon, A., del Cerro, M. C., Ortega, E., Perez-Laso, C., Rodriguez-Zafra, M., & Beyer, C. (1999). The development of brain sex differences: A multisignaling process. *Behavior and Brain Research, 105,* 69–80.

Stattin, H., & Magnusson, D. (1990). *Pubertal maturation in female development.* Hillsdale, NJ: Erlbaum.

Stoff, D. M., Breiling, J., & Maser, J. D.(1997). *Handbook of antisocial behavior.* New York: Wiley.

Sunblad, C., & Eriksson, E. (1997). Reduced extracellular levels of serotonin in the amygdala of androgenized rats. *European Neuropsychopharmacology, 7,* 253–259.

Susman, E. J. (1997). Modeling developmental complexity in adolescence: Hormones and behavior in context. *Journal of Research on Adolescence, 7,* 283–306.

Susman, E. J. (1998). Biobehavioural development: An integrative perspective. *International Journal of Behavioral Development, 22,* 671–679.

Susman, E. J., Dorn, L. D., & Chrousos, G. P. (1991). Negative affect and hormone levels in young adolescents: Concurrent and longitudinal perspectives. *Journal of Youth and Adolescence, 20,* 167–190.

Susman, E. J., Dorn, L. D., Inoff-Germain, G., Nottelmann, E. D., & Chrousos, G. P. (1997). Cortisol reactivity, distress behavior, behavior problems, and emotionality in young adolescents: A longitudinal perspective. *Journal of Research on Adolescence, 7,* 81–105.

Susman, E. J., & Finkelstein, J. W. (2001). Biology, development and dangerousness. In L. Pagani & G. F. Pinard (Eds.), *Contributors of clinical assessment of dangerousness: Empirical contributions* (pp. 23–46). New York: Cambridge University Press.

Susman, E. J., Inoff-Germain, G. E., Nottelman, E. D., Cutler, G. B., Loriaux, D. L., & Chrousos, G. P. (1987). Hormones, emotional dispositions and aggressive attributes in young adolescents. *Child Development, 58,* 1114–1134.

Susman, E. J., Finkelstein, J. W., Chinchilli, V. M., Schwab, J., Liben, L. S., D'Arcangelo, M. R., Meinke, M. S., Demers, L. M., Lookingbill, G., Kulin, H. E. (1998). The effect of sex hormone replacement therapy on behavior problems and moods in adolescents with delayed puberty. *Journal of Pediatrics, 133,* 521–525.

Susman, E. J., & Magnusson, D. (2003). *Psychobiology of persistent antisocial behavior.* Manuscript submitted for publication.

Susman, E. J., & Petersen, A. C. (1992). Hormones and behavior in adolescence. In E. R. McAnarney, R. E. Kreipe, D. P. Orr, & G. D. Comerci (Eds.), *Textbook of adolescent medicine* (pp. 125–130). New York: Saunders.

Tschann, J. M., Adler, N., Irwin, C. E., Jr., Millstein, S. G., Turner, R. A., & Kegeles, S. (1994). Initiation of substance use in early adolescence: The role of pubertal timing and emotional distress. *Health Psychology, 13,* 326–333.

Udry, R. J., & Talbert, L. M. (1988). Sex hormone effects on personality at puberty. *Journal of Personality and Social Psychology, 54,* 291–295.

Vanyukov, M. M., Moss, H. B., Plail, J. A., Blackson, T., Mezzick, A. C., & Tarter, R. E. (1993). Antisocial symptoms in preadolescent boys and in their parents: Associations with cortisol. *Psychiatric Research, 46,* 9–17.

Virkkunen, M. (1985). Urinary free cortisol secretion in habitually violent offenders. *Acta Psychiatrica Scandinavica, 72,* 40–44.

Virkkunen, M., Nuutila, A., Goodwin, F. K., & Linnoila, M. (1987). Cerebrospinal fluid monoamine metabolite levels in male arsonists. *Archives of General Psychiatry, 44,* 241–247.

Virkkunen, M., Rawlings, R., Tokola, R., Poland,, R. E., Guidotti, A., Nemeroff, C., Bissette, G., Kalogeras, K., Karonen, S. L., & Linnoila, M. (1994). CSF biochemistries, glucose metabolism, and diurnal activity rhythms in alcoholic, violent offenders, fire setters, and healthy volunteers. *Archives of General Psychiatry, 51,* 20–27.

Yehuda, R., & Meyer, J. S. (1984). A role for serotonin in the hypothalmic–pituitary–adrenal response to insulin stress. *Neuroendocrinology, 38,* 25–32.

Zoccolillo, M. (1993). Gender and the development of conduct disorder. *Development and Psychopathology, 5,* 65–78.

# CHAPTER 3

# All Things Interpersonal

## Socialization and Female Aggression

Carolyn Zahn-Waxler *and* Nicole Polanichka

Many forms of antisocial behavior are less prevalent in females than in males (Earls, 1987; Eme & Kavanaugh, 1995). However, other forms of antisocial behavior do not differ by gender, and criminal behavior in all major offense categories is increasing at a rapid rate in females (Budnick & Shields-Fletcher, 1998). The gender gap narrows when self-reports of deviant acts are used (e.g., drug use, school-related offenses, and property and violent crimes against family members). In a high-risk sample of boys and girls (Tiet, Wasserman, Loeber, McReynolds, & Miller, 2001), while boys were more physically aggressive than girls, boys and girls did not differ on stealing, lying, and substance use. Some forms of aggression more common to females than males are indirect, subtle, and occur in the context of interpersonal relationships (Crick, 2003).

An important contemporary issue concerns whether the same developmental models apply to males and females. Some argue that there are fundamental differences in etiology and expression of antisocial patterns for boys and girls, while others emphasize the similarities, including similar developmental trajectories. This debate is currently reflected in the question of whether "childhood-onset" and "adolescent-onset" subtypes of conduct disorder (CD) described by the *Diagnostic and Statistical Manual of Mental Disorders*, fourth edition (DSM-IV; American Psychiatric Association, 1994) apply to females as well as males. In males, these two subtypes have distinct etiological pathways and developmental courses.

"Childhood-onset type" is diagnosed in children who meet at least one criterion of CD prior to the age of 10. These children are at increased risk for a severe and persistent course of the disorder, with antisocial behavior that escalates in adolescence and continues into adulthood. It is linked to cognitive and neurological deficits, comorbid attention-deficit/hyperactivity disorder (ADHD), poor parenting, parental antisocial behavior, and other features of family dysfunction. Youth with "adolescent-onset CD" tend not to show this pattern and are more likely to desist offending by young adulthood. Silverthorn and Frick (1999) propose that girls' antisocial behavior rarely begins in childhood. Rather, there is a single "delayed-onset" developmental trajectory for antisocial girls, who share many of the same risk factors as childhood-onset males. Moffitt and Caspi (2001), in contrast, propose that both life-course persistent (early-onset) and adolescence-limited forms apply to males and females. Fergusson and Horwood (2002) report that risk factors appear to operate similarly on male and female offending trajectories. Socialization of sex differences in antisocial patterns recently has begun to receive research attention.

Adverse family environments are implicated in mental and physical health problems across childhood, adolescence, and adulthood. Family environments characterized by conflict and aggression and by relationships that are unsupportive and neglectful create vulnerabilities that interact with genetic risk factors in children to disrupt adaptive functioning (Repetti, Taylor, & Seeman, 2002). The goal of this chapter is to identify environmental factors that contribute to antisocial behaviors in females, as well as experiences that mitigate against aggression in females.

Two different socialization issues relevant to female aggression need to be addressed. One concerns experiences that contribute to girls' characteristic restraint from behaviors that injure others and violate their rights. The other concerns experiences that shape antisocial patterns in girls. We know more about the former than the latter, that is, why females more than males accept and adhere to the norms and rules of their cultures. Explanations for sex differences in antisocial behavior will need to take into account both why (1) antisocial behaviors, particularly physical violence and criminal behavior, are less common in females, and (2) why some females show these behaviors despite gender-based biological and environmental constraints. Research on conscience and internalization confirms what many parents already believe—that girls, on average, are more receptive to their socialization messages than are boys.

## PROCESSES, FORMS, AND
## FUNCTIONS OF SOCIALIZATION

Socialization is the process by which a human being, beginning in infancy, acquires the habits, beliefs, and accumulated knowledge of society
through education and training for adult status (also known as encultur-
ation). It is not necessarily a contradiction to refer to the socialization of
antisocial behavior, as this is what happens in deviant peer subcultures.
This does, however, foreshadow some of the complexities that surround
this topic. All cultures create abundant opportunities for social learning,
development, and change in children. In addition to parents as socialization figures, there are siblings, other relatives, peers, teachers, institutions, subcultures, and society. Initially, influence centers within the family. But soon most children enter nursery school, day care, and then
elementary school, where they experience additional environmental influences. Messages about societal expectations for appropriate female
and male behavior also reach children early in life, through television,
books, and movies.

Socialization has been conceptualized and measured in many ways,
mostly in parents and other caregivers. These processes range from
proximal to distal, as well as from specific to global in form. They include gender- or sex-role modeling, direct tuition (instruction), and other
aspects of modeling, reward, and punishment that contribute to social
(and antisocial) learning. Parental cognitions reflected in perceptions,
expectations, attitudes, and attributions about different behaviors in
girls and boys may create biases and diatheses toward gender-based patterns. General discipline and control practices also may differ (e.g., authoritarian, authoritative, and permissive styles; physical control vs. psychological control), as may more specific techniques and practices (e.g.,
monitoring, love withdrawal, spanking). Parenting has been conceptualized as well in terms of the affective relationship with the child.

Forms of child maltreatment (physical abuse, sexual abuse, neglect)
can be construed as global negative environmental influences on children's development. Another factor concerns quality of the relationship
between parents. Marital discord and parental anger are risk factors for
aggression, as are single parenthood, poverty, violent neighborhoods,
and other adverse conditions that affect the quality of home life. All of
the socialization processes described can be considered environmental
factors, as they reflect different constellations of affective, behavioral,
and cognitive stimuli that impinge upon the child. At the same time,
many are embedded in parental personality and/or psychopathology that
reflect dispositions and are partly determined by genetic factors. They
also interact with child dispositions that have some biological bases.

Scholarly articles, chapters, and handbooks provide a wealth of information about dimensions of parenting that influence many aspects of children's development and functioning (Bornstein, 2002; Bugental & Goodnow, 1998; Collins, Maccoby, Steinberg, Hetherington, & Bornstein, 2000; Maccoby & Martin, 1983; Parke & Buriel, 1998). In this chapter we examine ways in which parenting and other aspects of socialization inform us about gender differences in antisocial patterns in children and adolescents. The focus is primarily on parental socialization, both because caregivers have considerable influence on their children and because they have been studied the most.

Several questions arise. Are girls and boys socialized differently, and if so, how? Are certain socialization practices used more often with girls and others with boys? Does this affect the extent of antisocial behavior and the form of developmental trajectories (as well as desistance from deviance)? Do girls and boys interpret similar socialization experiences differently? Are there physical, physiological, and/or constitutional differences that also affect how these experiences impinge upon boys and girls? Do differences in the social and emotional lives of girls and boys influence different expressions and forms of antisocial behavior?

## PERSPECTIVES ON ANTISOCIAL BEHAVIOR

Psychiatry, criminology, and psychology have different views of antisocial behavior and environmental influences. In psychiatry, serious antisocial behavior is a diagnosable disease; for example, CD is defined categorically as either present or absent. Moreover, either it co-occurs with other disruptive behavior disorders (ADHD, oppositional defiant disorder), or it does not; similarly, comorbidity with anxiety and mood disorders is either present or absent. In the juvenile justice system, serious antisocial behaviors, too, are defined categorically as illegal, criminal acts against other individuals or society. Within a psychological framework, aggression and delinquency more often are viewed as dimensions that range from normal to subclinical to clinical levels.

Socialization research within psychiatric and criminality frameworks has tended to focus on broad, global risk and protective factors related to relatively serious forms of aggression in older children and youth. Psychological approaches have tended to focus on fewer, more narrowly defined and precisely measured aspects of socialization, on less severely impaired children and youth, and on younger as well as older children and youth. In recent decades there has been increased emphasis on research that merges the different perspectives. Within a developmental psychopathology framework, the etiology of adaptive and maladaptive patterns are studied simultaneously in both normative and non-normative, often longitudinal, samples. We draw from each of these literatures to provide summaries and generalizations regarding socialization and female aggression. Since research on antisocial behavior in females is relatively recent, there is not a large body of literature on environmental contributions to their aggression.

## SOCIALIZATION IN EARLY CHILDHOOD

Research reviews initially revealed surprisingly few systematic differences in the treatment of girls and boys in general. There are now some pertinent studies based on rigorous, extensive observations of child-rearing practices, discipline, and family dynamics in early childhood. Mainly these studies consider the role of mothers and are based on normative samples. Little is known about fathers who—as studies of other aspects of their parenting have shown—treat their sons and daughters more differently than do mothers (Lytton & Romney, 1991; Siegal, 1987). This suggests that fathers might play an important role in the antisocial behavior of their daughters and sons. Many parents encourage sex-typed activities in their children. In the extreme, this might cause some children to adopt some of the negative qualities associated with these roles, that is, aggression/noncompliance in boys and submission/compliance in girls. Parents use more power-assertive techniques and physical punishment with boys than girls. This can be interpreted as boys being treated more harshly. However, parents may be "harder" on girls in other ways, which include pressure to *anticipate* the consequences of negative acts and high expectations for mature interpersonal behavior.

Mothers more often show disapproval when their infant daughters display anger (i.e., by frowning), but support the expression of anger in male infants (i.e., by showing empathy) (Malatesta & Haviland, 1982). Mothers more often accept anger and retaliation as an appropriate response to another's anger in 2- to 3-year-old sons, but encourage daughters to resolve anger by reestablishing the damaged relationship (Fivush, 1989, 1991). Mothers appear to show greater authenticity in their expressions of anger toward daughters than sons in preschool children at risk for conduct problems (Cole, Teti, & Zahn-Waxler, 2003).

Mothers of 2-year-olds require their girls more than boys to relinquish toys to guests (Ross, Tesla, Kenyon, & Lollis, 1990). This may contribute to daughters feeling less entitled, and less likely when there is a struggle, to try to keep things that they want. Parents of 3-year-olds are more likely to override and negate the verbal assertions of their daughters than those of their sons (Kerig, Cowan, & Cowan, 1993).

Mothers of 2-year-olds more often reason with their daughters than sons, pointing out the harmful consequences for others of their disruptive behavior, even though the girls are not showing less aggression than boys at that age (Smetana, 1989). One year later, however, the girls did show less aggression, possibly because of the mothers' early teachings.

Teachers more often ignore misbehavior of preschool girls than that of boys, who sometimes receive positive attention (Fagot, 1984a, 1984b; Fagot & Hagan, 1985). When day care teachers observe misbehavior, they are more likely to coax or beg 2- to 6-year-old boys than girls to behave, and are less likely to use firm directives and follow through on requests to boys, even though boys showed more aggression, hostility, and noncompliance than girls (Arnold, McWilliams, & Arnold, 1998). This greater laxness with boys was causally implicated in their high rates of misbehavior.

These and other studies (Zahn-Waxler, 2000) of young children suggest that girls are oversocialized and boys are undersocialized regarding appropriate social behaviors. They illustrate why (1) girls are more likely than boys to mask their anger (Underwood, Coie, & Herbsman, 1992) and (2) girls tend to anticipate negative consequences of their aggression, even though they show less of it, while boys find aggression rewarding and ego enhancing (Perry, Perry, & Weiss, 1989). Socialization practices directed toward girls often reflect pressures to be prosocial, suppress anger, and curtail aggression. Because girls already are advanced in these domains, strong parental efforts here often may be misdirected. Many girls may become overly anxious, sensitive, and socially attuned, whereas boys may become increasingly unconcerned about their misbehavior.

Still other environmental conditions can foster gender-stereotypical patterns. Parental depression, for example, has been associated with externalizing problems, particularly in boys. However, parental depression may lead to role reversal in girls who act as caregivers to parents and behave in a oversocialized manner (Zahn-Waxler, Duggal, & Gruber, 2002). Five-year-old daughters of depressed mothers were less likely to recommend aggressive solutions to peer conflict, relative to other children, whereas sons of depressed mothers were more likely to advocate aggression (Hay, Zahn-Waxler, Cummings, & Iannotti, 1992).

Although the preschool period is a time when sex differences in aggression are nonexistent or just unfolding, parents already treat these behaviors and angry emotions differently in girls and boys. There are relatively few longitudinal studies, particularly with risk samples, and prediction of individual differences in aggression *within* groups of males and females has not been a focus. Recent research with young boys indicates that serious, chronic aggression can emerge in the first few years of life and that negative socialization experiences (e.g., harshness, stress, and unresponsiveness in parents) predict its continued expression over time (Campbell, Shaw, & Gilliom, 2000; Shaw, Bell, & Gilliom, 2000; Shaw, Owens, Giovannelli, & Winslow, 2001; Wakschlag & Hans, 1999).

There are, however, young girls who are at risk for serious antisocial behavior (Zahn-Waxler, Iannotti, Cummings, & Denham, 1990) and show it at a quite young age (Cole et al., 2003; Denham, Workman, et al., 2000). In these studies, harsh, negative parenting predicted children's later disruptive behaviors. However, preschool children's aggression decreased over early and middle childhood if parents were able to regulate their own anger, express support, use modulated and respectful control, as well as engage in other aspects of more proactive parenting (Cole et al., 2003; Zahn-Waxler et al., 1990). Parental risk and protective factors mainly operated similarly for girls and boys. However, in more recent work with one of these samples (Cole et al., 2003), parenting led to different patterns for girls and boys over time. Maternal anger contributed to the exacerbation of boys' but not girls' conduct problems. Greater authenticity and less ambivalence in mothers' expressions of anger toward daughters than sons may have helped to deter girls' aggression.

Other studies, based mainly on more normative, less high-risk samples also have reported interactions between parental discipline, gender, and aggression. McFadyen-Ketchum, Bates, Dodge, and Pettit (1996) found that mothers' coercive behaviors and lack of affection predicted (1) increases in boys' physical aggression and disruptive behaviors from kindergarten to third grade but (2) decreases in the aggressive, disruptive behaviors of girls. In other studies (Crick, in press; Nelson & Crick, 2002), fathers' use of control strategies (behavioral or psychological or both) predicted girls' (but not boys') use of physical or relational aggression. A similar pattern emerged in a study of mainland Chinese mothers and fathers and their young boys and girls (Yang et al., in press). These and other studies (e.g., Denham et al., 2000) highlight the importance of the socializing role of fathers. Research by Campbell (1999) suggests that parental influence depends upon the child's sex and form of aggression (relational vs. overt) and, that it encourages gender normative expressions of aggression.

## SOCIALIZATION IN MIDDLE CHILDHOOD AND ADOLESCENCE

In older children and youth, similar socialization experiences also can affect the antisocial behavior of girls and boys differently. In a study of youth at three time points (Davies & Windle, 1997), family discord played a greater role in the development of conduct problems in girls than in boys. In another longitudinal study (Windle, 1992), stressful life events and low family support predicted problem behaviors for adolescent girls but not boys. In work by Griffin, Botvin, Scheier, Diaz, and Miller (2000) with sixth-grade children, parental monitoring was related to less delinquency in boys and girls, and less drinking in boys. Eating family dinners together was linked to less aggression in both boys and girls, and to less delinquency in girls. Similarly, frequent parental checking of homework was linked to less aggression in girls only. Girls may be more sensitive than boys to positive parenting in ways that reduce their antisocial behavior.

Onset of delinquent behaviors before age 12 years was related to higher rates of more serious acts over a longer period of time for both boys and girls (Tolan & Thomas, 1995). Early onset appeared to spur later criminal involvement, but the contribution was small once psychosocial factors were considered. For girls, family factors, school achievement, and acceptance were more important in determining the extent of delinquent patterns. Criminal involvement was best explained by boys' participation in deviant peer groups. In two large-scale, longitudinal studies (Eron, 1992), males and females responded differently to child-rearing practices in ways linked to different levels of aggression and differential prediction of aggression in females and males over time.

Keenan, Loeber, and Green (1999) have summarized findings on the child-rearing environments of high-risk older children and adolescents. Several child-rearing practices such as poor supervision, lack of parental warmth, and discipline styles that are either overly permissive or overly harsh and coercive have been correlated with disruptive or delinquent behavior in mainly male samples. Based on a meta-analytic study, Loeber and Stouthamer-Loeber (1986) proposed four paradigms relevant to the development of conduct problems: neglect, conflict, deviant attitudes, and disruptions in parenting. Family conflict was particularly relevant to the etiology of aggression and neglect for the etiology of covert conduct problems. Antisocial girls appear to be more sensitive to disruptions in the social environment, particularly at home. Since attachment to the home environment is especially strong for girls, stressors and disruptions here can substantially affect girls' behavioral and emotional functioning.

Adolescent antisocial girls and female criminals have more dysfunctional family backgrounds than antisocial boys (Cloninger & Guze, 1970; Henggeler, Edwards, & Borduin, 1987). For example, mother–adolescent dyads and parents in families of female delinquents had higher rates of conflict than their counterparts in families of male delinquents. Moreover, fathers of female delinquents were more neurotic than the fathers of male delinquents. Parental psychopathology is more common for females than males with conduct problems, and mothers contribute to perpetuation of deviance in female delinquents (Lewis et al., 1991). Childhood history of sexual abuse is associated with conduct problems in both females and males (Kendall-Tackett, Williams, & Finkelhor, 1993). Female delinquents, however, are more likely than males to come from violent, abusive homes (Lewis et al., 1991). Often they become enmeshed in violent relationships, perpetuating family traditions of violence and showing abuse and neglect to their own offspring. Antisocial adolescent girls have poor adult outcomes, including psychiatric illness, continued arrests, and comorbid internalizing problems (Loeber & Keenan, 1994).

By early adolescence, pubertal development plays a unique role in how females' psychological problems are experienced and expressed. Normatively, girls reach puberty before boys, and early-maturing girls (relative to other girls) are at increased risk for both externalizing and internalizing problems (e.g., Caspi, Lynam, Moffitt, & Silva, 1993; Ge, Conger, & Elder, 1996; Graber, Lewinson, Seeley, & Brooks, 1997). Adverse family environments are thought to accelerate puberty for girls (Belsky, Steinberg, & Draper, 1991). Moreover, family conflict and father absence in childhood have been shown to predict an earlier age of menarche (Moffitt, Caspi, Belsky, & Silva, 1992).

Girls with early conduct problems are at later risk for teenage pregnancy (Woodward & Fergusson, 1999). This is explained in part by family and social factors, including relatively disadvantaged family backgrounds and girls' tendencies to engage in risk-taking behaviors prior to adolescence. Becoming a parent at a very young age unleashes complex dynamics and difficult life circumstances. Often there is no direct counterpart for antisocial males. In fact, they are young parents as well but tend to have less involvement and responsibility in the lives of their offspring.

## PEER SOCIALIZATION

This chapter emphasizes adults as socializers who can either contribute to or minimize antisocial behavior in their offspring, since this is where research has centered. Here we provide examples of peer socialization and emphasize the need for further work on this topic. Variations in peer relationships also reflect different aspects of socialization, including relationship quality, modeling of antisocial behavior, and different forms of punishment and maltreatment, such as bullying and exclusion. As children reach adolescence and young adulthood, they play a greater role in creating their environments—in the form of peer networks, friendships, romantic relationships, and marriages. Since children's friendships are often segregated by gender until late childhood and adolescence, young girls have limited exposure to and approval of physical aggression in peer relationships. Even after increased exposure, consequences of aggression can differ for females and males (Xie, Cairns, & Cairns, 1999). In inner-city, African American adolescents, aggression in girls undermined social membership, whereas for boys, aggression was promoted in the most prominent peer social networks.

The peer environment can modify the deleterious effects of early pubertal development on females' externalizing and internalizing problems (e.g., Caspi et al., 1993). Conduct problems in girls were a function of the availability of antisocial male partners. Early-developing girls who attended all-girl schools rather than coeducational schools were not at increased risk. The differential effects for antisocial males and females of having an antisocial mate provide another example (Moffitt, Caspi, Rutter, & Silva, 2001). Antisocial individuals often are attracted to each other, due in part to biologically based propensities. But their living environments appear to affect females and males differently. The antisocial behavior of females involved with an antisocial partner at 21 years persisted into adulthood. For males, an antisocial partner had no effect on persistence. Since antisocial males tend to perpetrate aggression and criminal behavior in groups, girls who become involved with them may be exposed to a network of antisocial males, creating continued occasions and pressures to participate.

## CHILD CHARACTERISTICS

Environmental and biological contributions to antisocial behavior are considered in separate chapters in this volume. However, person and environment are mutually and interactively influential in determining developmental outcomes (Cairns, 1997; Hood, 1996). Here we consider some characteristics more common to females than males that influence their aggression and socialization experiences. Understanding how socialization affects aggression in females ultimately requires that their environments be studied in relation to more biologically based underpinnings.

Several mechanisms have been used to explain lower rates of disruptive behavior in females than males (Zahn-Waxler, 1993). Genetic influence on antisocial behavior is inferred from studies of twins, siblings, adoptees, and intergenerational similarities. Biological processes linked to aggression include hormonal (e.g., testosterone) and biochemical (e.g., serotonin) variations; frontal-lobe function; temperament; activity level; psychophysiology (e.g., autonomic arousal); and physical strength and muscle mass. Females differ from males on a number of these dimensions. One important distinguishing quality is the strong interpersonal orientation more common to females, where interdependency is valued and others are seen as integrally connected to the self (Cross & Madson, 1997). Positive bonds may act as a social control that prevents crime and other forms of antisocial behavior. It can help to explain females' low aggression, the kinds of aggression shown, how they are socialized, and how they interpret experiences.

Strong affiliative tendencies are seen more often in girls than boys even in childhood, in conjunction with other qualities likely to create lower risk for aggression (see reviews by Brody, 1999; Keenan & Shaw, 1997; Zahn-Waxler, 2000). Girls show more empathy, guilt, and remorse, as well as more prosocial, reparative, and internalizing behaviors that often accompany these emotions. They are more anxious and fearful in many contexts. Girls exert more control over negative emotions (e.g., in masking anger and disappointment). They are more compliant, have greater difficulty influencing others, and show better self-regulation than boys. Most of these factors also indicate that what others think and feel about them matters greatly to girls.

In longitudinal studies of early empathy (observed in several hundred 1- to 3-year-old children), girls more often than boys respond to distress victims in ways that reflect concern for others (Zahn-Waxler, 2000). These early sex differences are probably not entirely the product of socialization, as female infants are more responsive than male infants to the distress cries of other infants, even in the first days of life (Hoffman, 1977). That is not to say that socialization is unimportant. But it does suggest possible biological underpinnings that predispose young girls to care more about others and their problems. Empathy is one powerful force that limits expressions of aggression.

A strong interpersonal orientation reflects core qualities that females bring to their social exchanges, including how they respond to stress. Shelley Taylor and colleagues (2000) have questioned the universal applicability of the human stress response, originally construed by Cannon as fight–flight. While fight–flight responses to stress are likely to stimulate physical aggression and are more common in males, human females' responses often reflect a pattern that Taylor and colleagues refer to as tend-and-befriend. Tending involves nurturant activities that protect the self and offspring, promote safety, and reduce distress. Befriending creates and maintains social networks that are also protective. The biobehavioral mechanism that underlies the tend-and-befriend process appears to be linked to the attachment/caregiving system.

Neuroendocrine evidence implicates oxytocin in conjunction with female reproductive hormones and endogeneous opioid peptide mechanisms. Oxytocin is a hormone that enhances relaxation, reduces fearfulness, and decreases sympathetic activity, all of which are antithetical to the fight–flight response. Hence it is thought to be adaptive for physical and mental health.

There are also costs (Zahn-Waxler, Cole, & Barrett, 1991). Caregiving can be burdensome, social relationships can engender dependencies, and affiliation may create reluctance to assert oneself or to fight in contexts where it would be appropriate. Tending and befriending may reduce physical aggression but create risk for depression. Relational aggression reflects a darker side of interpersonal concerns, and it is seen more often in girls than boys, beginning in the preschool years (Crick, Casas, & Mosher, 1997). Caring and social behaviors that reflect tending and befriending are more common in girls than boys early in life, well before reproductive hormones and oxytocin levels differentiate them. Interpersonal themes are also common in the symbolic play and scripts of young girls (Maccoby, 2002; Zahn-Waxler, Gruber, Usher, Belouad, & Cole, 2004).

Aggressive children's socialization themes in narratives and symbolic play also reflect the salience of interpersonal relationships for girls (Zahn-Waxler, Polanichka, & Brand, 2004). By early grade school, both aggressive girls and boys perceived parental figures as punitive more often than nonaggressive children. But the antisocial girls also perceived more parental rejection and withdrawal than nonaggressive children or antisocial boys, suggesting concerns about abandonment and loss of love. Such internalized fears may fuel girls' efforts to curtail behaviors that threaten close, intimate relationships, foreshadowing later sex differences. Rejection sensitivity (Purdie & Downey, 2000) may lead to peer rejection which may, in turn, lead to associations with rejected, deviant peers.

## REFLECTIONS, PROJECTIONS, AND RECOMMENDATIONS

Based on the extant literature, several conclusions about environmental contributions to antisocial behavior in females are offered. Normatively, beginning early in life, girls are afforded a greater degree of protection than boys and are treated in ways that heighten social awareness and sensitivity to the needs, rights, and welfare of others. While this can contribute to lower levels of aggression in females than males, it can also lead to lack of assertion and appropriate aggression. Under optimal conditions, however, efforts to sensitize children to others' emotions and experiences can be one aspect of positive parenting that enhances adaptive social development in children—in relationships with families and friends, in reaching out to less familiar others, and in becoming good citizens in their communities.

While proactive socialization typically has been studied in nonclinical populations, a few studies have begun to examine its significance for risk groups in reducing aggression. In normative samples, parental responsiveness, involvement, and reciprocity are linked consistently to fewer negative behaviors in offspring (reviewed by Maccoby & Martin, 1983). Proactive maternal involvement (anticipatory guidance, supportive and affectively positive educative patterns) has been linked to fewer behavior problems in 4 year olds (Pettit & Bates, 1989) and fewer problems in preschool children and adolescents (Miller, Cowan, Cowan, Hetherington, & Clingempeel, 1993). It also has been shown to reduce aggression over time for infants and young children at risk (Denham et al., 2000; Wakschlag & Hans, 1999; Zahn-Waxler et al., 1990). While proactive parenting in the form of support, structure, and responsiveness does not differ for girls and boys, girls appear more receptive than boys to positive socialization.

The risk literature has emphasized negative socialization experiences that encourage antisocial behavior. Here negative, punitive parenting is construed broadly to include parental violence, abuse, neglect, and psychopathology as well as specific harsh discipline and child rearing practices. Greater negative environmental disturbance is required to elicit antisocial and criminal behavior in females than males. Cumulatively, the effects of both positive and negative socialization on girls can be understood in terms of their strong interpersonal orientation. This personal focus carries with it both strengths and vulnerabilities. It limits infliction of physical harm, but heightens risk for subordination, dependence, and aggression expressed indirectly and in the context of relationships. It also may relate to females' greater tendency to experience anxiety, depression, and guilt, as well as for their externalizing problems to more often be comorbid with internalized distress than for males. This comorbidity, not often studied in research on antisocial behavior, could have a profound influence on how females' hostile impulses and behaviors are experienced, expressed, and even socialized.

Substantial progress has been made in theory and research on socialization of children and adolescents, particularly regarding the role of parents. Based on new approaches, current findings on parental influences provide more sophisticated and less deterministic explanations than before (Collins et al., 2000). Newer approaches include (1) behavior genetics designs that estimate (and sometimes directly measure) environmental influences; (2) studies that examine how children of different temperaments respond to similar environments; (3) experimental studies of changes in children's behavior resulting from exposure to parents' behavior, after controlling for initial child characteristics; and (4) research on interactions between parenting and nonfamilial environmental contexts that consider influences beyond the parent–child dyad.

This general progress has not extended to research on socialization and antisocial behavior in females. Few of the more sophisticated research designs have been used to study similarities and differences in environmental influences on aggression in females and males. Several conceptual and methodological constraints in high-risk research make it difficult to identify differential socialization influences on forms and frequencies of female and male aggression. Environmental and genetic influences are difficult to disentangle. Socialization measures are often restricted to parental report, based on small numbers of items, and are rough proxies for the environments children experience. Because childhood onset is so rare in females, small sample sizes make it difficult to detect socialization influences. Socialization data are often retrospective, and trajectory designs are not always longitudinal. Many studies that test hypotheses about etiological differences in female and male aggression were not initially designed for this purpose. Finally, with the emphasis on parental socialization, several other influences have been understudied. Relatively little is known about the roles of institutions and the media, and more generally of the larger societal and cultural forces that encourage different normative and non-normative behaviors in girls and boys.

Issues also remain regarding assessment of antisocial and disruptive behavior problems. Typically, measures are based on a number of different items. This is essential for reliability and validity. At the same time, females and males may endorse different items and different combinations of items. Identical quantitative scores could reflect important qualitative differences. This is a problem not just with respect to gender, but for the study of other aspects of individual differences in antisocial behavior as well. Similarly, there are different ways of reaching a psychiatric diagnosis of conduct disorder. For example, the status offenses more common to females and the physical violence more common to males also may have different socialization antecedents, biological underpinnings, and developmental pathways. Even if patterns of relationships between predictor and outcome variables appear similar for females and males, the fact that they differ on extent and types of antisocial behavior cannot be ignored.

The etiology of extreme cases, that is, violent, psychopathic females, remains a mystery. How were they socialized? How do they socialize?

Most of what is known comes from biographical accounts and memoirs of children raised by antisocial mothers (e.g., Rule, 1987; Walker & Schone, 2001). Systematic research on the extremes would be informative. It seems implausible that adverse environmental conditions alone could produce women who carry out heinous crimes, including, for example, murdering one's own children in order to be with a boyfriend who did not want children. Socialization may "work around the edges" in such instances, but factors other than how one was reared would be more likely candidates for study.

Differential socialization of emotions in girls and boys may alter the very emotions that underlie antisocial behavior patterns in the two sexes; this merits further study. Differential responses to different emotions in boys and girls could channel hostile impulses in different ways. Links between anger and aggression appear to be more direct for young boys than girls, with anger in girls being more closely associated with feelings of guilt, shame, and other internalizing emotions (Zahn-Waxler, 2000). Parents may play a role in shaping these different patterns in ways that help deter aggression in girls and encourage it in boys (as suggested by the data on early socialization).

Keenan and colleagues (1999) recommend that we do more than examine how well results from studies on the precursors, correlates, and risk factors for CD in boys apply to girls. Research should also delve more deeply into the biopsychosocial experience of the individual. We have emphasized the role of a strong interpersonal orientation in females, but other important biological, psychological, social-emotional, and environmental factors also remain to be considered in research based on improved conceptual, methodological, and analytic frameworks. Keenan and colleagues note that since girls are at lower risk for CD, it is appropriate to explore the apparent "protective" effect of gender and whether it is always protective. Are girls who are at lower risk for CD at higher risk for depression? Or does the lower risk for CD signal the existence of protective factors that promote mental health? Are there different subsets of individuals for whom particular patterns apply, and what are the different etiologies?

From a developmental perspective, early depression may contribute to later antisocial behavior (Obeidallah & Earls, 1999), or certain types of early antisocial patterns may contribute to later depression, particularly in girls (Crick, 2002, personal communication). Again, what are the different etiologies, including environmental processes that contribute to these differences? Understanding these different processes in the context of the known high comorbidity of externalizing and internalizing problems, particularly in females, would help to identify causal factors. Both similarities and differences in risk and protective factors implicated in antisocial development of girls and boys would be expected. It is important not to shut the door too early by proclaiming that these factors are either the same *or* different for girls and boys.

We wish to underscore the importance of including both females and males in research designs. Understanding of antisocial behavior in both females and males can best be achieved in this manner. Despite many years in which only males were studied, we are far from having definitive answers about their antisocial development, even given the vast amount of research that has been conducted. Research on both males and females is inevitably hampered whenever the conceptual framework and research design is based on only one sex. Lessons learned from past mistakes will benefit all those who suffer from disruptive behavior problems, as well as those affected by their suffering.

## REFERENCES

American Psychiatric Association. (1994). *Diagnostic and statistical manual of mental disorders* (4th ed.). Washington, DC: Author.

Arnold, D. H., McWilliams, L., & Arnold, E. H. (1998). Teacher discipline and child misbehavior in daycare: Untangling causality with correlational data. *Developmental Psychology, 34*, 276–287.

Belsky, J., Steinberg, L., & Draper, P. (1991). Childhood experience, interpersonal development, and reproductive strategy: An evolutionary theory of socialization. *Child Development, 62*(4), 647–670.

Bornstein, M. H. (Ed.). (2002). *Handbook of parenting.* Mahwah, NJ: Erlbaum.

Brody, L. R. (1999). *Gender, emotion and the family.* Cambridge, MA: Harvard University Press.

Budnick, K. J., & Shields-Fletcher, E. (1998). *What about girls?* (OJJDP Fact Sheet #84). Washington, DC: United States Department of Justice, Office of Justice Programs, Office of Juvenile Justice and Delinquency Prevention.

Bugental, D. B., & Goodnow, J. J. (1998). Socialization processes. In W. Damon & N. Eisenberg (Eds.), *Handbook of child psychology* (5th ed., Vol. 3, pp. 389–462). New York: Wiley.

Cairns, R. B. (1997). Socialization and sociogenesis. In D. Magnusson (Ed.), *The lifespan development of individuals: Behavioral, neurobiological, and psychosocial perspectives: A synthesis* (pp. 277–295). New York: Cambridge University Press.

Campbell, J. J. (1999). Familial antecedents to children's relational and overt aggression. *Dissertation Abstracts International, 60*(6-B), 2980.

Campbell, S. B., Shaw, D. S., & Gilliom, M. (2000). Early externalizing behavior problems: Toddlers and preschoolers at risk for later maladjustment. *Development and Psychopathology, 12*, 467–488.

Caspi, A., Lynam, D., Moffitt, T. E., & Silva, P. A. (1993). Unraveling girls' delinquency: Biological, dispositional, and contextual contributors to adolescent misbehavior. *Developmental Psychology, 29,* 19–30.

Cloninger, C. R., & Guze, S. B. (1970). Female criminals: Their personal, familial, and social backgrounds. *Archives of General Psychiatry, 23,* 554–558.

Cole, P. M., Teti, L. O., & Zahn-Waxler, C. (2003). Mutual emotion regulation and the stability of conduct problems between preschool and early school age. *Development and Psychopathology, 15*(1), 1–18.

Collins, W. A., Maccoby, E. E., Steinberg, L., Hetherington, E. M., & Bornstein, M. H. (2000). Contemporary research on parenting: The case for nature and nurture. *American Psychologist, 55,* 218–232.

Crick, N. R. (2003). A gender-balanced approach to the study of childhood aggression and reciprocal family influences. In A. C. Crouter & A. Booth (Eds.), *Children's influence on family dynamics: The neglected side of family relationships* (pp. 229–235). Mahwah, NJ: Erlbaum.

Crick, N. R., Casas, J. F., & Mosher, M. (1997). Relational and overt aggression in preschool. *Developmental Psychology, 33,* 579–588.

Cross, S., & Madson, L. (1997). Models of the self: Self-constructs and gender. *Psychological Bulletin, 122,* 5–37.

Davies, P. T., & Windle, M. (1997). Gender-specific pathways between maternal depressive symptoms, family discord, and adolescent adjustment. *Developmental Psychology, 33,* 657–668.

Denham, S. A., Workman, E., Cole, P. M., Weissbrod, C., Kendziora, K. T., & Zahn-Waxler, C. (2000). Prediction of externalizing problems from early to middle childhood. *Development and Psychopathology, 12*(1), 23–45.

Earls, F. (1987). Sex differences in psychiatric disorders: Origins and developmental influences. *Psychiatric Developments, 1,* 1–23.

Eme, R. F., & Kavanaugh, L. (1995). Sex differences in conduct disorder. *Journal of Clinical Psychology, 24,* 406–426.

Eron, L. D. (1992). Gender differences in violence: Biology and/or socialization? In K. Björkqvist & P. Niemelä (Eds.), *Of mice and women: Aspects of female aggression* (pp. 89–97). San Diego, CA: Academic Press.

Fagot, B. I. (1984a). The consequences of problem behavior in toddler children. *Journal of Abnormal Child Psychology, 12,* 385–396.

Fagot, B. I. (1984b). Teacher and peer reactions of boys and girls' play styles. *Sex Roles, 11,* 691–702.

Fagot, B. I., & Hagan, R. (1985). Aggression in toddlers: Responses to the assertive acts of boys and girls. *Sex Roles, 12,* 341–351.

Fergusson, D. M., & Horwood, L. J. (2002). Male and female offending trajectories. *Development and Psychopathology, 14,* 159–177.

Fivush, R. (1989). Exploring sex differences in the emotional content of mother-child conversations about the past. *Sex Roles, 20,* 675–691.

Fivush, R. (1991). Gender and emotion in mother–child conversations about the past. *Journal of Narrative and Life History, 1,* 325–341.

Ge, X., Conger, R. D., & Elder, G. H. (1996). Coming of age too early: Pubertal influences on girls' vulnerability to psychological distress. *Child Development, 67,* 3386–3400.

Graber, J. A., Lewinsohn, P. M., Seeley, J. R., & Brooks, J. (1997). Is psychopathology associated with the timing of pubertal development? *Journal of the American Academy of Child and Adolescent Psychiatry*, *36*, 1768–1776.

Griffin, K. W., Botvin, G. J., Scheier, L. M., Diaz, T., & Miller, N. L. (2000). Parenting practices as predictors of substance use, delinquency, and aggression among urban minority youth: Moderating effects of family structure and gender. *Psychology of Addictive Behaviors*, *14*, 174–184.

Hay, D. F., Zahn-Waxler, C., Cummings, E. M., & Iannotti, R. J. (1992). Young children's views about conflict with peers: A comparison of the daughters and sons of depressed and well women. *Journal of Child Psychiatry*, *33*(4), 669–683.

Henggeler, S. W., Edwards, J., & Borduin, C. M. (1987). The family relations of female juvenile delinquents. *Journal of Abnormal Child Psychology*, *15*, 199–209.

Hoffman, M. L. (1977). Sex differences in empathy and related behaviors. *Psychological Bulletin*, *34*, 712–722.

Hood, K. E. (1996). Intractable tangles of sex and gender in women's aggressive development: An optimistic view. In D. M. Stoff & R. B. Cairns (Eds.), *Aggression and violence: Genetic, neurobiological, and biosocial perspectives* (pp. 309–335). Mahwah, NJ: Erlbaum.

Keenan, K., Loeber, R., & Green, S. (1999). Conduct disorder in girls: A review of the literature. *Clinical and Child Family Psychology Review*, *2*, 3–19.

Keenan, K., & Shaw, D. (1997). Developmental and social influences on young girls' early problem behavior. *Psychological Bulletin*, *121*, 95–113.

Kendall-Tackett, K. A., Williams, L. M., & Finkerlhor, D. (1993). Impact of sexual abuse on children: A review and synthesis of recent empirical studies. *Psychological Bulletin*, *113*, 164–180.

Kerig, P. K., Cowan, P. A., & Cowan, C. P. (1993). Marital quality and gender differences in parent–child interaction. *Developmental Psychology*, *29*, 931–939.

Lewis, D. O., Yeager, C. A., Cobham-Portorreal, C. S., Klein, N., Showalter, C., & Anthony, A. (1991). A follow-up of female delinquents: Maternal contributions to the perpetuation of deviance. *Journal of the American Academy of Child and Adolescent Psychiatry*, *30*, 197–201.

Loeber, R., & Keenan, K. (1994). The interaction between conduct disorder and its comorbid conditions: Effects of age and gender. *Clinical Psychology Review*, *14*, 497–523.

Loeber, R., & Stouthamer-Loeber, M. (1986). Family factors as correlates and predictors of juvenile conduct problems and delinquency. In M. Tonry & N. Morris (Eds.), *Crime and justice: An annual review of research* (pp. 29–149). Chicago: University of Chicago Press.

Lytton, H., & Romney, D. (1991). Parents' differential socialization of boys and girls. A meta-analysis. *Psychological Bulletin*, *109*, 287–296.

Maccoby, E. E. (2002). Gender and group process: A developmental perspective. *Current Directions in Psychological Science*, *11*, 54–58.

Maccoby, E. E., & Martin, J. A. (1983). Socialization in the context of the family: Parent–child interaction. In P. H. Mussen (Series Ed.) & E. M. Hetherington (Vol. Ed.), *Handbook of child psychology: Vol. 4. Socialization, personality, and social development* (4th ed., pp. 1–101). New York: Wiley.

Malatesta, C. Z., & Haviland, J. (1982). Learning display rules: The socialization of emotion expression in infancy. *Child Development, 53,* 991–1003.

McFadyen-Ketchum, S. A., Bates, J. E., Dodge, K. A., & Pettit, Y. S. (1996). Pattern of change in early childhood aggressive-disruptive behavior: Gender differences in predictions from early coercive and affectionate mother–child interactions. *Child Development, 67,* 2417–2433.

Miller, N. B., Cowan, P. A., Cowan, C. P., Hetherington, E. M., & Clingempeel, W. G. (1993). Externalizing in preschoolers and early adolescents: A cross-study replication of a family model. *Developmental Psychology, 29,* 3–18.

Moffitt, T. E., & Caspi, A. (2001). Childhood predictors differentiate life-course persistent and adolescence-limited antisocial pathways among males and females. *Development and Psychopathology, 13,* 355–375.

Moffitt, T. E., Caspi, A., Belsky, J., & Silva, P. A. (1992). Childhood experience and the onset of menarche: A test of a sociobiological model. *Child Development, 63,* 47–58.

Moffitt, T. E., Caspi, A., Rutter, M., & Silva, P. A. (2001). *Sex differences in antisocial behaviour: Conduct disorder, delinquency, and violence in the Dunedin longitudinal study.* Cambridge, UK: Cambridge University Press.

Nelson, D. A., & Crick, N. R. (2002). Parental psychological control: Implications for childhood physical and relational aggression. In B. K. Barber (Ed.), *Intrusive parenting: How psychological control affects children and adolescents* (pp. 161–189). Washington, DC: American Psychological Association.

Obeidallah, D. A., & Earls, F. J. (1999, July). *Adolescent girls: The role of depression and the development of delinquency.* Washington, DC: U.S. Department of Justice, Office of Justice Programs, National Institute of Justice Research Preview.

Parke, R. D., & Buriel R. (1998). Socialization in the family: Ethnic and ecological perspectives. In W. Damon & N. Eisenberg (Eds.), *Handbook of child psychology* (5th ed., Vol. 3, pp. 463–552). New York: Wiley.

Perry, D. G., Perry, L. C., & Weiss, R. J. (1989). Sex differences in the consequences that children anticipate for aggression. *Developmental Psychology, 25,* 312–319.

Pettit, G. S., & Bates, J. E. (1989). Family interaction patterns and children's behavior problems from infancy to four years. *Developmental Psychology, 25,* 413–420.

Purdie, V., & Downey, G. (2000). Rejection sensitivity and adolescent girls' vulnerability to relationship-centered difficulties. *Child Maltreatment, 5,* 336–347.

Repetti, R. L., Taylor, S. E., & Seeman, T. E. (2002). Risky families: Family social environments and the mental and physical health of offspring. *Psychological Bulletin, 128,* 330–366.

Ross, H., Telsa, C., Kenyon, B., & Lollis, S. (1990). Maternal intervention in toddler-peer conflict: The socialization of principles of justice. *Developmental Psychology, 26,* 994–1003.

Rule, A. (1987). *Small sacrifices.* New York: Penguin.

Shaw, D. S., Bell, R. Q., & Gilliom, M. (2000). A truly early starter model of antisocial behavior revisited. *Clinical Child and Family Psychology Review, 3,* 155–172.

Shaw, D. S., Owens, E. B., Giovannelli, J., & Winslow, E. B. (2001). Infant and toddler pathways leading to early externalizing disorders. *Journal of the American Academy of Child and Adolescent Psychiatry, 40*, 36–43.

Siegal, M. (1987). Are sons and daughters treated more differently by fathers than mothers? *Developmental Review, 7*, 183–209.

Silverthorn, P., & Frick, P. J. (1999). Developmental pathways to antisocial behavior: The delayed-onset pathway in girls. *Development and Psychopathology, 11*, 101–126.

Smetana, J. G. (1989). Toddlers' social interactions in the context of moral and conventional transgressions in the home. *Developmental Psychology, 25*, 499–509.

Taylor, S. E., Klein, L. C., Lewis, B. P., Gruenewald, T. L., Gurung, R. A. R., & Updegraff, J. A.(2000). Biobehavioral responses to stress in females: Tend-and-befriend, not fight-or-flight. *Psychological Review, 107*, 411–429.

Tiet, Q. Q., Wasserman, G. A., Loeber, R., McReynolds, L. S., & Miller, L. S. (2001). Developmental and sex differences in types of conduct problems. *Journal of Child and Family Studies, 10*, 181–197.

Tolan, P. H., & Thomas, P. (1995). The implications of age of onset for delinquency risk II. Longitudinal data. *Journal of Abnormal Child Psychology, 23*, 157–181.

Underwood, M. K., Coie, J. D., & Herbsman, C. R. (1992). Display rules for anger and aggression in school-age children. *Child Development, 63*, 366–380.

Walker, K., & Schone, M. (2001). *Son of a grifter: The twisted tale of Sante and Kenny Kimes, the most notorious con artists in America: A memoir by the other son.* New York: Morrow/Avon.

Wakschlag, L. S., & Hans, S. L. (1999). Relations of maternal responsiveness during infancy to the development of behavior problems in high-risk youths. *Developmental Psychology, 35*, 569–579.

Windle, M. (1992). A longitudinal study of stress buffering for adolescent problem behaviors. *Developmental Psychology, 28*, 522–530.

Woodward, L. J., & Fergusson, D. M. (1999). Early conduct problems and later risk of teenage pregnancy in girls. *Development and Psychopathology, 11*, 127–141.

Xie, H., Cairns, R. B., & Cairns, B. D. (1999). Social networks and configurations in inner-city schools: Aggression, popularity, and implications for students with EBD. *Journal of Emotional and Behavioral Disorders, 7*, 147–155.

Yang, C., Hart, C. H., Nelson, D. A., Porter, C. L., Olsen, S. F., Robinson, C. C., & Jin, S. (in press). Associations among Chinese fathering, children's negative emotionality, and aggression. In R. Day & M. Lamb (Eds.), *Reconceptualizing and measuring fatherhood.* Mahwah, NJ: Erlbaum.

Zahn-Waxler, C. (1993). Warriors and worriers: Gender and psychopathology. *Development and Psychopathology, 5*, 79–89.

Zahn-Waxler, C. (2000). The development of empathy, guilt, and internalization of distress: Implications for gender differences in internalizing and externalizing problems. In R. Davidson (Ed.), *Anxiety, depression, and emotion: Wisconsin symposium on emotion* (Vol. 1, pp. 222–265). New York: Oxford University Press.

Zahn-Waxler, C., Cole, P.M., & Barrett, K. (1991). Guilt and empathy: Sex differences and implications for the development of depression. In K. Dodge & J. Garber (Eds.), *Emotional regulation and dysregulation* (pp. 243–272). New York: Cambridge University Press.

Zahn-Waxler, C., Duggal, S., & Gruber, R. (2002). Parental psychopathology. In M. H. Bornstein (Ed.), *Handbook of parenting: Vol. 4. Social conditions and applied parenting* (2nd ed., pp. 295–327). Mahwah, NJ: Erlbaum.

Zahn-Waxler, C., Gruber, R., Usher, B., Belouad, F., & Cole, P. M. (2004). *Young children's representations of conflict and distress: A longitudinal study of boys and girls with disruptive behavior problems.* Manuscript under review.

Zahn-Waxler, C., Iannotti, R. J., Cummings, E. M., & Denham, S. A. (1990). Antecedents of problem behaviors in children of depressed mothers. *Development and Psychopathology, 2,* 271–291.

Zahn-Waxler, C., Polanichka, N., & Brand, A. (2004). *Young children's perceptions of parenting: Developmental patterns and predictive validity.* Unpublished manuscript.

# PART II

# AGGRESSION AND VICTIMIZATION AMONG GIRLS IN CHILDHOOD

# CHAPTER 4

# Relational Aggression in Early Childhood

## "You Can't Come to My Birthday Party Unless ... "

Nicki R. Crick, Jamie M. Ostrov, Karen Appleyard, Elizabeth A. Jansen, *and* Juan F. Casas

For several decades, studies of childhood aggression have focused primarily on forms of aggression most typical of boys (e.g., physical aggression). In recent years, however, researchers have begun to explore the types of aggressive behaviors that are most salient for girls. One form of aggression that has been identified as particularly important for girls is relational aggression (Crick & Grotpeter, 1995). In contrast to physical aggression, which harms others through damage (or the threat of damage) to physical well-being, relational aggression harms others through damage (or the threat of damage) to relationships (Crick, Werner, et al., 1999). Relational aggression includes both direct and indirect acts, such as threatening to end a friendship unless a peer complies with a request, using social exclusion or the "silent treatment" to control or punish others, and spreading nasty rumors about someone so that others will reject him or her. Relative to the relationally aggressive behaviors exhibited by school-age children and adolescents, those behaviors most common among young children are more likely to be direct (e.g., "You can't come to my birthday party unless ... ") and focused on the immediate social exchange (e.g., covering the ears to signal ignoring or the "silent treatment" as a peer is speaking).

Although significant progress has been made in our understanding of relational aggression in recent years, relatively little attention has been paid to young children. This is a significant area of inquiry due to its important implications for early prevention and intervention efforts, and for advancing our knowledge of the early development of relational aggression. Our goal for this chapter is to provide an overview of existing empirical findings on relational aggression among young children as well as ideas for advancing and encouraging future work in this area. Specific objectives include (1) consideration of current theories regarding the aggressive behaviors exhibited by young girls and their implications for research on relational aggression; (2) description of the types of relationally aggressive behaviors that are most common during early childhood; (3) description of assessment procedures used to assess relational aggression in young children; (4) consideration of evidence regarding the harmful nature of relational aggression; (5) review of potential factors in a developmental model of relational aggression during early childhood; and (6) an overview of future directions and challenges for research.

## THEORETICAL VIEWS OF YOUNG GIRLS' AGGRESSIVE BEHAVIOR

In tandem with the recent empirical interest in the behavioral problems of girls, theoretical efforts in this area have also burgeoned. In general, two distinct hypotheses have been proposed regarding the aggressive behavior problems of young girls (for a review, see Crick & Zahn-Waxler, 2003). In the first hypothesis, it has been posited that girls do not experience significant aggressive or conduct problems during early childhood (Keenan & Shaw, 1997; Moffitt & Caspi, 2001; Silverthorn & Frick, 1999). Generally, these theorists have proposed that the majority of aggressive girls do not develop aggressive behavior problems until much later than early childhood. This view has been described as the "Benign Childhood" hypothesis (Crick & Zahn-Waxler, 2003). The majority of theorists who espouse this perspective have targeted the adolescent years as the developmental period most relevant for the initiation of behavioral problems among females. Other theorists have focused on middle childhood as the developmental period during which girls first develop aggressive behavior problems (Bjorkqvist, Lagerspetz, & Kuakianen, 1992). Not surprisingly, this approach has limited empirical efforts that focus on the aggressive behavior patterns of girls in early childhood.

In sharp contrast to the tenet described in the first hypothesis, other theorists have posited that a significant number of girls *do* exhibit aggressive behavior problems during early childhood (e.g., Crick, Casas, & Mosher, 1997; Feshbach, 1969; Ostrov & Keating, 2004). These investigators have proposed that young girls' aggressive acts have been overlooked due to the failure to assess forms of aggression most common among girls during these early years. Studies of relational aggression have been based on this perspective. Research has demonstrated that relationally aggressive acts are relatively common in early childhood and can be reliably and validly identified in children as young as 2½ years of age (Crick, Ostrov, Cullerton-Sen, Appleyard, & Jansen, 2003). Furthermore, observational studies have shown that, during the preschool years, girls are significantly more relationally aggressive than boys (Crick et al., 2003; Ostrov & Keating, 2004; Ostrov, Woods, Jansen, Casas, & Crick, in press). These findings support the hypothesis that a substantial number of aggressive girls can be identified in early childhood if indices of hostile behavior that are salient to girls are included in assessments of aggression.

## MANIFESTATIONS OF RELATIONAL AGGRESSION IN EARLY CHILDHOOD

The earliest studies of relational aggression have been concerned with, among many other things, what these behaviors look like during the preschool period. At this point there have not been any studies that have assessed relational aggression prior to age 2½. This does not imply that relationally aggressive behaviors are nonexistent before age 2½ but rather that valid assessments may be more difficult to obtain while toddlers are still achieving important developmental milestones (for an expanded discussion, see Crick, Werner, et al., 1999).

Studies of relational aggression during the preschool years have found that these behaviors are quite common in young children's interactions (Crick et al., 1997; McNeilly-Choque, Hart, Robinson, Nelson, & Olsen, 1996). These studies have also highlighted the fact that relational aggression during these years is still relatively unsophisticated. During this period, preschoolers are just beginning to gain an understanding of various social skills, so when they engage in relational aggression they tend to do so in relatively simple, concrete ways (e.g., telling a peer that he or she can't come to their birthday party unless certain conditions are met). In an earlier chapter (Crick, Werner, et al., 1999), we had posited that relational aggression would most often be direct in nature during early childhood, reflecting children's cognitive, linguistic, and social abilities. However, more recent observational work (Ostrov & Keating, 2004; Ostrov et al., in press), has shown that in fact preschoolers are already beginning to use complicated indirect behaviors that are more rudimentary in nature. For example, gossiping and rumor spreading can be seen in young children's interactions in both structured and unstructured environments.

Another important characteristic of relational aggression in preschool is that it tends to be enacted "in the moment," in response to immediate problems. That is, the use of relational aggression tends to be a reaction to children's present situations rather than a response to a perceived transgression in the past. As work in this area continues, more light, ideally, will be shed on when children begin to routinely hold grudges, an "ability" that most likely serves to prolong anger and emotional distress among those children involved in the particular incident.

## ASSESSMENT OF PRESCHOOLERS' RELATIONAL AGGRESSION: CURRENT ISSUES AND ADVANCES

One of the fundamental issues for defining and understanding aggression in early childhood concerns identifying and utilizing appropriate assessment strategies. A number of approaches have been employed during early childhood including observation, peer reports, teacher reports, and parent reports. The continued use of these instruments may offer key insights into the development of relational aggression during early childhood, and these tools may be used to assess the utility and effectiveness of intervention and prevention efforts in a myriad of social contexts. The following sections will briefly review some of these innovative research tools with a focus on the developmental appropriateness of these early childhood measures of relational aggression.

### Observation

Most empirical work on relational aggression in young children has relied on peer and teacher reports, and only a few studies have incorporated observational approaches to specifically assess relational forms of aggression (see Archer, in press).

#### Naturalistic Observations

The focal child approach (Arsenio & Lover, 1997; Fagot & Hagan, 1985; Laursen & Hartup, 1989) appears to be one of the easiest methods to administer in a classroom or playground setting and may offer the most insight into the developmental progression of relationally aggressive behaviors. Past researchers adopting this method have observed a focal child for 10-minute intervals across 5 to 8 independent sessions, during 2 to 3 months of observation, recording both the behaviors that he or she delivers to peers (aggression) and those that he or she receives from peers (victimization) (see Ostrov & Keating, 2004). Observers are able to record children's behavior unobtrusively in a variety of environments (i.e., classroom, gym, playground), and children's aggression scores reflect their behavior across multiple days, times, settings, and peer groups in order to obtain a relatively valid assessment of their natural peer interactions (Pellegrini, 1996, 2001). The valid assessment of relational aggression requires that observers be in close proximity to participants so that they can readily hear their conversations (i.e., because many acts of relational aggression are verbal and/or subtle in nature). Although this proximity runs the risk of affecting children's behavior, fortunately there are a number of steps that can be taken to reduce participant reactivity (e.g., spending considerable time in the classroom prior to observations) (Pelligrini, 2001; Reid, Baldwin, Patterson, & Dishion, 1988). Observations of preschoolers' relationally aggressive behaviors during free play have been found to correlate significantly with teacher reports of the same behaviors (Crick et al., 2003; McNeilly-Choque et al., 1996; Ostrov & Keating, 2004). As an example, results of our ongoing longitudinal study of relational aggression during early childhood, the "Preschool PALS Project," has revealed significant correlations between teachers and observers (e.g., physical aggression, $r = .60$, $p < .001$; relational aggression, $r = .48$, $p < .001$; Crick et al., 2003). Favorable reliability of these approaches has also been revealed in each of these studies.

## Semistructured Situations

In addition to naturalistic approaches, observational techniques designed to assess young children's relationally aggressive behavior have also included semistructured, analogue situations (Ostrov & Keating, 2004; Ostrov et al., in press). These developmentally appropriate observational methods are designed to elicit and capture (via videotape) the types of peer interactions that naturally occur in children's play environments in a relatively time- and cost-efficient manner. Based on past resource-utilization studies, Ostrov and Keating (2004) designed a developmentally appropriate and ecologically valid coloring task for use with preschool children. This coloring task was designed as a limited-resource utilization task in which the presence of preferred colorful crayons was restricted during the coloring of various age-appropriate pictures. The sessions were videotaped and later coded for relational aggression, physical aggression, and other social behaviors (e.g., prosocial behavior). Researchers have included dyads and triads of same- and opposite-gender children in the coloring task (for details, see Ostrov & Keating, 2004; Ostrov et al., in press). Favorable psychometric properties have been demonstrated for raters' coding of preschoolers' aggressive behavior elicited within these situations (e.g., high interobserver reliability, cross-context stability, agreement with teacher reports, etc.; see Crick et al., 2003; Ostrov & Keating, 2004; Ostrov et al., in press). In addition, it is possible to achieve relatively low levels of participant reactivity using this paradigm (Ostrov et al., in press), which supports the external validity of the task (Reid et al., 1988).

## Peer Reports

Peer reports of social behavior have been used with young children in several studies of relational aggression (e.g., Crick et al., 1997, 2003; McNeilly-Choque et al., 1996). Findings from these studies indicate that young children, aided by pictures of their classmates and practice items, are able to provide reliable and valid information concerning a host of constructs, including peer acceptance and relational aggression, particularly when a peer rating approach is used (see Denham et al., 2000; Hart et al., 2000), a method in which children rate each classmate on the behavior of interest. Peer nomination approaches have also been used with young children in recent research (e.g., Crick et al., 1997; Sebanc, Pierce, Cheatham, & Gunnar, 2003; Walden, Lemerise, & Smith, 1999). In this approach, children are asked to point to several children who exhibit the characteristic described by the item (e.g., physical and relational aggression, etc.; Crick et al., 1997). We have found that, when assessing relational aggression, both peer rating and peer nomination techniques are readily understandable by children as young as 3 years old, although children younger than 3 years old have had difficulty understanding these types of procedures (Hymel, 1983). Furthermore, particularly when peer ratings are used, peer reports correspond rather well with information yielded by other informants (teachers, observations; Crick et al., 2003; Wu, Hart, Draper, & Olsen, 2001).

## Teacher Reports

Teacher report methods of aggression and antisocial behavior have been used quite extensively with preschool children (e.g., Willoughby, Kupersmidt, & Bryant, 2001). The Preschool Social Behavior Scale for Teachers Form (PSBS-TF; Crick et al., 1997) and the Preschool Peer Victimization Measure for Teachers Form (PPVM-TF; Crick, Casas, & Ku, 1999) have been developed to measure relational (and physical) forms of aggression and victimization in early childhood (for a review, see Crick, Werner, et al., 1999). Adapted versions of these teacher reports have been used successfully in several cross-cultural studies (e.g., Hart, Nelson, Robinson, Olsen, McNeilly-Choque, 1998; Hart et al., 1999; Russell, Hart, Robinson, & Olsen, 2003).

## Parent Reports

Parent reports may be an alternate source of reliable information about young children's aggressive behavior; however, relatively few studies have explored this issue (Denham et al., 2000), and to our knowledge no studies have yet examined parent reports of relational aggression for this age group. In particular, parents may be able to provide important information about behaviors that occur among siblings and neighborhood children, and their perspective warrants consideration in future research.

## IS RELATIONAL AGGRESSION HARMFUL?

To demonstrate that, like physical aggression, relational aggression is harmful to the perpetrators and the victims, a number of studies have attempted to assess the hurtfulness of these acts. Evaluation of the harmfulness of relationally aggressive behaviors among young children has tended to follow three avenues: (1) assessment of children's perceptions of the harm inflicted by relationally aggressive behaviors; (2) evaluation of the association between relational victimization (i.e., being the frequent target of relationally aggressive behaviors) and social–psychological adjustment; and (3) evaluation of the relation between relational aggression and social–psychological adjustment.

## Children's Perceptions of Harm

The results of several studies demonstrate that children believe that relational aggression is a hurtful behavior that often occurs in their peer groups. However, almost all of the studies assessing the children's perceptions of the harmfulness of relational aggression have focused on middle childhood and adolescence (see Crick, Werner, et al., 1999). For example, Crick, Bigbee, and Howes (1996) found that 9- to 12-year-old children reported relational aggression as the most common hurtful behavior instigated in the interactions of girls' peer groups, whereas, in boys' peer groups, physical aggression was the most frequently cited hurtful behavior. Similarly, in a study of 9- to 13-year-old sibling pairs, relational aggression was cited as the most frequent mean behavior that occurred within the dyad, regardless of age or gender (O'Brien & Crick, 1997). Older adolescents also describe relational aggression as a mean behavior commonly occurring within peer groups (Morales, Crick, Werner, & Schellin, 2002). Findings from these studies indicate that school-aged children and adolescents view relationally aggressive behaviors as hostile, mean, and harmful (i.e., "aggressive").

In one of the few studies of young children's perceptions of aggressive behaviors, McNeilly-Choque and colleagues (1996) found that, like older children, preschool children associated relational aggression with anger. In a study recently conducted within our own research lab, we assessed preschoolers' perceptions of the harm caused by relational aggression by using a combination of open-ended and forced-response interview questions (Jansen, Ostrov, Woods, Casas, & Crick, 2004). The 3- to 5-year-old participants were asked about a limited-resource coloring task that they had just completed with two peers (Ostrov et al., in press). Following his or her open-ended description of the situation, each child was asked a series of eight forced-choice interview questions pertaining to the child's perceptions about how upsetting several types of behaviors were for the recipient. These included physical aggression (e.g., pinching) and relational aggression (e.g., saying, "I won't be your friend anymore unless you give me that crayon"). All questions followed the format: "When they are coloring, some kids _____ [state a physically aggressive or relationally aggressive behavior]. When a kid gets _____ [restate behavior], how do you think that kid would feel? Not sad at all, a little sad, or very sad?" A series of three schematic drawings depicting a happy face, a neutral face, and a frowning face were shown to the child to accompany the response choices (Arsenio & Kramer, 1992; Hart et al., 1998). Children either verbally responded or pointed to the face that corresponded with their answer choice.

Results of this study showed that the majority of boys and girls rated both physically and relationally aggressive acts as distressing. There were no significant differences in level of distress between relational and physical aggression items and no gender differences. The relatively high mean levels of distress reported for relational (74% of participants rated these behaviors as making a person feel very sad) and physical aggression (83% of participants rated these behaviors as making a person feel very sad) indicated that both subtypes of aggression were viewed as harmful by preschool children. Taken together, these results highlight the need to continue to study relationally aggressive behaviors in preschoolers since there is evidence that children as young as 3 years of age find these behaviors to be emotionally upsetting. It will be important to replicate these findings with preschoolers and extend this work to children under the age of 3.

## Relational Victimization and Social–Psychological Adjustment

The hurtful nature of relationally aggressive acts also has been evaluated by examining the association between relational victimization (i.e., being the frequent target of relational aggression) and social–psychological adjustment. The majority of studies in this area have focused on school-aged children and adolescents. These studies provide consistent evidence that relational victimization is associated with significant adjustment problems, including depressive symptoms, social anxiety, loneliness, peer rejection, and externalizing difficulties (e.g., Crick & Bigbee, 1998; Crick & Grotpeter, 1996; Crick & Nelson, 2002; Linder, Crick, & Collins, 2002; Schafer, Werner, & Crick, 2002). Although relational victimization has rarely been studied in early childhood, initial evidence indicates that the correlates may be similar to those found in older children. Specifically, relational victimization among preschoolers has been shown to be related significantly to poor peer relationships and to rejection by peers, internalizing problems, and a lack of prosocial skills (Crick, Casas, & Ku, 1999). These findings are consistent with the hypothesis that, even among young children, relationally aggressive behaviors are distressful and hurtful for the victims.

## Relational Aggression and Social–Psychological Adjustment

The potential harmfulness of relational aggression also has been evaluated through exploration of the social–psychological adjustment status of the perpetrators of these behaviors. Similar to research on relational victimization, the majority of studies in this area have targeted middle childhood and adolescence. Findings for these age groups indicate that relationally aggressive children are at risk for continuing their use of relationally aggressive behaviors in the future, and are also likely to exhibit other adjustment problems including peer rejection, internalizing difficulties, and externalizing problems (e.g., Crick, 1996, 1997; Putallaz, Kupersmidt, Grimes, DeNero, & Coie, 1999; Rys & Bear, 1997; Tomada & Schneider, 1997).

Several studies have focused on the early childhood period. As has been found for older children, individual differences in the use of relationally aggressive behaviors have been shown to be relatively stable over time for preschoolers with $r = .45$, $p < .001$, for observations of relational aggression and $r = .69$, $p < .001$, for teacher reports over the course of an academic year (Crick et al., 2003)—indicating that young relationally aggressive children are at risk for continued engagement in these behaviors. Other studies also have shown that young relationally aggressive children are at risk for peer rejection, feelings of loneliness, and depressive symptoms (Crick et al., 1997, 2003; McNeilly-Choque et al., 1996).

These findings, combined with those described previously regarding young children's perceptions of relational aggression and the association between relational victimization and adjustment in early childhood demonstrate that young children view relationally aggressive acts as mean and hurtful, and that both the victims and the perpetrators are at risk for serious adjustment problems. This evidence suggests the importance of a research focus on strategies that might prevent and reduce levels of relational aggression and relational victimization among young children.

## TOWARD A MODEL OF RELATIONAL AGGRESSION DURING EARLY CHILDHOOD

The research discussed in the previous sections makes it fairly clear that relational aggression occurs and is detrimental in early childhood and that we have made progress in developing reliable and valid measures for assessing these behaviors during this developmental period. Given the accumulating findings outlined previously, the next step would be to more clearly define the developmental trajectories of relationally aggressive children and to determine the types of factors that might put children at risk for these behaviors. Although there is no well-specified developmental model of relational aggression, certain areas of research in relational aggression may be identified as likely to be particularly informative in developing such a model. A multicontextual model of development would address child, family, peer, and broader systems of influence (e.g., schools, neighborhoods, etc.).

Research on the development and maintenance of aggressive behavior problems has highlighted the validity of social information-processing models of the social behaviors of children (see Crick & Dodge, 1994). Although most of the research on social information processing has focused on physical aggression, several studies have shown that relationally aggressive children exhibit social-cognitive biases that are likely to contribute to the development and maintenance of their relationally aggressive behavior patterns (Crick & Werner, 1998). Specifically, relationally aggressive children exhibit hostile attribution biases for relational provocation situations (Crick, 1995; Crick et al., 2003; Leff, Kupersmidt, & Power, 2003). Similar findings have also been obtained that illustrate the presence of social-cognitive biases among young children. Casas and Crick (2004) found that relationally aggressive preschoolers evaluated the use of relational aggression in relational conflict stories significantly more positively than they evaluated its use in instrumental conflict stories. Therefore it is conceivable that social information processing, hostile attribution biases, and peer status coupled with these social-cognitive biases may influence the development of relational aggression even during early childhood.

In addition to social information processing, children's perspective-taking abilities may also be highly relevant to understanding the developmental trajectories of relational aggression (Nguyen & Frye, 1999). In the past, researchers have found that preschoolers possessing perspective-taking capabilities displayed socially expressive, sympathetic, and prosocial behaviors toward children experiencing distress during play and tended to be accepted by peers (Saarni, Mumme, & Campos, 1998). Thus, perhaps these social-cognitive skills may also be an important factor in relationally aggressive behavior. That is, in order to understand that relationally aggressive behaviors would be harmful to another person, children may need to have the requisite perspective-taking capabilities to know how such behaviors would affect the recipient. In addition, an ability to detect positive and negative affect or emotions may be associated with onset of relational aggression (Denham & Couchoud, 1990; Dunn & Hughes, 1998; Lemerise & Arsenio, 2000). To date, this has not been empirically explored with respect to relational aggression.

Similarly, other cognitive factors such as language development may play a significant role in relationally aggressive behaviors (Bonica, Yershova, Arnold, Fisher, & Zeljo, 2003). Although to date there has been little research focused on the topic, it will be useful to explore the influences of language development on the development of relational aggression. Many relationally aggressive acts require relatively sophisticated verbal skills (e.g., "I won't come to your birthday party unless you do this right now"), whereas others do not require such verbal production skills (e.g., ignoring or nonverbal social exclusion). Further research is needed to clarify the association between relational aggression and language skills, as existing studies have yielded mixed findings (Bonica et al., 2003; Crick, Werner, et al., 1999; Estrem, 2003). In addition, developmental findings that suggest that girls' verbal fluency occurs earlier than similar language capacities in male peers further suggests the importance of future attempts to ascertain how (and whether) children's verbal ability relates to relational aggression (Bonica et al., 2003).

The development of gender roles, gender schemata, and gender attitudes may also be important for the development of relational aggression (Liben & Bigler, 2002). The work of Fagot and colleagues (Fagot, Leinbach, & Hagan, 1986) highlights that physical aggression is decreasing in girls at the same time that gender-role expectations are increasing. It is possible that, in contrast to physical aggression, relational aggression increases among girls as they develop a firmer understanding of female gender roles. Peer-group-specific gender norms may also influence the types of behavior in which children engage (Maccoby, 1988, 2002) and the consequences of those behaviors. There is evidence that children who engage in gender non-normative types of aggression (i.e., physically aggressive girls and relationally aggressive boys) are significantly more maladjusted than children who engage in gender-normative aggressive behaviors (Crick, 1997). This work suggests that gender norms may be particularly important for understanding the outcomes of aggressive behavior.

Peer and sibling influences may also play a significant role in the development of relational aggression (Coie & Dodge, 1998). Along these lines, in a recent study with school-age children it was demonstrated that nonaggressive children who befriended relationally aggressive peers were relatively more likely to become relationally aggressive themselves in the future (Werner & Crick, in press). Furthermore, sibling research with older children has demonstrated that relational aggression is the most frequent form of aggression exhibited by siblings toward each other, a situation that may provide for the learning of these behaviors within the family context (for a review, see Crick, Werner, et al., 1999). The role of learning, modeling, and reinforcement of relational aggression in the context of peer and sibling relationships offers promise for informing a developmental model of relational aggression.

There is also evidence that family interactions and parent–child relationship factors (e.g., developmentally inappropriate parental expectations, parent–child coercive interactions, high family stress, etc.,) can affect physically aggressive behaviors in children (Coie & Dodge, 1998; Reid & Eddy, 1997). A parent–child relationship focus may be important for understanding the development of relational aggression during a variety of developmental periods, but especially during early childhood (Casas, Crick, Ostrov, Woods, & Jansen, 2004; Grotpeter, 1996; Nelson & Crick, 2002). More distal risk factors such as parental psychopathology and substance use, family discord, socioeconomic status, neighborhood instability/community violence, and difficulties with extended family and workplace relationships may also contribute to the onset and persistence of aggression in early childhood and across the lifespan (Reid & Eddy, 1997). However, the association of these factors with the development of relational aggression has not yet been explored.

## FUTURE DIRECTIONS, FUTURE CHALLENGES, AND CONCLUSIONS

Although information about the development of relational aggression in early childhood is increasing at a relatively rapid pace, a host of significant research questions have yet to be explored. One of the most significant challenges for future research will be to identify, at a relatively young age, individuals who are most likely to be at risk for engaging in high levels of relational aggression. The identification of precursors and risk factors associated with the onset and maintenance of relationally aggressive behaviors will be critically important for the formation of effective intervention or prevention programs.

Future studies should address how cognitive factors such as language abilities (e.g., Bonica et al., 2003), coping strategies, social information processing mechanisms (e.g., Casas & Crick, 2004; Crick, 1995; Crick et al., 2003; Crick & Werner, 1998), perspective-taking abilities, and emotional competence relate to the development of relational aggression and victimization. Additionally, it will be important to explore a variety of other proximal and distal risk and protective factors in young children in future investigative efforts targeting relational aggression. These are likely to include culture (e.g., Hart et al., 1998), socioeconomic status (e.g., McNeilly-Choque et al., 1996), stress reactivity (e.g., Dettling, Gunnar, & Donzella, 1999), family factors (e.g., Hart et al., 1998), social dominance patterns, play styles, attachment, and the role of the media. By studying many of these diverse factors concurrently and prospectively throughout early childhood, we may better understand factors that contribute to the early development of relationally aggressive behavior problems.

There are also a number of methodological challenges for the future. It is recommended that future work be dedicated to refining and adapting current measurement techniques for use with children younger than age 3. Qualitative methods may be useful to identify the range and diversity of relationally aggressive behaviors exhibited by children in toddlerhood. For example, focus groups with teachers and parents of toddlers may provide information that could inform the development of teacher, peer, parent, and observational measures appropriate for very young children. Such approaches may also be helpful for evaluating the range and diversity of relationally aggressive behaviors among young children in other cultures.

In future research, it will also be important to assess young children's relationally aggressive behavior in multiple contexts. Thus far, these assessments have been limited to the school setting. To generate a more complete picture of the range and diversity of relationally aggressive acts in early childhood it will be necessary to include additional settings such as home, neighborhood, and day care contexts. This is particularly important for young children, as they often spend significantly less time at school than older children, and less time at school than in other settings. Accordingly, it is recommended that future studies continue to explore the use of multi-informants to assess relational aggression in early childhood.

Clearly, our collective future agenda for research on relational aggression in early childhood is both challenging and exciting. It is also significant because it holds promise for clarifying theoretical and empirical questions regarding the prevalence, onset, and development of aggressive behavior, particularly among females.

## ACKNOWLEDGMENTS

Preparation of this chapter was supported by grants from the National Institute of Mental Health (No. MH63684) and the National Science Foundation (No. BCS-0126521) to Nicki R. Crick, and by Eva O. Miller Graduate Fellowships to Jamie M. Ostrov and Karen Appleyard. We thank Crystal Cullerton-Sen for comments and suggestions on an earlier draft. We are also grateful to the directors, teachers, parents, and children who participated in the research described in this chapter.

## REFERENCES

Archer, J. (in press). Sex differences in aggression in real-world settings: A meta-analytic review. *Review of General Psychology*

Arsenio, W. F., & Kramer, R. (1992). Victimizers and their victims: Children's conceptions of the mixed emotional consequences of moral transgressions. *Child Development, 63*, 915–927.

Arsenio, W. F., & Lover, A. (1997). Emotions, conflicts and aggression during preschoolers' free play. *British Journal of Developmental Psychology, 15*, 531–542.

Bjorkqvist, K., Lagerspetz, K., & Kaukianen, A. (1992). Do girls manipulate and boys fight? Developmental trends in regard to direct and indirect aggression. *Aggressive Behavior, 18*, 117–127.

Bonica, C., Yershova, K., Arnold, D. H., Fisher, P. H., & Zeljo, A. (2003). Relational aggression and language development in preschoolers. *Social Development, 12*, 551–562.

Casas, J. F., & Crick, N. R. (2004). *Response evaluation processes and relational aggression in preschool.* Manuscript in preparation.

Casas, J. F., Crick, N. R., Ostrov, J. M., Woods, K. E., & Jansen, E. A. (2004). *Early parenting and children's use of relational aggression in preschool.* Manuscript in preparation.

Coie, J. D., & Dodge, K. A. (1998). Aggression and antisocial behavior. In W. Damon & N. Eisenberg (Eds.), *Handbook of child psychology: Vol. 3. Social, emotional, and personality development* (5th ed., pp. 779–862). New York: Wiley.

Crick, N. R. (1995). Relational aggression: The role of intent attributions, provocation type, and feelings of distress. *Development and Psychopathology, 7*, 313–322.

Crick, N. R. (1996). The role of overt aggression, relational aggression, and prosocial behavior in children's future social adjustment. *Child Development, 67*, 2317–2327.

Crick, N. R. (1997). Engagement in gender normative versus non-normative forms of aggression: Links to social-psychological adjustment. *Developmental Psychology, 33*, 610–617.

Crick, N. R., & Bigbee, M. A. (1998). Relational and overt forms of peer victimization: A multi-informant approach. *Journal of Consulting and Clinical Psychology, 66*, 337–347.

Crick, N. R., Bigbee, M. A., & Howes, C. (1996). Gender differences in children's normative beliefs about aggression: How do I hurt thee? Let me count the ways. *Child Development, 67*, 1003–1014.

Crick, N. R., Casas, J. F., & Ku, H. C. (1999). Physical and relational peer victimization in preschool. *Developmental Psychology, 35*, 376–385.

Crick, N. R., Casas, J. F., & Mosher, M. (1997). Relational and overt aggression in preschool. *Developmental Psychology, 33*, 579–588.

Crick, N. R., & Dodge, K. A. (1994). A review and reformulation of social information processing mechanisms in children's social adjustment. *Psychological Bulletin, 11*, 74–101.

Crick, N. R., & Grotpeter, J. K. (1995). Relational aggression, gender, and social-psychological adjustment. *Child Development, 66*, 710–722.

Crick, N. R., & Grotpeter, J. K. (1996). Children's treatment by peers: Victims of relational and overt aggression. *Development and Psychopathology, 8*, 367–380.

Crick, N. R., Grotpeter, J. K., & Bigbee, M. A. (2002). Relationally and physically aggressive children's intent attributions and feelings of distress for relational and instrumental peer conflicts. *Child Development, 73*, 1134–1142.

Crick, N. R., & Nelson, D. A. (2002). Relational and physical victimization within friendships: Nobody told me there'd be friends like these. *Journal of Abnormal Child Psychology, 30*, 599–607.

Crick, N. R., Ostrov, J. M., Cullerton-Sen, C., Appleyard, K., & Jansen, E. A. (2003, April). *A longitudinal examination of relational and physical aggres-*

*sion in early childhood*. Paper presented at the biennial meeting of the Society for Research in Child Development, Tampa, FL.

Crick, N. R., & Werner, N. E. (1998). Response decision processes in relational and overt aggression. *Child Development, 69,* 1630–1639.

Crick, N. R., Werner, N. E., Casas, J. F., O'Brien, K. M., Nelson, D. A., Grotpeter, J. K., & Markon, K. M. (1999). Childhood aggression and gender: A new look at an old problem. In D. Bernstein (Ed.), *Nebraska Symposium on Motivation* (pp. 75–141). Lincoln: University of Nebraska.

Crick, N. R., & Zahn-Waxler, C. (2003). Gender and developmental psychopathology: Current progress and future challenges. *Development and Psychopathology, 15,* 719–742.

Denham, S. A., Workman, E., Cole, P. M., Weissbrod, C., Kendziora, K., Zahn-Waxler, C. (2000). Prediction of externalizing behavior problems from early to middle childhood: The role of parental socialization and emotion expression. *Development and Psychopathology, 12,* 23–45.

Dettling, A. C., Gunnar, M. R., & Donzella, B. (1999). Cortisol levels of young children in full-day childcare centers: Relations with age and temperament. *Psychoneuroendocrinology, 24,* 519–536.

Dunn, J., & Hughes, C. (1998). Young children's understanding of emotions within close relationships. *Cognition and Emotion, 12,* 171–190.

Estrem, T. L. (2003). *Relational and physical aggression among preschoolers: The effect of language skills and gender.* Unpublished doctoral dissertation, University of Minnesota.

Fagot, B. I., & Hagan, R. (1985). Aggression in toddlers: Responses to the assertive acts of boys and girls. *Sex Roles, 12,* 341–351.

Fagot, B. I., Leinbach, M. D., & Hagan, R. (1986). Gender labeling and the adoption of sex-typed behaviors. *Developmental Psychology, 22,* 440–443.

Feshbach, N. (1969). Sex differences in children's modes of aggressive behavior toward outsiders. *Merrill-Palmer Quarterly, 15,* 249–258.

Grotpeter, J. K. (1996). *Relational aggression, overt aggression, and family relationships.* Unpublished doctoral dissertation, University of Illinois at Urbana-Champaign.

Hart, C. H., Nelson, D. A., Robinson, C. C., Olsen, S. F., & McNeilly-Choque, M. K. (1998). Overt and relational aggression in Russian nursery-school-age children: Parenting style and marital linkages. *Developmental Psychology, 34,* 687–697.

Hart, C. H., Yang, C., Nelson, D., Robinson, C. C., Jin, S., Wu, P., Olsen, S. F., & Newell, L. D. (1999, April). *Subtypes of aggression in Chinese, Russia, and U.S. preschoolers: Sex and peer status linkages.* Paper presented at the biennial meeting of the Society for Research in Child Development, Albuquerque, NM.

Hart, C. H., Yang, C., Nelson, L. J., Robinson, C. C., Olsen, S. A., Nelson, D. A., et al. (2000). Peer acceptance in early childhood and subtypes of socially withdrawn behaviour in China, Russia, and the U.S. *International Journal of Behavior Development, 24,* 73–81.

Hymel, S. (1983). Preschool children's peer relations: Issues in sociometric assessment. *Merrill-Palmer Quarterly, 29,* 237–260.

Jansen, E. A., Ostrov, J.M., Woods, K. E, Casas, J. F., & Crick, N. R. (2004). *Preschool children's perceptions of physical and relational aggression: What makes a kid sad?* Manuscript in preparation.

Keenan, K., & Shaw, D. (1997). Developmental and social influences on young girls' problem behavior. *Psychological Bulletin, 121,* 95–113.

Laursen, B., & Hartup, W. W. (1989). The dynamics of preschool children's conflicts. *Merrill-Palmer Quarterly, 35,* 281–297.

Leff, S. S., Kupersmidt, J. B., & Power, T. J. (2003). An initial examination of girls' cognitions of their relationally aggressive peers as a function of their own social standing. *Merrill-Palmer Quarterly, 49,* 28–53.

Lemerise, E. A., & Arsenio, W. F. (2000). An integrated model of emotion processes and cognition in social information processing. *Child Development, 71,* 107–118.

Liben, L. S., & Bigler, R. S. (2002). The developmental course of gender differentiation: Conceptualizing, measuring, and evaluating constructs and pathways. *Monographs of the Society for Research in Child Development, 67,* i–viii, 1–147.

Linder, J., Crick, N. R., & Collins, W. A. (2002). Relational aggression and victimization in young adults' romantic relationships: Association with perceptions of parent, peer, and romantic relationship quality. *Social Development, 11,* 69–86.

Maccoby, E. E. (1988). Gender as a social category. *Developmental Psychology, 24,* 755–765.

Maccoby, E. E. (2002). Gender and group process: A developmental perspective. *Current Directions in Psychological Science, 11,* 54–58.

McNeilly-Choque, M. K., Hart, C. H., Robinson, C. C., Nelson, L., & Olsen, S. F. (1996). Overt and relational aggression on the playground: Correspondence among different informants. *Journal of Research in Childhood Education, 11,* 47–67.

Moffitt, T. E., & Caspi, A. (2001). Childhood predictors differentiate life-course persistent and adolescent-limited antisocial pathways among males and females. *Development and Psychopathology, 13,* 355–375.

Morales, J., Crick, N. R., Werner, N., & Schellin, H. (2002). *Adolescents' normative beliefs about aggression: What we do to be hurtful and mean.* Manuscript in preparation.

Nelson, D. A., & Crick, N. R. (2002). Parental psychological control: Implications for childhood physical and relational aggression. In B. K. Barber (Ed.), *Intrusive parenting: How psychological control affects children and adolescents* (pp. 161–188). Washington DC: American Psychological Association Books.

Nguyen, L., & Frye, D. (1999). Children's theory of mind: Understanding of desire, belief, and emotion with social referents. *Social Development, 8,* 70–92.

O'Brien, K., & Crick, N. R. (1997). *Relational and physical aggression in sibling relationships: From hitting and kicking to ignoring and excluding, siblings do it all.* Manuscript in preparation.

Ostrov, J. M., & Keating, C. F. (2004). Gender differences in preschool aggression during free play and structured interactions: An observational study. *Social Development, 13,* 255–277.

Ostrov, J. M., Woods, K. E., Jansen, E. A., Casas, J. F., & Crick, N. R. (in press). An observational study of delivered and received aggression, gender, and social–psychological adjustment in preschool: "This white crayon doesn't work . . . " *Early Childhood Research Quarterly.*

Pellegrini, A. D. (1996). *Observing children in their natural worlds: A methodological primer.* Mahwah, NJ: Erlbaum.

Pellegrini, A. D. (2001). Practitioner review: The role of direct observation in the assessment of young children. *Journal of Child Psychology and Psychiatry and Allied Disciplines, 42,* 861–869.

Putallaz, M., Kupersmidt, J., Grimes, C. L., DeNero, K., & Coie, J. D. (1999, April). *Overt and relational aggressors, victims, and gender.* Paper presented at the biennial meeting of the Society for Research in Child Development, Albuquerque, NM.

Reid, J. B., Baldwin, D. V., Patterson, G. R., & Dishion, T. J. (1988). Observations in the assessment of childhood disorders. In M. Rutter, A. H. Tuma, & I. S. Lann (Eds.), *Assessment and diagnosis in child psychopathology.* New York: Guilford Press.

Reid, J. B., & Eddy, J. M. (1997). The prevention of antisocial behavior: Some considerations in the search for effective interventions. In D. M. Stoff, J. Breiling, & J. D. Maser (Eds.), *The handbook of antisocial behavior* (pp. 343–356). New York: Wiley.

Russell, A., Hart, C. H., Robinson, C. C., & Olsen, S. F. (2003). Children's sociable and aggressive behavior with peers: A comparison of the U.S. and Australia, and contributions of temperament and parenting style. *International Journal of Behavioral Development, 27,* 74–86.

Rys, G. S., & Bear, G. G. (1997). Relational aggression and peer rejection: Gender and developmental issues. *Merrill-Palmer Quarterly, 43,* 87–106.

Saarni, C., Mumme, D., & Campos, J. (1998). Emotional development: Action, communication, and understanding. In N. Eisenberg (Vol. Ed.) & W. Damon (Series Ed.), *The handbook of child psychology: Vol. 3. Social, emotional, and personality development* (5th ed., pp. 237–309). New York: Wiley.

Schafer, M., Werner, N. E., & Crick, N. R. (2002). Relational victimization, physical victimization, and bullying among German school children. *British Journal of Psychology, 20,* 281–306.

Sebanc, A., Pierce, S. Cheatham, C., & Gunnar, M. R. (2003). The friendship features of preschool children: Links with prosocial behavior and aggression. *Social Development, 12,* 91–106.

Silverthorn, P., & Frick, P. J. (1999). Developmental pathways to antisocial behavior: The delayed-onset pathway in girls. *Development and Psychopathology, 11,* 101–126.

Tomada, G., & Schneider, B. H. (1997). Relational aggression, gender, and peer acceptance: Invariance across culture, stability over time, and concordance among informants. *Developmental Psychology, 33,* 601–609.

Walden, T., Lemerise, E., & Smith, M. C. (1999). Friendship and popularity in preschool classrooms. *Early Education and Development, 10,* 351–371.

Werner, N. E., & Crick, N. R. (in press). Peer relationship influences on the development of relational and physical aggression during middle childhood: The roles of peer rejection associated with aggressive friends. *Social Development.*

Willoughby, M., Kupersmidt, J., & Bryant, D. (2001). Overt and covert dimensions of antisocial behavior in early childhood. *Journal of Abnormal Child Psychology, 29,* 177–187.

Wu, X., Hart, C. H., Draper, T. W., & Olsen, J. A. (2001). Peer and teacher sociometrics for preschool children: Cross-informant concordance, temporal stability, and reliability. *Merrill-Palmer Quarterly, 47,* 416–443.

# CHAPTER 5

# Girls Who Bully

## A Developmental and Relational Perspective

Debra Pepler, Wendy Craig,
Amy Yuile, *and* Jennifer Connolly

Bullying is a relationship problem because it is a form of aggression that unfolds in the context of a relationship. Within a bully–victim relationship, the child who bullies is in a position of power relative to the victim. This power advantage may arise from many aspects of the relationship—differential in size, strength, age, social status—or through familiarity with the other's vulnerabilities. As bullying unfolds over time, the power differential in the relationship becomes increasingly consolidated. Although girls do not report bullying to the same extent as boys (Charach, Pepler, & Ziegler, 1995; Olweus, 1993), there is substantial evidence that some girls are involved in using their power aggressively. In this chapter, we examine the nature and context of girls' bullying to address three questions: Is bullying only found in childhood or is it a problem in adolescence too? Do children who bully experience problems in their peer relationships? Are relationship problems related to the extent of involvement in bullying? We compare girls' bullying to that of boys to bring attention to the risks associated with involvement in this form of aggression within salient relationships and social contexts.

Generally, girls' aggressive problems are thought to be less prevalent and serious than those of boys (Keenan, 2001; Offord, Lipman, & Duku, 2001). It is not surprising, therefore, that the theoretical models and empirical foundation for understanding the development of aggression have been based on research on aggressive boys. The purpose of the present chapter is neither to debate gender differences in aggression nor to deflect concerns for male aggression, but to highlight the risks, processes, and outcomes in the development of girls' aggression. Accordingly, we have focused on the interactions of aggressive girls within the primary social context of peer relationships to begin to understand the development of their problems.

## A CONCERN FOR GIRLS WHO BULLY

Girls' aggressive problems are generally found to be less prevalent and serious than those of boys (Moffitt, Caspi, Rutter, & Silva, 2001; Offord et al., 2001). Girls' involvement in delinquency and criminal behavior is also less prevalent than that of boys (Statistics Canada, 1998). Data on the prevalence of bullying reflect similar trend. On self-report measures of bullying, the prevalence of girls reporting bullying is about a third of that of boys. On a survey of students in grades 4–8, 8% of girls acknowledged bullying others more than once or twice a term, compared to 23% of boys (Charach et al., 1995). Our naturalistic observations of bullying on the school playground, however, suggest that the discrepancy between girls' and boys' involvement in bullying may not be as great as self-reports imply. We observed girls' bullying at a rate of 2.7 episodes per hour and boys' bullying at a rate of 5.2 episodes per hour (Craig & Pepler, 1997). In a subsequent observational study, the ratio was similar: Girls were observed to bully in 107 (35%) episodes and boys were observed to bully in 199 (65%) episodes (Pepler, Craig, O'Connell, & Atlas, 1998). The form of girls' bullying differs somewhat from that of boys. Girls are more likely to use social forms of aggression than boys (Smith, Pepler, & Craig, 2003). Girls' use of power and aggression may include malicious gossip and exclusion. These forms of social aggression can be carried out covertly, with a low probability of detection. Boys are more likely than girls to assert their power through physical aggression; however, girls do resort to physical forms of aggression when provoked (Smith et al., 2003). Similar to other patterns of aggression (Bjorkqvist, Osterman, & Kaukiainen, 1992), there are some gender differences in bullying, but substantial overlap in the distributions of girls and boys on social and physical forms of bullying.

Although girls' bullying has drawn minimal research attention, we contend that, similar to boys (Farrington, 1993), it places girls at risk for a range of problems in adolescence and adulthood. In particular, the relationship context of bullying raises concerns for girls involved in this form of aggression because styles of interaction may become consolidated through these negative peer experiences. Girls who bully may be establishing patterns of power and aggression in the context of both same-sex and opposite-sex relationships. Our naturalistic observations revealed that girls were involved in bullying boys and other girls at approximately equal rates: In our first study, 52% of the victims of girls' bullying were boys and 48% were girls (Craig & Pepler, 1997). In our second study, we observed that girls bullied boys in 45% and other girls in 55% of the episodes in which girls were the aggressors (Pepler et al., 1998). In both studies, boys were much more likely to bully other boys than to bully girls. The episodes in which boys bullied girls represented 14% and 19% in the first and second observational studies, respectively. Some episodes involving girls bullying boys appear to be attention-seeking in intent and may represent a form of pre-courtship with interest and positive intent embedded in negative interaction. Thorne (1993) noted this pattern of interaction between girls and boys in her playground observations: "The ambiguities of borderwork [separation into same-sex peer groups] allow the signalling of sexual or romantic, as well as aggressive, meanings, and the two often mix together" (p. 81). Girls who attract boys' attention by calling them names, physically attacking them, or taking their belongings may be learning how effective these strategies can be compared to positive strategies, such as starting a conversation. Using aversive strategies to attract boys' attention places girls who bully at risk for establishing a dangerous precedent for subsequent dating relations. We are seeing evidence of this in our early adolescent study. Girls and boys who bully are more likely to report being aggressive and victimized in early adolescent romantic relationships compared to children who do not report engaging in bullying (Connolly, Pepler, Craig, & Taradash, 2000). Similar patterns of girls' aggression toward male partners were also found among late adolescents and young adults (Capaldi & Gorman-Smith, 2003; Moffitt et al., 2001).

## BULLYING IN CHILDHOOD AND EARLY AND MIDDLE ADOLESCENCE

Over the past decade, we have conducted research on aggression and victimization with students in elementary, middle school, and high school. For this chapter, we have examined data from cross-sectional samples of students in three studies. The first study was conducted in elementary schools with students in grades 1–6. There were 56 girls and 34 boys in grade 1 (6 years old), 56 and 62 boys in grade 2 (7 years old), 71 girls and 71 boys in grade 3 (8 years old), 79 girls and 77 boys in grade 4 (9 years old), 79 girls and 65 boys in grade 5 (10 years old), and 63 girls and 63 boys in grade 6 (11 years old).

In our second study of early adolescents, we assessed children in the top three grades of kindergarten–grade 8 elementary schools. There were students in the middle school years: grade 6 (11 years old; 163 girls and 151 boys), grade 7 (12 years old; 187 girls and 233 boys), and grade 8 (13 years old; 245 girls and 271 boys). The third study focused on high school and involved students in grade 9 (14 years old; 132 girls and 161 boys), grade 10 (15 years old; 167 girls and 157 boys), grade 11 (16 years old; 160 girls and 166 boys), and grade 12 (17 years old; 138 girls and 66 boys). Approximately three quarters of the students were from Euro-Canadian and middle-class backgrounds, and two-parent families, although there was considerable variability in socioeconomic status.

## Is Bullying Only a Childhood Problem?

To determine the prevalence of bullying among girls and boys, we used an adaptation of Olweus's (1989) student questionnaire for all of our studies. Figure 5.1 presents the prevalence of bullying at least once in the past 2 months from grade 1 through grade 12, for both girls and boys. In this figure, we have indicated the proportion of children who report bullying others and those who report both bullying and being victimized by their peers. We classified children in four mutually exclusive groups, according to their answers on an adapted version of the bullying questionnaire (Olweus, 1989). Bullies were identified as those children who reported bullying others in the past 2 months and were not victimized. Victims were identified as those children who reported being victimized in the past 2 months and did not bully others. Bully/victims were identified as those children who reported that they had both bullied others and been victimized in the past 2 months. Comparison children were those who reported that they had not bullied and had not been victimized in the past 2 months. Within this chapter on bullying, we focus on those children who reported this form of aggression compared to those not involved in bullying. Data on the victimized children are not included in this discussion of aggression.

As can be seen, bullying is not just a problem in elementary school, but also a problem for adolescents when they enter high school. Up to grade 4 (9 years old), an equal proportion of girls and boys report bullying others at least once during the past 2 months. The proportion of girls who reported bullying declined steadily across the grades, with the exception of a significant increase in bullying at the school transition into grade 9. For girls, the proportion who report both bullying others and being victimized by peers increases during the pubertal transition years.

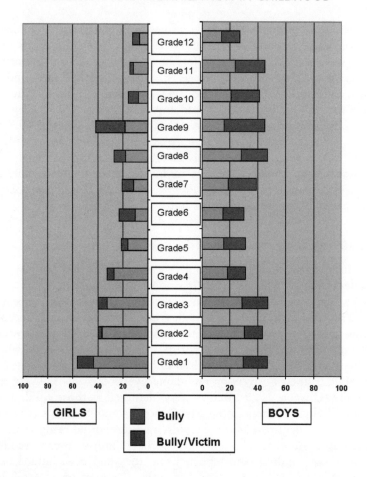

**FIGURE 5.1.** The percentage of girls and boys reporting bullying and both bullying and being victimized in the past 2 months.

## Do Children Who Bully Experience Problems in Peer Relationships?

If bullying is a relationship problem, then children who bully others might be expected to have difficulties within peer relationships. We were able to examine this hypothesis within our three studies, albeit somewhat differently for the three developmental stages.

### Childhood

In our study of elementary school children, we assessed the quality of peer relationships through sociometric ratings. For the sociometric ratings, children indicated on a 5-point scale how much they liked to play with each of their classmates, and the data were scored according to the recommendations of Asher and Dodge (1986). We compared bullies, bully/victims, and comparison children on relationship difficulties as reflected in the sociometric data. Girls who reported that they bullied (and were not victimized) were most likely to be neglected (26%) or average (28%), followed by rejected (21%), then popular (19%) according to peer ratings. Boys who reported that they bullied were most likely to be rejected (32%), followed by neglected (21%) and popular (21%). For the children who reported being bully/victims, both girls (38%) and boys (36%) were most likely to be rejected. The children who were caught in the dynamic of both bullying and victimization received more negative nominations (boys: mean = .36, $SD$ = .12; girls: mean = .40, $SD$ = .20, measured in standardized scores) than comparison children (girls: mean = 0, $SD$ = .06; boys: mean = −.15, $SD$ = .07). The bully/victims also had fewer best-friend nominations (girls: mean = −.32, $SD$ = .12; boys: mean = −.29, $SD$ = .13) than comparison children (girls: mean = .12, $SD$ = .06; boys: mean = 0, $SD$ = .07) cases. Taken together, these patterns suggest that both girls and boys in elementary school who use power and aggression in their relationships with peers are at risk for peer-relationship difficulties. Although girls and boys who bully may use different forms of aggression, both experience difficulties in the quality of peer relationships. The patterns for the girls and the boys identified as bully/victims are comparable and suggest significant problems in developing friendships and sustaining positive relationships with peers. These girls and boys tended to be rejected by the peer group at a stage of life when peer relationships are central to the development of social skills and relationship formation.

## Early and Middle Adolescence

During the early and middle adolescent stages, we assessed the quality of girls' and boys' relationships in a similar manner utilizing the Inventory of Peer and Parent Attachment (Armsden & Greenberg, 1987) and the Networks of Relationships Inventory (Furman & Buhrmester, 1985).

As with the data from elementary school students, we compared bullies, bully/victims, and comparison children on the qualities of peer relationships. For the students in the middle school and high school studies, we examined the scales associated with closeness and conflict in friendships. Closeness was examined with scales assessing trust, commitment, alienation, intimacy, and activities. The group means for these closeness scales are provided in Table 5.1. On the closeness scales, there was a significant main effect for the bully groups, $F(15, 3101)$ = 3.94, $p < .001$, lambda$^2$= .017, which was qualified by an interaction with

TABLE 5.1. Mean Scores for Middle School Students on Quality of
Peer Relationships

| | Bully | | Bully/victim | | Comparison | |
|---|---|---|---|---|---|---|
| | Boys ($n$ = 143) | Girls ($n$ = 80) | Boys ($n$ = 120) | Girls ($n$ = 61) | Boys ($n$ = 294) | Girls ($n$ = 375) |
| Trust | 3.96 (.64) | 4.40 (.64) | 3.75[c] (.80) | 4.09[c] (.59) | 4.05 (.68) | 4.34 (.65) |
| Commitment | 3.87 (.86) | 4.22 (.80) | 3.76[e] (.94) | 3.91[e] (.84) | 3.98 (.80) | 4.23 (.82) |
| Alienation | 2.31 (.86) | 1.74 (.59) | 2.24 (.80) | 2.36[a] (.78) | 2.03 (.86) | 1.89 (.72) |
| Intimacy | 3.36 (1.04) | 4.19 (1.06) | 3.12[d] (1.04) | 3.87[d] (.85) | 3.24 (1.04) | 3.82 (.96) |
| Activities | 3.67[b] (.89) | 3.92[b] (.86) | 3.37 (.83) | 3.59 (.79) | 3.50 (.89) | 3.55 (.91) |
| Conflict | 2.30[f] (.54) | 2.13[f] (.44) | 2.31[f] (.43) | 2.35[f] (.49) | 2.06 (.46) | 2.08 (.47) |
| Aggression during conflict | 2.16[f] (.83) | 1.90[f] (.73) | 2.14[f] (.70) | 2.05[f] (.77) | 1.75 (.73) | 1.74 (.65) |

Note. Standard deviations are in parentheses.

[a]Girls who were bully/victims reported more alienation than boys who were bully/victims.

[b]Youth in the bully group reported more activities with friends than bully/victims and comparison students.

[c]Youth in the bully/victim group reported less trust and affection in their relationships than all other groups.

[d]Youth in the bully/victim group reported less intimacy than bullies.

[e]Youth in the bully/victim group reported less commitment in relationships than victims and comparison students.

[f]Youth in the bully and bully/victim group reported more conflict with friends and more aggression during conflict with friends than comparison students.

gender, $F(15, 3101)$ = 1.86, $p < .05$, lambda$^2$ = .008. Girls who were bully/victims reported more alienation than boys who were bully/victims; however, within all other groups of children, boys reported more alienation than girls. The high level of alienation reported by girls who both bully and were victims may represent their cognitive dissonance between placing a high value on friendships and being marginalized in the peer group without positive friendships. Those in the bully group reported engaging in more activities with their friends than bully/victims and comparison children. Children in the bully/victim group reported less trust and affection in their friendships than all other groups of students. Bully/victims also reported less intimacy than children in the bully group, and less commitment with friends than victims and comparison students. Children who bully (both bullies and bully/victims) reported feeling more alienation from friends than comparison students.

For the middle school students, the conflict questions comprised three scales: conflicts in relationships with friends, aggression during conflict with friends, and conflict with positive resolution. For the middle school students, there was a significant multivariate effect for the bully groups on conflict with friends, which did not differ by gender, $F(9, 2913) = 6.64$, $p < .001$, lambda$^2$ = .016. Girls and boys who bullied or who were bully/victims reported more conflict with their friends than comparison students; students who were bully/victims reported the highest levels of conflict with friends. A similar pattern was found for aggression in conflicts with friends: Both girls and boys who were either bullies or bully/victims reported more aggression in conflicts with friends than victimized and comparison students. There were no group differences reported in positive conflict resolution with friends. There were also no significant gender by group interactions.

In high school, the patterns for closeness and conflict with friends were quite similar to those in middle school, with the bully/victims appearing to have the most strained relationships. The means for the high school students' closeness and conflict scales are presented in Table 5.2. On the closeness scales, there was a significant main effect for the bully groups, $F(15, 2559) = 3.32$, $p < .001$, lambda$^2$ = .018, which was not qualified by an interaction with gender. Girls and boys who were bully/victims reported less trust, less commitment, and more alienation than comparison students. Those in the bully group also reported less commitment in their friendships than comparison students. There were no group differences, however, in the reported intimacy and activities with friends.

There was a significant multivariate effect for the high school bully groups on conflict with friends, which was not differentiated by gender, multivariate $F(6, 2152) = 7.48$, $p < .001$, lambda$^2$ = .020. In high school, girls and boys who reported both bullying and being victimized experienced the greatest conflicts with friends and were significantly higher than all other groups. The bully/victims reported significantly more aggression during conflicts than bullies, and comparison students.

For the high school students, data were also available on the quality of romantic relationships, using the same scales for closeness and conflict. There were no bully group differences on measures of closeness (i.e., the extent of activities with romantic partners, trust with romantic partners, commitment, intimacy, or alienation). There was, however, a significant bully status by gender interaction for trust and alienation in romantic relationships, $F(15, 774) = 1.93$, $p < .05$, lambda$^2$ = .033. The means for scales for boys and girls in the two bully groups and comparison group are presented in Table 5.3. In general, girls reported higher levels of trust in their romantic relationships than boys. Girls and boys who bullied others, however, reported simi-

TABLE 5.2. Mean Scores for High School Students on Quality of Peer Relationships

| | Bully | | Bully/victim | | Comparison | |
|---|---|---|---|---|---|---|
| | Boys ($n$ = 104) | Girls ($n$ = 61) | Boys ($n$ = 112) | Girls ($n$ = 56) | Boys ($n$ = 251) | Girls ($n$ = 426) |
| Trust | 4.03[b] (.74) | 4.41[b] (.54) | 3.84[a] (.74) | 4.42[a] (.57) | 4.05 (.74) | 4.44 (.61) |
| Commitment | 3.92 (.84) | 4.30 (.72) | 3.81[a] (.90) | 4.21[a] (.89) | 4.04 (.91) | 4.37 (.73) |
| Alienation | 2.02 (.63) | 1.75 (.57) | 2.12[a] (.72) | 1.85[a] (.74) | 1.87 (.75) | 1.78 (.71) |
| Intimacy | 3.47 (.97) | 4.13 (.99) | 3.31 (1.08) | 4.35 (.71) | 3.44 (1.08) | 4.16 (.82) |
| Activities | 3.73 (.80) | 4.03 (.88) | 3.60 (.87) | 4.04 (.84) | 3.61 (.94) | 3.77 (.89) |
| Conflict | 1.73 (.52) | 1.76 (.53) | 1.96[c] (.77) | 1.94[c] (.63) | 1.56 (.52) | 1.63 (.48) |
| Aggression during conflict | 1.87 (.66) | 1.71 (.60) | 2.13[c] (.87) | 1.90[c] (.66) | 1.62 (.62) | 1.55 (.53) |

Note. Standard deviations are in parentheses.

[a] Youth in the bully/victim group reported less trust, less commitment, and more alienation than comparison students.

[b] Youth in the bully group reported less commitment in friendships than comparison students.

[c] Youth in the bully/victim group reported more conflict with friends and more aggression during conflict with friends than all other groups.

lar levels of trust in romantic relationships: Girls who bullied had the lowest trust scores and boys who bullied had the highest trust scores. Girls generally reported lower or equivalent levels of alienation than boys. Again, the difference in this pattern emerged for the bully group: Girls who bullied others reported greater alienation in their romantic relationships than boys who bullied.

On the conflict scales, there was a significant bully status by gender interaction for conflict in romantic relationships and aggression during conflict in romantic relationships, $F(6, 798) = 2.26$, $p < .05$, lambda$^2$ = .017. The means for the responses on the conflict scales given by boys and girls in each bully group are presented in Table 5.3. Girls who bullied other students reported higher levels of aggressive conflict with their romantic partner than boys who bullied. Girls and boys who both bullied and were victimized reported similar levels of aggression during conflicts within romantic relationships. Among comparison students in romantic relationships, girls reported higher levels of aggressive conflict than boys.

TABLE 5.3. Mean Scores for High School Students on Quality of
Romantic Relationships

| | Bully | | Bully/victim | | Comparison | |
|---|---|---|---|---|---|---|
| | Boys ($n$ = 56) | Girls ($n$ = 25) | Boys ($n$ = 51) | Girls ($n$ = 23) | Boys ($n$ = 102) | Girls ($n$ = 426) |
| Trust | 4.15[a] (.61) | 4.29[a] (.62) | 3.57 (1.06) | 4.52 (.27) | 3.85 (1.06) | 4.33 (.73) |
| Commitment | 3.41 (1.10) | 3.42 (.89) | 3.15 (1.02) | 3.38 (.89) | 3.33 (1.23) | 3.66 (1.05) |
| Alienation | 1.85 (.79) | 2.15[b] (.63) | 2.20 (.99) | 1.75 (.56) | 1.84 (.72) | 1.87 (.75) |
| Intimacy | 3.47 (1.02) | 3.58 (1.15) | 3.17 (1.17) | 3.67 (.90) | 3.42 (1.24) | 3.92 (1.05) |
| Activities | 3.50 (.90) | 3.58 (.98) | 3.41 (1.09) | 3.61 (1.03) | 3.43 (1.04) | 3.63 (.94) |
| Conflict | 1.53 (.57) | 1.67 (.56) | 1.73 (.86) | 1.58 (.56) | 1.49 (.63) | 1.64 (.60) |
| Aggression during conflict | 1.44[c] (.57) | 1.72[c] (.70) | 1.71 (.99) | 1.57 (.61) | 1.42[c] (.65) | 1.61[c] (.65) |

Note. Standard deviations are in parentheses.

[a] In general, girls reported higher levels of trust than boys; however, girls who bullied reported lower trust scores than other girls and boys who bullied reported higher trust scores than other boys.

[b] In general, girls reported lower or similar levels of alienation as boys; however, girls who bullied reported higher levels of alienation than boys who bullied.

[c] Girls in the bully and comparison groups reported higher levels of aggressive conflict with their romantic partners than boys in these respective groups.

## Are Relationship Problems Related to the Extent of Involvement in Bullying?

We were interested in whether the extent of involvement in bullying was associated with difficulties in relationships. To explore this question, three levels of involvement were identified by students' reports of how often they bullied others: never, low frequency (once or twice in the last 2 months), and high frequency (several times to more than once a week in the last 2 months). Since we were interested in the extent of involvement in bullying, we combined the bully and bully/victim groups for these analyses. The distribution of these two groups between the two bullying frequency groups indicates that those children who were bully/victims were relatively evenly divided between the low (60%) and high (40%) frequency groups. The children who were in the bully group were more likely to be categorized as low frequency (74%) than high frequency (26%). Table 5.4 displays the number of boys and girls in middle school and high school who reported bullying at these levels of fre-

TABLE 5.4. Reported Levels of Bullying in Middle and High School by Frequency

| | Peer relationships | | | | Romantic relationships | |
| | Middle school (grades 6–8) | | High school (grades 9–12) | | High school (grades 9–12) | |
| Bullying | Boys | Girls | Boys | Girls | Boys | Girls |
|---|---|---|---|---|---|---|
| Never | 387 | 443 | 312 | 470 | 123 | 154 |
| Low frequency | 180 | 112 | 133 | 93 | 60 | 35 |
| High frequency | 77 | 26 | 90 | 23 | 51 | 13 |

quency. Peer relationships were assessed among middle and high school students; romantic relationships were assessed among the subset of high school students for whom we had these data.

We compared the three groups (never, low frequency, and high frequency) on the qualities of peer relationships by examining the scales associated with closeness and conflict in friendships. For the middle school students, there was a multivariate effect for gender with trust and intimacy in peer relationships, $F(5, 1131) = 11.35$, $p < .001$, lambda$^2$ = .045. In general, girls in middle school reported more trust and intimacy in their friendships than boys. There was a significant multivariate effect for the frequency groups on trust, alienation, and commitment with friends, which did not differ by gender, $F(10, 2262)$ = 3.86, $p < .001$, lambda$^2$ = .017. The means for the responses on the closeness scales given by boys and girls in each bullying frequency group are presented in Table 5.5. Girls and boys who bullied (both low or high frequency) reported less trust, more alienation, and less commitment with their friends than comparison students. Thus, in middle school, the extent of bullying (i.e., low vs. high frequency) was not associated with different levels of difficulties with closeness in peer relationships.

Conflict was also assessed among students who bullied at different frequencies. For the middle school sample, a multivariate effect for gender was found related to conflict with resolution, $F(3, 1205) = 4.57$, $p < .01$, lambda$^2$ = .011. The means for the responses on the conflict scales given by boys and girls in each bullying frequency group are presented in Table 5.5. Girls, in general, reported greater resolution of conflicts with friends. There was a significant multivariate effect for bullying frequency groups on conflict with friends and aggression during conflicts, $F(6, 2410) = 7.35$, $p < .001$, lambda$^2$ = .018. Boys and girls who bullied at either a low or high frequency reported significantly more conflict in their friendships compared to students who never bullied others.

TABLE 5.5. Mean Scores for Middle School Students on Quality of Peer Relationships by Bullying Frequency Groups

| | Never | | Low frequency | | High frequency | |
|---|---|---|---|---|---|---|
| | Boys ($n$ = 388) | Girls ($n$ = 448) | Boys ($n$ = 181) | Girls ($n$ = 114) | Boys ($n$ = 81) | Girls ($n$ = 26) |
| Trust | 4.03 (.68) | 4.33 (.66) | 3.89 (.68) | 4.26 (.63) | 3.79 (.83) | 4.30 (.65) |
| Commitment | 3.99 (.80) | 4.20 (.83) | 3.86 (.85) | 4.12 (.77) | 3.73 (1.01) | 3.99 (1.04) |
| Alienation | 2.05 (.82) | 1.92 (.76) | 2.29 (.80) | 1.98 (.75) | 2.23 (.92) | 2.08 (.70) |
| Intimacy | 3.25 (1.04) | 3.80 (.97) | 3.18 (1.04) | 4.04 (.87) | 3.43 (1.02) | 4.10 (.93) |
| Activities | 3.45 (.89) | 3.56 (.91) | 3.44 (.85) | 3.78 (.83) | 3.74 (.90) | 3.76 (.92) |
| Conflict with friends | 2.08 (.46) | 2.09 (.46) | 2.28 (.45) | 2.20 (.49) | 2.38 (.58) | 2.34 (.58) |
| Aggression during conflict with friends | 1.80 (.73) | 1.74 (.63) | 2.09 (.72) | 1.92 (.73) | 2.28 (.88) | 2.18 (.82) |

Note. Standard deviations are in parentheses. Scale range: 1 ("never true") to 5 ("always true").

Aggression during conflicts increased as the frequency of bullying increased: Students who bullied at a high frequency reported more aggression than those who bullied at a low frequency, and students who bullied at a low frequency reported more aggression during conflicts than students who never bullied.

For high school students, there was a multivariate effect for frequency of bullying on activities, trust, and commitment with friends, $F(10, 1874) = 2.67$, $p < .01$, lambda$^2$ = .014. The means for the responses on the closeness scales given by boys and girls in each bullying frequency group are presented in Table 5.6. High school students who bullied with high frequency reported engaging in more activities than students who bullied at low frequency and students who never bullied. Similar to the middle school sample, adolescents in high school who bullied at a low or high frequency reported less trust and less commitment in their friendships than students who never bullied. During both early and middle adolescence, students who reported bullying at any level were more likely to have poorer-quality relationships with their friends than students who never bullied. There was a multivariate effect for gender on closeness in peer relationships, $F(5, 937) = 11.35$, $p < .001$, lambda$^2$ = .057. Overall, girls in high school reported more trust, com-

TABLE 5.6. Mean Scores for High School Students on Quality of Peer Relationships by Bullying Frequency Groups

|  | Never | | Low frequency | | High frequency | |
|---|---|---|---|---|---|---|
|  | Boys ($n$ = 318) | Girls ($n$ = 481) | Boys ($n$ = 133) | Girls ($n$ = 94) | Boys ($n$ = 90) | Girls ($n$ = 23) |
| Trust | 4.04 (.72) | 4.44 (.60) | 3.93 (.72) | 4.43 (.55) | 3.94 (.79) | 4.34 (.54) |
| Commitment | 4.04 (.87) | 4.37 (.72) | 3.88 (.86) | 4.27 (.81) | 3.84 (.89) | 4.19 (.79) |
| Alienation | 1.92 (.76) | 1.79 (.71) | 2.01 (.60) | 1.84 (.66) | 2.17 (.78) | 1.64 (.60) |
| Intimacy | 3.46 (1.05) | 4.16 (.82) | 3.22 (.99) | 4.18 (.93) | 3.65 (1.03) | 4.46 (.57) |
| Activities | 3.58 (.92) | 3.75 (.88) | 3.52 (.79) | 3.98 (.85) | 3.87 (.86) | 4.26 (.86) |
| Conflict with friends | 1.59 (.53) | 1.63 (.49) | 1.77 (.54) | 1.85 (.59) | 1.96 (.81) | 1.83 (.57) |
| Aggression during conflict with friends | 1.66 (.64) | 1.56 (.53) | 1.90 (.68) | 1.80 (.63) | 2.17 (.90) | 1.83 (.67) |

*Note.* Standard deviations are in parentheses. Scale range: 1 ("never true") to 5 ("always true").

mitment, intimacy, and activities, as well as less alienation, with their friends than boys.

For reports from high school students, a multivariate effect for gender was found with aggression during conflicts with friends, $F(2, 1096) = 11.59$, $p < .001$, lambda$^2$ = .021. The means for the responses on the conflict scales given by boys and girls in each bullying frequency group are presented in Table 5.6. Boys, in general, reported using aggression in conflicts with friends more often than girls. There was a significant multivariate effect for bullying frequency groups on conflict with friends and aggression during conflicts, $F(4, 2192) = 6.77$, $p < .001$, lambda$^2$ = .012. As was found in the middle school sample, boys and girls who bullied at either a low or high frequency reported significantly more conflict overall in their friendships compared to students who never bullied others. Again, there was a pattern of increasing aggression during conflicts as the frequency of bullying increased. Students who bullied at the highest frequency reported the highest level of aggressive behaviour during conflicts with friends, relative to adolescents who never bullied or bullied at a low frequency. Those who reported bullying once or twice (i.e., low frequency) indicated higher levels of aggression than peers who never bullied others.

Among the high school girls, 42% of the bullies, 34% of the bully/victims, and 33% of the comparison students reported having a romantic relationship. Among the boys, 55% of the bullies, 43% of the bully/victims and 38% of the comparison high school students reported having a romantic partner. Closeness and conflict in romantic relationships among high school students were examined. A significant gender effect was found for intimacy between romantic partners, $F(5, 284) = 4.00$, $p < .01$, lambda$^2$ = .066. The means for the responses on the closeness scales given by boys and girls in each bullying frequency group are presented in Table 5.7. Overall, girls reported higher levels of intimacy within romantic relationships than boys. This gender difference may represent girls' greater interest in relationships in general and in romantic relationships during adolescence. There was a trend for bullying frequency groups on commitment with romantic partner, $F(10, 568) = 1.69$, $p = .08$, lambda$^2$ = .029. The data suggest that students who reported bullying at a high frequency also report somewhat lower levels of commitment in their romantic relationships than other students. From the perspective of bullying as a relationship problem, this may suggest that those students who use aggression to assert control and achieve power over their peers tend to be less committed and concerned about their romantic relationships. Contrary to expectations, there were no bullying frequency group differences or gender differences on the extent of conflict with romantic partners, aggression during conflict, or conflict with resolution within romantic relationships.

TABLE 5.7. Mean Scores for High School Students on Quality of Romantic Relationships by Bullying Frequency Groups

| | Never | | Low frequency | | High frequency | |
|---|---|---|---|---|---|---|
| | Boys ($n = 126$) | Girls ($n = 162$) | Boys ($n = 57$) | Girls ($n = 33$) | Boys ($n = 51$) | Girls ($n = 32$) |
| Trust | 3.84 (.99) | 4.34 (.71) | 4.02 (.74) | 4.38 (.60) | 3.74 (1.01) | 4.37 (.37) |
| Commitment | 3.29 (1.17) | 3.67 (1.04) | 3.51 (1.10) | 3.59 (.98) | 3.04 (.99) | 3.06 (.49) |
| Alienation | 1.93 (.82) | 1.86 (.74) | 1.74 (.77) | 2.14 (.63) | 2.33 (.94) | 1.75 (.57) |
| Intimacy | 3.39 (1.21) | 3.94 (1.03) | 3.37 (1.08) | 3.71 (1.09) | 3.30 (1.12) | 3.39 (.98) |
| Activities | 3.37 (1.09) | 3.60 (.92) | 3.30 (1.09) | 3.53 (1.01) | 3.70 (.93) | 3.78 (.94) |

Note. Standard deviations are in parentheses. Scale range: 1 ("never true") to 5 ("always true").

## CONCLUSIONS

In considering the nature and consequences of girls' bullying for this chapter, we posed three questions: Is bullying just a childhood behavior problem? Do children who bully experience problems in their peer relationships? Are relationship problems related to the extent of bullying? All of these questions point to the central thesis of the chapter: Bullying is a relationship problem; therefore, children who bully are at risk for difficulties in relationships contemporaneously and in the future. The risks for girls who bully may be substantial because relationships are of central importance in the lives of girls and women (Maccoby, 1998; Underwood, 2003) and strain in these relationships may cause significant distress. From a developmental perspective, we are concerned that patterns of bullying established in childhood and adolescence may become consolidated as a foundation for future relationships. The present research, which is based on students' self reports of bullying, provides an initial step in answering these questions about the nature and importance of bullying from a developmental perspective.

### Is Bullying Just a Childhood Behavior Problem?

The bullying prevalence data for girls and boys highlight two important developmental issues. First, boys are more likely than girls to report bullying their peers at almost every grade level. This pattern is similar to the gender differences in physical aggression (e.g., Broidy et al., 2003; Cairns & Cairns, 1994; Crick & Grotpeter, 1995). The exception to this discrepancy is following the school transition from grade 8 to grade 9, when the percentage of girls who report both bullying and being victimized jumps up sharply. The transition to a new school context with a larger peer group may be a vulnerable time for girls who are establishing themselves in a new social context. At this point, girls may be using bullying not only to establish a position of status within the new social context, but also to establish their sense of belonging and acceptance (Underwood, 2003). Girls' bids for dominance and belonging in the transition to high school may come at a substantial relationship cost: This is the grade at which the proportion of girls who report both bullying others and being victimized by their peers is highest.

The second developmental issue is the trend for lower levels of bullying for both girls and boys as they reach the end of high school. The percentages of girls and boys who report bullying their peers at the end of high school are about half of the percentages at the end of elementary school. At first glance, it may appear as if bullying is a problem behavior that children "just grow out of"'; however, our analyses of other forms of using power and aggression suggest that the behavior diversifies for a proportion of troubled youth, rather than disappearing. Our studies of bullying in adolescence indicate that girls and boys who bully their peers are more likely to sexually harass and exhibit dating aggression than those who do not report bullying (Connolly et al., 2000; McMaster, Connolly, Pepler, & Craig, 2002). Interventions to reduce the problems of bullying in elementary school may prevent the formation of an aggressive relationship style and the escalation of bullying behaviors into sexual harassment and dating aggression.

## Do Children Who Bully Experience Problems in their Peer Relationships?

If bullying represents a problem in establishing healthy relationship styles with peers, then girls and boys who bully should experience significant difficulties in their peer relationships. Our data suggest that although the prevalence of bullying among girls is generally less than that of boys, the quality of their peer relationships is equally jeopardized. Contrary to the patterns of problems associated with some other forms of aggression (Crick & Grotpeter, 1995), there were few gender differences, suggesting that bullying is a relationship problem that has concurrent problems for both boys and girls. The peer problems faced by children who bully are evident across childhood, early adolescence, and middle adolescence. At each stage, the children who report both bullying others and being victimized by their peers experience the most troubling peer-relationship problems.

Children who bully others may be trying to establish a place for themselves in the peer group. They use bullying to establish power over others and, in the process, are often at the center of attention within the peer group (Craig & Pepler, 1997; O'Connell et al., 1999). In some respects, bullying is a bid for leadership and status, albeit a negative one. For both girls and boys who bully others without the cost of being victimized themselves, the profile of their peer relationships is ambivalent. For example, in early adolescence, they report spending more time in activities with peers than other children, suggesting they are well integrated into a peer group. These friendships however, may be problematic. These same children report more conflict in their friendships than comparison children. Problems also emerge in the context of romantic relationships, which in these analyses were more marked for girls. Girls who bullied reported higher levels of aggression in conflicts with their romantic partners compared to boys. The style of negative leadership that they have adopted in peer interactions may enable them to maintain peer contacts, but creates relationship contexts that are challenging. These girls and boys may not have developed the positive conflict resolution strategies that are required for mature, balanced friendships.

The children who report both bullying and victimization are at greatest risk for negative peer experiences at all stages of development. In elementary school, both the girls and boys who are bully/victims have the least number of best-friend nominations and are most likely to be actively rejected by their classmates. In early adolescence, girls who are bully/victims report higher alienation in their friendships than other girls. Both girls and boys who are bully/victims report less closeness and more conflict within their friendships than other children. In middle adolescence, a similar pattern arises, with bully/victims reporting less positive and more negative qualities in their friendships. Within romantic relationships, this group of girls and boys experienced aggression in their conflicts with romantic partners. The pattern of difficulties for children involved in bullying both as the perpetrator and the victim suggests that this group of children may not have established the requisite social skills to sustain positive relationships with peers. Without the capacity for positive relationships, these children may be at particularly high risk for relationship problems in their later roles as spouses, parents, and employees. Given that peer and romantic relationships are of central importance to children's development, it is essential to identify these children and provide them with the necessary support to build positive relationships during childhood and adolescence. Unless these children develop relationship capacity, they will be lacking a firm foundation for their relationships throughout adulthood.

## Are Relationship Problems Related to the Extent of Bullying?

Bullying is a behavior that many children engage in from time to time. In our first observational study, we were surprised to find that the children identified by their teachers as socially competent engaged in bullying on the school playground at the same rate as the children identified as aggressive (Craig & Pepler, 1997). The final question for this chapter relates to the social costs of bullying and whether they vary by the extent to which children engage in this problem behavior. We were able to compare the reports of peer relationships for groups of children who reported bullying others frequently, occasionally, and never.

The patterns of peer relationships were remarkably similar for children in early and middle adolescence. For both boys and girls, any involvement in bullying (low and high groups) during early and middle adolescence was associated with less closeness and more conflict in relationships. The adolescents who acknowledged frequently bullying their peers reported higher levels of aggression during conflicts with friends compared to the low and never groups. These girls and boys also tended to have lower-quality romantic relationships. Therefore, we should be concerned for the qualities of peer relationships of all children who use aggression to establish power over their peers through bullying. This approach to peer interactions bodes poorly for establishing positive, trusting, low-conflict relationships with friends during a period of life when peer relationships are of utmost importance. The group of adolescents who frequently bully may have learned to use aggression effectively to dominate others and resolve conflicts. This group of girls and boys may be at greatest risk for carrying their interactional style combining power and aggression forward into their adult relationships.

Bullying is a relationship problem—both girls and boys who bully are at risk for difficulties in their peer relationships throughout childhood and adolescence. Although girls do not generally report bullying at as high a rate as boys, those girls who bully experience levels of relationship problems similar to boys who bully. Girls tend to rely less on physical means of bullying and more on social forms of bullying, such as social exclusion and gossip (Owens, Shute, & Slee, 2000; Underwood, 2003). As such, it may be much more difficult to detect and intervene in situations of girls' bullying compared to those of boys. Nevertheless, given the negative relationship outcomes, it is incumbent on us to continue to research these problem behaviors for girls and to develop strategies to assess and intervene to reduce girls' bullying. The consequences of bullying are just as serious for girls as for boys, as evidenced by the quality of concurrent relationships. The social costs of bullying may be even more serious for girls than for boys in adulthood relationships when, as women, their social skills are called upon to promote positive marital relationships and to promote their own children's healthy social development.

## REFERENCES

Armsden, G. C., & Greenberg, M. T. (1987). The inventory of parent and peer attachment: Relationships to well-being in adolescence. *Journal of Youth and Adolescence, 16,* 427–454.

Asher, S., & Dodge, K. (1986). Identifying children who are rejected by their peers. *Developmental Psychology, 22,* 444–449.

Bjorkqvist, K., Osterman, K., & Kaukiainen, A. (1992). The development of direct and indirect aggressive strategies in males and females. In K. Bjorkqvist & P. Niemela (Eds.), *Of mice and women: Aspects of female aggression* (pp. 51–64). San Diego, CA: Academic Press.

Broidy, L. M., Nagin, D. S., Tremblay, R. E., Bates, J., Brame, B., Dodge, K., Fersusson, D., Horwood, J., Loeber, R., Laird, R., Lynam, D., Moffitt, T. E., & Pettit, G. (2003). Developmental trajectories of childhood disruptive behaviors and adolescent delinquency: A six-site, cross-national study. *Developmental Psychology, 39*, 222–245.

Cairns, R. B., & Cairns, B. D. (1994). *Lifelines and risks: Pathways of youth in our time*. Cambridge, UK: Cambridge University Press.

Capaldi, D. M., & Gorman-Smith, D. (2003). The development of aggression in young male/female couples. In P. Florsheim (Ed.), *Adolescent romantic relations and sexual behavior: Theory, research and practical implications* (pp. 243–278). Hillsdale, NJ: Erlbaum.

Charach, A., Pepler, D., & Ziegler, S. (1995). Bullying at school: A Canadian perspective. *Education Canada, 35*, 12–18.

Connolly, J., Pepler, D. J., Craig, W. M., & Taradash, A. (2000). Dating experiences and romantic relationships of bullies in early adolescence. *Journal of Maltreatment, 5*, 299–310.

Craig, W. M., & Pepler, D. J. (1997). Observations of bullying and victimization in the schoolyard. *Canadian Journal of School Psychology, 13*, 41–60.

Crick, N. R., & Grotpeter, J. K. (1995). Relational aggression, gender, and social-psychological adjustment. *Child Development, 66*, 710–722.

Farrington, D. P. (1993). Understanding and preventing bullying. *Crime and Justice, 17*, 381–458.

Furman, W., & Buhrmester, D. (1985). Children's perceptions of the qualities of the personal relationships in their social networks. *Developmental Psychology, 21*, 1016–1024.

Keenan, K. (2001). Uncovering preschool precursors to problem. In R. Loeber & D. P. Farrington (Eds.), *Child delinquents: Development, intervention, and service needs* (pp. 117–134). Thousand Oaks: Sage.

Maccoby, E. E. (1998). *The two sexes: Growing up apart, coming together. Family and public policy*. Cambridge, MA: Belknap Press/Harvard University Press.

McMaster, L., Connolly, J., Pepler, D. J., & Craig, W. M. (2002). Peer to peer sexual harassment among early adolescents. *Development and Psychopathology, 14*, 91–105.

Moffitt, T. E., Caspi, A., Rutter, M., & Silva, P. A. (2001). Cambridge, UK: Cambridge University Press.

O'Connell, P., Pepler, D. J., & Craig, W. M. (1999). Peer involvement in bullying: Insights and challenges for intervention. *Journal of Adolescence, 22*, 437–452.

Offord, D. R., Lipman, E. L., & Duku, E. K. (2001). Epidemiology of problem up to age 12 years. In R. Loeber & D. P. Farrington (Eds.), *Child delinquents: Development, intervention, and service needs* (pp. 95–116). Thousand Oaks, CA: Sage.

Olweus, D. (1989). *Student Bully Victim Questionnaire*. Unpublished manuscript, University of Bergen, Bergen, Norway.

Olweus, D. (1993). Victimization by peers: Antecedents and long-term outcomes. In K. H. Rubin & J. B. Asendorf (Eds.), *Social withdrawal, inhibition, and shyness in children* (pp. 315–341). Hillsdale, NJ: Erlbaum.

Owens, L. D., Shute, R., & Slee, P. (2000). "Guess what I just heard!": Indirect aggression among teenage girls in Australia. *Aggressive Behavior, 26,* 67–83.

Pepler, D. J., Craig, W. M., O'Connell, P., & Atlas, R. (1998, July). *Observations of bullying on the school playground.* Paper presented at the 10th biennial meeting of the International Society for the Study of Behavioural Development, Berne, Switzerland.

Smith, C., Pepler, D., & Craig, W. (2003, April). *Observations of girls' aggression on the school playground.* Paper presented at the biennial meetings of the Society for Research in Child Development, Tampa, FL.

Statistics Canada. (1998). *Canadian Crime Statistics* (1997, No. 85-002-XPE, Vol. 18.11).

Thorne, B. (1993). *Gender play: Girls and boys in school.* New Brunswick, NJ: Rutgers University Press.

Underwood, M. K. (2003). *Social aggression among girls.* New York: Guilford Press.

# CHAPTER 6

# A Behavioral Analysis of Girls' Aggression and Victimization

Martha Putallaz, Janis B. Kupersmidt, John D. Coie,
Kate McKnight, *and* Christina L. Grimes

There has been a plethora of writings recently in both the popular media and research literature casting girls in a light usually not ascribed to them. All attest that it is necessary to amend the age-old adage, "Sugar and spice and everything nice." Apparently girls now warrant the additional description, "But behind the scene, they're really mean." Aggression is no longer considered the exclusive domain of boys. In addition to the hitting, pushing, verbal assault, and physical intimidation characteristic of overt aggression, attention now is being given to other, often hidden, forms of aggression involving social manipulation, ostracism, rumors, and exclusionary behaviors harmful to social relationships and thought to be more relevant to the social world of girls. The public has been peppered with writings with such compelling titles as *Best Friends, Worst Enemies* (Thompson & Grace, 2001), *Odd Girl Out* (Simmons, 2002), *Queen Bees & Wannabes* (Wiseman, 2002), *Mom, They're Teasing Me* (Thompson, Cohen, & Grace, 2002), and *You Can't Say You Can't Play* (Paley, 1992), to name but a few.

Many of these popular authors credit these newfound perspectives to reflections on personal experience, either of their own or that of their daughters. Simmons (2002), for example, writes of her remembered personal experience at age 8 of being victimized by a popular friend at school named Abby and later of her own recalled complicity in the group exclusion of Anne, a close friend. Thompson (Thompson &

Grace, 2001) recalls his daughter's 13th birthday party, her hurt feelings, and his own felt helplessness when one of the invited girls manipulated the social dynamics to exclude his daughter.

The purpose of the present chapter is to present findings relevant to aggression and victimization among girls from a comprehensive observational study of middle childhood girls' peer relationships. The chapter begins with a brief review of the relevant literature and issues concerning aggression, particularly the more covert form of aggression, with a focus on the middle-childhood age period. This review is not intended as an exhaustive review of the literature, but rather as a context for the study that is presented. For more extensive accounts of the literature, the reader is referred to several excellent reviews which provide thorough discussions of the topic (Coie & Dodge, 1998; Crick et al., 1999; Underwood, 2003).

## DEFINITION

There is heated debate among researchers as to how the more covert form of aggression should be defined, what the most appropriate label for it should be, and precisely what should be encompassed within this aggression construct. Consequently, this more hidden form of aggression has been studied under such terms as "indirect aggression" (Lagerspetz, Björkqvist, & Peltonen, 1988), "relational aggression" (Crick & Grotpeter, 1995), and "social aggression" (Cairns, Cairns, Neckerman, Ferguson, & Gariepy, 1989; Galen & Underwood, 1997). (More complete discussions of this conceptual debate can be found in Crick et al., 1999; Underwood, 2003; Underwood, Galen, & Paquette, 2001; Xie, Cairns, & Cairns, 2002.) Although it has complicated comparisons across studies, the definitional debate has succeeded in broadening the construct and elaborating the various components necessary to fully understand the dynamics of aggression among girls. As Maccoby (Chapter 1, this volume) states, this debate "has called our attention to two main points: Girls are not as unaggressive as we have believed, and there are qualitatively different forms in which aggression is expressed during childhood and youth. Therefore, we need to follow the development of more forms of expressing aggression than the direct forms that have been mainly studied until recently. These are compelling points that require our close attention" (p. 13).

Across the various definitions and conceptualizations, certain important theoretical elements emerge. This type of aggression (1) uses relationships or the social community to inflict harm, (2) can involve nonconfrontational tactics, making it difficult for the victim to know the identity of the perpetrator or even if an attack occurred with certainty (e.g., rumors, social exclusion, social alienation), (3) can involve direct confrontational strategies that can cause harm to relationships (e.g., threatening to withdraw friendship, telling someone he or she is not welcome to join a group activity, and (4) includes both verbal and nonverbal behaviors. Recently, Crick and colleagues (1999) defined relational aggression as "behaviors that harm others through damage (or threat of damage) to relationships or feelings of acceptance, friendship, or group inclusion (e.g., giving someone the silent treatment to punish them or to get one's way; using social exclusion as a form of retaliation; or threatening to end a friendship unless the friend complies with a request)" (p. 75). Included in this definition are all hostile acts in which relationships serve as the vehicle of harm, regardless of the direct or indirect nature of the behaviors. Adopting this definition in the current chapter, relational aggression then is considered to involve any interpersonal behavior negatively influencing a child's relationship with a peer or peers, and may be conceptualized as either an indirect or a direct act of aggression, depending on how it is delivered.

Although conceptualized as distinct components of aggression, overt aggression and relational aggression appear to be related constructs. Most studies consistently report moderate to high correlations between overt and relational aggression (Crick, 1996; Crick & Grotpeter, 1995; Crick et al., 1999, McNeilly-Choque, Hart, Robinson, Nelson, & Olsen, 1996; Olsen, 1996; Putallaz, Kupersmidt, Grimes, DeNero, & Coie, 1999; Putallaz, Rhule, Kupersmidt, Grimes, McKnight, & Coie, 2001; Tomada & Schneider, 1997). This high concordance has been found regardless of differences in measurement or informant (peer, teacher, observer).

## PROFILE OF RELATIONALLY AGGRESSIVE CHILDREN AND VICTIMS

Exactly who are the children most likely to engage in relational aggression and whom do they target? Is there a profile that can be discerned from the literature to help us in our understanding of this type of aggression and victimization? Simmons (2002), the author of one of the popular books listed earlier, contends that those most likely to use relational aggression are popular girls, particularly when their status is threatened or when they fear loss or social isolation. The relational aggressor is likened to a "skilled politician, methodically building a coalition of other girls willing to throw their support behind her" (p. 80), and, in fact, popularity is defined by Simmons as "the ability of one girl to turn her friends against someone else" (p. 82). The girls most likely to be victimized, according to Simmons, are those she describes as "all that," meaning that they possess the attributes most likely to threaten other girls (e.g., they are pretty, popular, smart, thin, best dressed, pose a relationship threat). Covert aggression, she contends, allows the perpetrators to continue to be seen as "good girls," girls who do not get angry, who do not engage in overt conflict or direct confrontation, girls who are not mean, and who have close relationships.

Another author of a popular book, Thompson (Thompson & Grace, 2001), also describes girls as frequent users and victims of relational aggression, but evaluates their position in the social hierarchy somewhat differently. He describes the aggressor who manipulated the social dynamics at his daughter's party, for example, to be very much like his victimized daughter, not a "power-hungry villain," but instead an insecure middle schooler, someone who was not a part of the mainstream, not at the center of the cool group, but longed to be. She was simply someone who wanted to be certain that she had friends to sleep next to at his daughter's sleepover. Thompson contends that the victims of aggressive acts tend to be rejected children.

Although recent popular books proclaim relational aggression to be the weapon of girls, the research evidence is more mixed. Some reports indicate girls to be more relationally aggressive than boys (e.g., Crick & Grotpeter, 1995; Lagerspetz et al., 1988; Osterman et al., 1998; Xie et al., 2002), while others do not (e.g., Hart, Nelson, Robinson, Olsen, & McNeilly-Choque, 1998; Hughes, Cavell, & Thompson, 1998; Rys & Bear, 1997; Tomada & Schneider, 1997). In our own research involving an ethnically diverse sample of 1,828 fourth graders in 13 different public schools (Putallaz et al., 1999), we found that boys and girls were seen by peers as comparable in their use of relational aggression. In terms of victimization, boys were slightly more likely than girls to be seen by peers as victims of overt aggression, whereas girls were viewed as being somewhat more likely than boys to be victims of relational aggression.

It is also unclear from the research literature where relationally aggressive children fall in the social hierarchy. Children nominated by peers as highly relationally aggressive received more disliked nominations than their nonrelationally aggressive peers (Crick, 1996; Crick & Grotpeter, 1995). Crick and Grotpeter (1995) further reported that children viewed as controversial among their peers (i.e., they received high numbers of both "like most" and "like least" sociometric nominations from their peers) were seen as the most overtly and relationally aggressive children by their peers. Rejected children were seen as more relationally aggressive than their popular, average, or neglected peers. Similarly, Putallaz and colleagues (1999) found that both rejected and controversial children were seen by peers as engaging in both overt and relational aggression more than average children who, in turn, engaged in them more than popular children. Others have found that relationally aggressive children, especially by middle school age, tend to be central members of peer networks and to have high levels of intimacy in their friendship (e.g., Xie, Swift, Cairns, & Cairns, 2002). Relationally aggressive behavior may be especially evident when children have to re-establish their peer networks following a disruption such as a change in schools (see Pepler, Craig, Yuile, & Connolly, Chapter 5, this volume), and it may be more pronounced among older children. Consistent with this speculation, relational aggression is reported more frequently as the basis for peer conflicts among middle schoolers than among elementary school children (Xie, Cairns, & Cairns, 2002), and a greater proportion of relationally aggressive children are popular in middle and high schools than in elementary school (Rose, Lockerd, & Swenson, 2002).

More consensus exists among researchers that the victims of aggression are likely to be rejected. Rejected children were more likely to be the victims of both relational and overt aggression than were their more socially accepted peers (Crick & Grotpeter, 1996; Putallaz et al., 1999).

## FUNCTIONS OF RELATIONAL AGGRESSION

Much discussion has been devoted to the functions of relational aggression. The standard definition of aggression involves "behavior that is aimed at harming or injuring another person or persons" (Parke & Slaby, 1983, p. 550), and there is little doubt that this is a central tenet of overt aggression. Although it is clear that relational aggression also serves this purpose, it appears that relational aggression may serve other functions as well. After all, negative comments made about a girl who others do not know and never will meet are unlikely to have been delivered with the intent to harm the target's social relationships, the definition of relational aggression. The following exchange between unfamiliar girls in our study serves as an illustration:

ALICIA: And guess what? When my friend was here [referring to a girl in her prior familiar playgroup who is unknown to the girls in her present unfamiliar group], she pulled up her shirt and let them see her bra!

SUSAN: Ewwww! I don't know what was wrong with her.

BETSY: She musta had problems.

SUSAN: I know. Not little problems, but big problems.

Social interaction (and peer rejection) assumes heightened significance for girls relative to boys due to the greater emphasis placed on relationships and achievement in this domain for girls during the course of their socialization. As Maccoby (1990, 1998) has long posited, boys are socialized into an individual achievement framework, whereas girls are socialized to be relationship focused, measuring their success in terms of their relationships. Social interaction for girls is likely to have the dual purposes of forming connections with others as well as providing information concerning their relative social position within the group. If social interaction is about the nature of connection between participating girls, then exclusion and inclusion are likely to have very significant and unique meaning in girls' social lives. If inclusion is an important goal for girls, then exclusion serves a strategic social purpose, as it provides a mechanism for establishing group structure and a means of building and affirming bonds between members through the exclusion of others.

Girls are described as forming close, intimate friendships with a small subset of girls, typically one or two, with these friendships being marked by the sharing of confidences and self-disclosures rather than participation in group activities or group games (Berndt, 1986; Gottman & Mettetal, 1986; Waldrop & Halverson, 1975). Gottman and Mettetal (1986) reported that self-disclosure among girls was preceded by a period of negative evaluation gossip. They speculated that such gossip might serve to affirm the bond between gossipers due to their mutual rejection of another party, as well as inform them of the norms that should not be violated so as to avoid rejection themselves. Indeed, girls' friendships are described as more exclusive than those of boys (Eder & Hallinan, 1978). Gossip also allows for emotional venting and social support to be offered.

However, such covert interpersonal behaviors such as gossip can carry salient emotional consequences for girls, particularly within the highly intimate context of female relationships. The breakups of girls' friendships are typically emotional, as confidences have been shared, with new friendships forming at the expense of old ones (Archer, 1992; Maccoby, 1990).

Given that girls are socialized to avoid interpersonal conflict and confrontation and to be nice to others (Maccoby, 1998), relational aggression is likely to be tacit. Overt, unsubtle exclusionary acts threaten the stability of the entire group, as well as put the exclusionary child at risk, as too overt exclusion may cause others to be wary of the agent of exclusion. Thus, girls are likely to be quite tacit and subtle in their aggression against others, unless that aggression is condoned by the group and accepted as normative behavior. Indeed we have observed such caution in our playgroup observations of fourth-grade girls. Girls often used disclaimers ("I don't mean to be mean but . . . " or "I hate to say it, but . . . ") or sought permission ("Can I ask a question?") before proceeding to engage in relational aggression. Girls sometimes put out feelers and monitored group reactions. When negative gossip appeared to be condoned by the group, the process was likely to escalate, as illustrated by the following transcript examples:

CRYSTAL: I'm not trying to be picking on her or nothing. I'm just saying she can be kind of . . .

TONYA: (*Finishes sentence, but inaudible.*)

CRYSTAL: I think she sleeps with her sister.

IVEY: Kate don't (*inaudible*) . . . Never mind. I'm not going to say it 'cause it is too mean.

CORA: She's stupid. I say it too.

IVEY: Y'all, can I ask y'all something?

CORA: What?

IVEY: Does anybody notice that, like, think that she really do be stinkin' sometimes?

ALISHA: Yes.

Given the relationship focus of girls, it is not surprising that girls report being more distressed by particular experiences of victimization than do boys, even though girls and boys report experiencing social aggression with equal frequency (Paquette & Underwood, 1999). Further, for girls, but not for boys, victimization by social aggression appears related negatively to global self-concept (Underwood, 2003). Clearly, there is a need not only to understand the different forms of aggression among girls, but also the most effective means for victims to deal with aggressive attacks, both relational and overt.

## THE NEED FOR OBSERVATIONAL RESEARCH ON RELATIONAL AGGRESSION

A variety of different methodologies have been employed to examine and explore this more covert form of aggressive behavior, including peer report (e.g., Bjorkqvist, Lagerspetz, & Kaukiainen, 1992; Crick, 1995; Crick, Bigbee, & Howe, 1996; Grotpeter & Crick, 1996; Lagerspetz et al., 1988), teacher report (e.g., Crick, 1996; Hart, Nelson, Robinson,

Olsen, & McNeilly-Choque, 1998), self-report, including question-naires, interviews, and narrative accounts (e.g., Cairns et al., 1989; Paquette & Underwood, 1999; Xie et al., 2002), and an analogue situation involving child confederates (Galen & Underwood, 1997), and great strides have been made in our understanding of this phenomenon. However, due to the complexity of capturing children's aggressive behavior, particularly its more indirect or covert form, this latter manner of aggression has remained largely unexplored using observational techniques. As a result, the theoretical development of the concept of relational aggression is occurring with minimal observational information.

However, observational information concerning aggression among females would seem to be especially important, as the form and function of girls' aggression is subtle and less overt than among boys. It would be a mistake to assume that all of the important dynamics critical to understanding aggression among girls would be captured by the reports of teachers, peers, and even the girls themselves. Participants or casual observers often miss key dynamics to group process. Other researchers have underscored the need for observational approaches to complement existing findings:

> Because of the possibility of bias from gender stereotypes and self-report in questionnaire studies, observational research may lead to very different conclusions about gender and aggression. . . . Only when researchers collect more of these kinds of observational data will we have clear answers to such basic questions as how frequently boys and girls engage in indirect/relational/social aggression, how many children are victimized, and whether these behaviors are related to subsequent psychopathology. (Underwood, Galen, & Paquette, 2001, p. 259)

## THE PRESENT RESEARCH

The current study attempts to help fill this void by using an observational research approach to capture the intricacies of aggressive interactions as well as the processes by which they unfold. Two cohorts of fourth-grade girls ($n = 248$) participated in both familiar and unfamiliar same-race, five-person playgroups which were composed of one rejected girl, one popular girl, and three average-status girls (a variant of Coie & Kupersmidt, 1983). The familiar playgroups were composed so as to create a microcosm reflective of the girls' group relations in the larger classroom. Groups of familiar peers met after school in the spring of the fourth grade; in the summer, the same girls were assigned to a playgroup with unfamiliar peers for an additional 5 days. All groups (48 familiar, 46 unfamiliar) met for 1 hour on 5 consecutive days and were videotaped as they participated in structured and unstructured activities, crafts, and games. During the third and fourth days of playgroup, each girl left the room to be interviewed individually and then reentered the ongoing playgroup interaction 5 minutes later, thus allowing each girl's entry skills as well as any changes in group dynamics during her absence to be observed.

## Coding

All verbal and nonverbal acts of aggression were coded as one of the three primary forms outlined in the typology by Coie and Dodge (1998). Direct or overt aggression included all physical and verbal aggression delivered directly to the victim. In contrast, indirect aggression included all acts of aggression communicated to a peer bystander and not delivered directly to the target of the aggression. Finally, property damage included any overt or covert attempt to alter, remove, relocate, or destroy an object possessed or claimed by another child.

Kupersmidt, Putallaz, Coie, and Grimes (2001) reported preliminary analyses of aggressive behaviors among the fourth-grade girls participating in familiar and unfamiliar playgroups. Across the 470 hours of playgroup interaction, 10,330 aggressive behaviors were identified and coded. Although this number may seem large at first glance, keep in mind that an individual act of aggression represents a single utterance or act (e.g., "I heard her talking about you," or a rolling of the eyes). Playgroups averaged 22 aggressive acts per hour or an average of about 4.5 aggressive acts per girl per hour (taking absences into account). The variability in aggression across groups was quite notable, with the frequency of aggressive acts ranging from 0 to 153 across playgroup sessions. Not surprisingly, aggression occurred almost twice as often in familiar groups than in unfamiliar groups (68% vs. 32%).

In terms of the type of aggression, direct acts of aggression occurred about twice as often as indirect acts (64% vs. 33%). Damaging another girl's property was a relatively infrequent event, occurring only 3% of the time. Direct verbal aggression (e.g., insults or threats) delivered directly to the victim was the most common subtype of aggression, encompassing 53% of all aggressive acts. Direct physical aggression occurred infrequently (12%). Interestingly, direct acts of relational aggression, including direct exclusion and relational threats (e.g., "You're not in our club," or "If you can't be nice, then I ain't playing with you")—behaviors characterizing direct relational aggression typical of girls—were also a relatively rare phenomenon, accounting for only 4% of aggressive acts.

Indirect forms of relational aggression occurred far more frequently among the girls, accounting for 33% of all aggressive acts. Indirect relational aggression was as likely to be delivered overtly (i.e., in the presence of the victim, who is referred to in third-party terms [e.g., "We'd be having a good time if it weren't for a certain someone"]) as delivered covertly (i.e., out of the victim's earshot or while she was out of the room). Interestingly, then, the total amount of relational aggression (both direct and indirect) was 36%. Thus, only about one-third of all of the girls' aggressive acts exhibited in the familiar and unfamiliar playgroup context could be classified as relational aggression. In this particular context, then, girls were far more overtly aggressive than covert in their aggressive behavior.

However, one cannot conclude from these data that relational aggression occurs less frequently than overt aggression. First, the opportunities for indirect relational aggression in our study were relatively rare, as each girl was absent from the group for only about 5 minutes on 2 of the 5 days. In naturally occurring relationships girls would be separated from each other with greater frequency and for longer periods of time, thus permitting more opportunity for covert relational aggressive acts. In fact, it is interesting that half of the indirect relational aggression was covert, given the large percentage of time girls spent together relative to the percentage of time some girl was absent. Further, in all likelihood victimized girls would probably be absent with a greater frequency from group interactions than their nonvictimized peers. In this study all of the girls left the room to be interviewed for an equal length of time. Second, in the natural setting girls would choose their interaction partners rather than be assigned to playgroups established by researchers. Leaving the interaction also was not as readily available an option as in the natural environment. Thus, girls might have found it more difficult to stifle negative affect or avoid someone they were annoyed with in the present study. However, that said, it is clear that girls' aggressive behavior is both direct and indirect and that relational aggression is an important form of aggression engaged in by girls. Girls' aggressive behavior is rich in form. The following transcript samples are provided to illustrate the manner in which the coding system was used as well as to illustrate the richness of the observational data.

### Transcript Sample—Direct Aggression: Verbal Insult

ELIZABETH: I haven't been here as long as you, Mary.
MARY: Uh-huh.

ELIZABETH: No, I haven't. I started after you, Mary.

MARY: What do you mean by that?

ELIZABETH: I started after you.

BRITTANY: Started . . . Time . . . After . . . Mary before, Elizabeth after. Use your thingy up here. (*Points to her head.*) It may be a peanut. (*Everyone laughs.*)

BETTY: I was just going to say that. You know it might be a peanut.

BRITTANY: (*Whispers something to Elizabeth.*) Don't be angry at her.

ELIZABETH: Mary, we just want to get along with you, but sometimes. . . .

BETTY: Sometimes she gets a little annoying, right?

BRITTANY: A little?

ELIZABETH: Sometimes you're hard to get along with.

BETTY: Yeah.

ELIZABETH: We're trying our best, Mary.

BETTY: Our best. A lot.

ELIZABETH: So is everyone in the class.

### Transcript Sample—Direct Aggression: Exclusion

GAYE: (*Singing Baby Spice song*)

AMY: But you're not Baby Spice.

GAYE: I know that. Who says I was in the club? 'Cause you kicked me out because you said that I wasn't average height and neither is Michelle.

AMY: Michelle is still in.

MEG: She's the manager.

GAYE: I know, but she's not your height and you kicked everyone out.

AMY: Ashley's not the same height as us and she's in the club.

MEG: Uh-huh.

GAYE: Why then?

AMY: I don't know. I'm not the boss.

MEG: I was, but not when you were around.

*Transcript Sample—Damaging or Taking
Another's Property*

(*Keisha leaves playroom.*)

ALISHA: Y'all dare me to mess up Keisha's thing?

CORINA: Leave her thing. Stop, Alisha.

ALISHA: I'm not going to mess it up for real. (*Takes stick from Savina and puts it in Keisha's sand art bottle.*) I'm just going to make it better.

(*Alisha, Corina, and Savina all laugh.*)

KRISTINA: Alisha, did you change that girl's thing [referring to Keisha's bottle]?

SAVINA: She just made it a little better. (*Laughs.*) She just made it a little better.

ALISHA: I just made it a little better.

(*Corina picks up Keisha's bottle and shakes it.*)

KRISTINA: Oh! Corina made it a little worse!

CORINA: Sorry.

KRISTINA: Corina changed it.

CORINA: I'm sorry, Camera. Please erase that.

*Transcript Sample—Direct Aggression:
Verbal Insult Followed by Indirect Aggression:
Overt Relational Aggression*

MELANIE: (*to Meg*) Here's one of your stupid white beads that I've been hunting on the floor for your Highness (*in her face*).

MEG: Get a life.

MELANIE: You.

MEG: I already have one.

SUSAN: You both need a life!

MEG: She's the one who needs one badly. I have a good life except for Melanie.

KELLY: Right now, we're all having a bad life because of you two.

MEG: Melanie's the one who doesn't have a life.

MELANIE: Meg's the one who's accusing me of taking her beads.

KELLY: All right! All right! Quit!

*Transcript Sample—Indirect Aggression:*
*Covert Relational Aggression*

(*Betty leaves.*)

LLYNN: I think she was a little bit mad (*talking about Betty*).

DIANE: That makes me mad, you know, 'cause I was trying to help her right? And she always gets an attitude.

LILA: I noticed that. She said, "You know, Diane, you're not the boss."

LLYNN: It would be good if Betty was here, if Betty wasn't here.

DIANE: The reason I didn't ride with you and Betty (*to the playgroup*) is because she always acts like you and she are best friends . . . well, like she's your best friend.

To this point we have considered the form aggression tends to take. This still leaves a large unanswered question: How should girls respond to aggression? To address this question, a different, more microanalytic approach to the study of aggression and victim responses is required, which we turn to next.

## EFFECTIVENESS OF VICTIM RESPONSES

Currently, there is a growing impetus from lay people highlighting the need to advise girls on how to respond to aggression. Even children offer suggestions to their victimized peers as to the best way to handle daily gossip and rumors. Recently, a local newspaper invited readers to write in and offer their suggestions as to how to handle gossip. The following entries appeared in an advice column titled "Rumors? About Me? How Readers Handle Bad Gossip" (2002, p. 11).

> *"I just smile kindly at the person who has been spreading rumors about me and say, 'Thanks for making me the center of your universe.'"* B., age 15; B.'s recommendation: Sarcasm.

> *"When I was the victim of a vicious rumor at school, I realized that you just have to take in stride. Gossip happens. In no time, like magic, the crowd is on to another juicy rumor. My advice: Forget it and get on with*

*your life, which I did."* M., age 15; M.'s recommendation: Ignore the rumors.

*"Some friends teamed up against me. They'd cut down what I'd done or gossip about what I was wearing. I never handled it well, always returning their nasty remarks with cruel ones of my own* [an example of what we researchers would call reactive aggression]. *But then I realized that was a mistake. When I confronted people and talked civilly, it caused far less pain. First, I'd say something like how boring a class was. That set the tone that I wasn't in the mood to argue. Later on, I'd ask, 'Why did you say something about me that was untrue?' But my tone was questioning—not angry. Generally the person said, 'I'm sorry' and didn't do it again."* G., age 14; G.'s recommendation: Initially de-escalate the situation and then later calmly confront the aggressor.

Sometimes peers, parents, teachers, authors, and clinicians offer suggestions to victimized girls, but such advice is presented in lieu of empirical support. In the following detailed examination of observed aggression among girls, we specifically looked at what the girls did in response to finding themselves the victim of an aggressive act and the effectiveness of those responses. Through sequential analyses we then sought to examine empirically which responses to aggression were most effective in terms of reducing the likelihood of continued aggression. Finally, we examined how sociometric status and ethnicity affected this process. Such data are a necessary prerequisite to the development of empirically based advice for girls who want to understand how to deal with aggression.

## MICROANALYTIC STUDY OF AGGRESSION AND VICTIMIZATION

To complement the larger investigation of aggression and victimization using the complete corpus of data, the behavior of a subsample of groups was explored to allow for a more microanalytic, frame-by-frame assessment of aggression (McKnight et al., 2003). This more fine-grained approach permitted sequential analyses to be performed, providing insight into the process of aggression and victimization and allowing the identification of predictable sequences of behavior (Bakeman & Guera, 1985). To capture this level of detail, five African American and five European American familiar groups were randomly selected from the total data set for the more in-depth investigation. The unfamiliar groups for each of the popular and rejected girls in these familiar groups also were included in order to investigate behavior across settings. Thus, the target sample was comprised of 30 playgroups representing the interactions of 117 fourth-grade girls (60 African American and 57 European American). Aggressive episodes were transcribed verbatim from the videotapes on the first and third days of the familiar and unfamiliar playgroups to provide a representative sampling of the data, resulting in 60 hours of observation in all.

This type of microanalytic approach allows for fleeting facial expressions and quickly delivered under-the-breath comments to be captured as well as ambiguous acts of aggression (i.e., acts where aggressive intent was unclear). These are the kinds of acts that would not be observed readily in the normal course of viewing a videotaped playgroup session, let alone while watching children interact in a naturalistic setting such as the playground. Approximately 91% of the aggression observed was coded as either ambiguous (12%) or mild (79%) in its affective intensity. About 9% of the observed aggression was rated severe in intensity. Thus, although aggression occurs with some regularity in girls' interactions, it is proportionally a small part of their repertoire, and rarely is exhibited in a very severe form.

An analysis conducted to determine whether the girls' sociometric status, ethnicity, or familiarity (controlling for socioeconomic status) predicted total aggression revealed only a main effect for familiarity and no main effects for race or status and no significant interactions. Aggression was more likely to occur among girls who knew each other regardless of their status or ethnicity.

We next examined whether the girls' sociometric status, ethnicity, or familiarity predicted their victimization (controlling for socioeconomic status). There was only a main effect for sociometric status. Popular girls and average girls were less likely to be the recipients of aggressive acts than were rejected girls. However, these results were qualified by a familiar group by status interaction and by a race by status interaction. Average girls were victimized less than rejected girls only in familiar groups. In unfamiliar groups rejected and average girls did not differ in terms of their rate of victimization. The effects of sociometric status on victimization were more exaggerated for European American girls than for African American girls. Popular European American girls received fewer aggressive acts than popular African American girls and rejected Euro-American girls received far more aggressive acts than rejected African American girls.

## Victim Response to Aggression

When confronted with aggression, how are victims likely to respond? The most common response to aggression was simply to ignore it, and girls did this about 60% of the time. Girls chose to confront the aggressor by challenging the attack, offering a rebuttal, continuing the targeted behavior, or encouraging a peer to take their side approximately 15% of the time. Girls also responded to the aggression with reactive aggression about 13% of the time. Finally, girls attempted to de-escalate or diffuse the aggressive episode through apologizing, altering their behavior, compromising, clarifying the situation, defending themselves, or by insulting or making a disparaging joke about themselves about 12% of the time.

## Reaction to Victim Response

What happens after a victim responds? More than a quarter of the time (27%), the victim's response was followed by another act of aggression by the aggressor. However, about 18% of the time the victim's response led the aggressor to try to de-escalate, resolve, or diffuse the aggression. About a quarter of the aggressive episodes simply ended following the victim's response (23%). About a third of the time one of the girls not involved in the aggressive exchange joined in to aid the aggressor either by becoming an aggressor herself, by reinforcing the aggressor, or by "adding fuel to the fire" and intensifying the episode (32%).

## Effectiveness of Victim Responses to Aggression

Victim responses next were analyzed to determine which were most likely to lead to positive outcomes (either the episode ended or the aggressor sought to diffuse or de-escalate the aggression) and which were most likely to lead to negative outcomes (continued aggression or others joining in the aggression). As can be seen in Figure 6.1, only the victim's attempts to de-escalate the aggression resulted in a positive outcome more than a negative outcome (57% of the time vs. 43%). The least effective strategy was to react aggressively, which led to continued aggression or to another girl joining in about 77% of the time. Confrontation and ignoring had similar consequences, with a negative outcome occurring 59% of the time and a positive outcome 40% of the time in both instances.

## Effects of Sociometric Status and Race

We next examined the effects of status and race on the consequences of victim responses to aggression. As can be seen in Figure 6.2, popular girls had less negative consequences for any behavior they employed following an aggressive act than did average girls who had less negative consequences for any response than rejected girls. For all girls though,

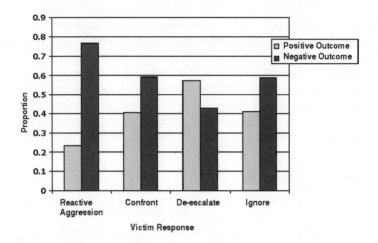

**FIGURE 6.1.** Consequences of victim responses to aggression.

the same pattern is evident: Attempting to de-escalate the aggression was the victim response least likely to result in a negative consequence; reacting aggressively was the response most likely to result in a negative outcome; and confronting the aggressor and ignoring the aggression fell in between.

Are there ethnicity differences with regard to the likelihood of negative outcomes following each of the four victim responses to aggression? European American girls had slightly less negative consequences for

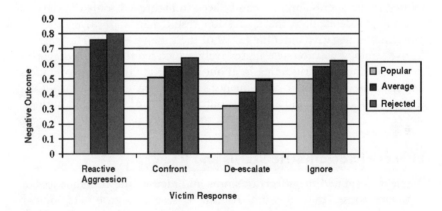

**FIGURE 6.2.** Effects of sociometric status on consequences of victim response to aggression.

their behavior than did African American girls, independent of the particular behavior in question (see Figure 6.3). However, again the same pattern held. Regardless of ethnicity, the victim's attempts to de-escalate the aggression were least likely to result in a negative outcome, and reactive aggression was most likely to do so, with confronting and ignoring the aggression falling in between.

An examination of familiarity revealed no differences across familiar and unfamiliar groups in terms of the consequences of a victim's response to aggression. Thus, the pattern appears to be fairly robust. Attempting to de-escalate or diffuse the aggression is better than ignoring or confronting, which are better than reactive aggression if the goal is a positive outcome (cessation or de-escalation of aggression by the aggressor).

Given the robustness of this pattern we decided to look one level deeper at the pattern of consequences for victim responses to aggression. Negative outcome was separated into continued aggression by the aggressor and joining into the aggression by another girl, while positive consequence was split into attempts to de-escalate the aggression by the aggressor and an end to the aggression altogether. Figure 6.4 shows the results of this more detailed analysis. Each victim response has a quite distinct pattern. Reactive aggression resulted in continued aggression 76% of the time and attempts to de-escalate 23% of the time. Only in 1% of the cases did the aggression sequence end following reactive aggression. All three other behaviors resulted in another girl joining the aggression at least 25% of the time. Ignoring was most likely to lead to another girl entering the aggression; this happened about 41% of the time.

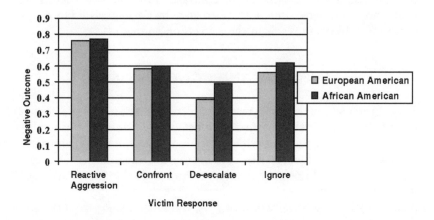

**FIGURE 6.3.** Effects of race on consequences of victim response to aggression.

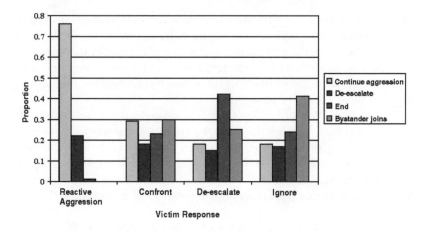

**FIGURE 6.4.** Consequences of victim response to aggression: A detailed view.

Confronting was more likely to lead to continued aggression, about 29% of the time, than were diffusion or ignoring, both 18%. Thus, while confrontation and ignoring were equally likely to lead to a negative consequence, the form of the consequence was different. Ignoring an aggressive act invites another girl to join the aggression, resulting in the victim facing two or more aggressors, whereas confronting the aggressor is more likely to result in continued aggression by the aggressor. On the positive consequence side, confronting and ignoring were equally likely to result in attempts to de-escalate by the aggressor (18%) or an end to the aggression episode (22%). In contrast, diffusion was slightly less likely to result in any attempt to de-escalate by the aggressor (15%), but much more likely to result in the aggression ending (42%).

## SUMMARY AND CONCLUSIONS

This chapter summarizes the results of a study that attempts to complement the broader literature through a behavioral assessment of the very subtle processes associated with aggression and affiliated victimization from a rich array of lenses. The patterns that emerge in the study present a picture that could only be developed through looking at data at both macroanalytic and microanalytic levels. Aggression appears to assume many forms in the social world of girls. Aggression is far from the most frequent behavior in girls' interaction, but girls aggressed often and in a wide variety of ways, especially among familiar peers. The majority of the girls' aggressive acts were acts of overt aggression, with relational aggression accounting for only one-third of their aggression. Although the aggressive acts were rarely severe, it is likely that their sheer frequency would have serious implications for victimized children.

The vast majority of aggressive acts by girls in the microanalytic study were rated by observers as being either mild or ambiguous in intensity. Ninety-one percent of the aggressive acts were of mild or ambiguous intensity, suggesting that research using more macroanalytic approaches would miss the majority of aggressive acts. Girls' aggression is subtle. Girls were often cautious when being aggressive, using disclaimers or seeking permission prior to an aggressive act. Thus, girls appeared to know the potential importance of the impact of their behavior for the victim and the prohibition against such behavior, and they sought to mitigate blame for the consequences by having their behavior condoned by the group prior to proceeding. Consistent with the notion that aggression is intended to have a strategic relational effect is the result that girls aggressed twice as often in familiar groups as in unfamiliar groups, as the group response of the familiar group to any aggressive overture would be well known. Thus, any intervention attempt aimed at reducing the level of aggression among girls would need to incorporate a group component aimed at increasing the level of acceptance and felt empathy among the girls while decreasing the likelihood that aggression, regardless of its subtlety, would be tolerated or condoned.

Considering the role of sociometric status in aggression, a surprising result arises. In contrast to studies using peer perceptions to identify aggressors, sociometric status was not related to the level of aggression among the girls in our more microanalytic observational study. If effective relational aggression has the feature of being done in a way that evades both responsibility and retaliation (at least some of the time), then competent relational aggressors would not be readily identifiable by their peers. Less socially competent children, however, would be obvious and ineffective in their use of relational aggression and would lack the necessary social base or power in the peer group to use relational aggression effectively. Peer perceptions of relational aggression, then, may be distorted by the impression peers have of the amount of overt aggression children display.

Consistent with the peer perception research, though, our observational research found that victimization was quite strongly related to sociometric status. Popular girls were less victimized than average girls who, in turn, were less victimized than rejected girls. This result again suggests the importance of victimization in the study of girls' aggression. Because of the negative relation between social competence and peer rejection, it is likely that rejected girls' social behavior makes them a likely target in the victimization process. Any attempt to decrease the level of aggressiveness among girls would need to include an individual component that would address the social skillfulness of victimized girls, thereby decreasing the likelihood that they would be targets of the aggressive acts of others.

Given the relation between victimization and rejection, it is important to consider how girls who are victimized respond to aggression and the consequences of these responses. The results of these data are striking. Girls appear to adopt responses that maximize the likelihood of continued aggression and the inclusion of others into the aggression toward the victim. Results indicated that only a direct effort at de-escalation leads to a positive outcome more often than a negative one for victims of aggression. However, girls attempted to diffuse or de-escalate the aggression only 12% of the time. Instead, girls ignored the aggression 60% of the time and confronted or escalated the aggression at least as often as they attempted diffusion. This pattern of victim responses and their consequences is robust across status, race, and familiarity of the group.

Given that the pattern is so clear, it is surprising that victims only attempt to de-escalate 12% of the time. Three possibilities suggest themselves. First, girls may not know the real consequences of their behavior and may believe that their behavior is the most efficacious. As Maccoby indicates, girls are socialized to avoid conflict and confrontation. Intuitively, girls may feel that any response to aggression creates further conflict, thus, the best strategy is to ignore the conflict. Unfortunately, this is not true. Rather than ending the conflict, ignoring aggression was most likely to cause a third party to enter the aggression. It was almost as if ignoring aggression represented an invitation to further aggression by others.

Furthermore, girls may have two alternative motives in addition to stopping the immediate aggression that drive their behavior when they confront or aggress back. Girls may be focused upon avoiding future aggression and believe that confrontation or escalation serves as a warning to aggressors to avoid similar aggression in the future; alternatively, girls may wish to save face in their peer group and hope that ignoring the aggression will minimize their loss of status or face in the group. Ignoring an aggressive act by a peer might permit a girl to save a sense of personal dignity. Both of these motives have more to do with ongoing interaction with peers than with the immediate consequences of the aggression. The findings described earlier in the study provide some hint of the long-term effects of these strategies, however. Rejected girls tend to be victims more than average or popular girls, suggesting that girls' typical response to aggression may contribute to a truly negative cycle. Rejected girls are more likely to be the recipients of aggressive acts. The most likely response is to attempt to ignore the aggression, thus maximizing the likelihood that others will enter the aggressive sequence, causing the girl to become further rejected. If this cycle is typical for repeated victims of aggression and a link to social rejection for girls, it requires thoughtful consideration about how to intervene as parents, teachers, and other socialization agents. Clearly the popular advice to just ignore aggressive behavior as it will go away needs reexamination. As this study suggests, it may not go away, but persist in very hurtful forms requiring intervention at both the individual as well as group level.

## ACKNOWLEDGMENT

This research was funded by Grant No. RO1 MH52843-05 from the National Institutes of Health.

## REFERENCES

Archer, J. (1992). Childhood gender roles: Social context and organization. In H. McGurk (Ed.), *Childhood social development: Contemporary perspectives* (pp. 31–61). Hove, UK: Erlbaum.

Bakeman, R., & Guera, V. (1985). *Analyzing interaction: Sequential analysis with SDIS and GSEQ.* Cambridge, UK: Cambridge University Press.

Berndt, T. J. (1986). Children's comments about their friendships. In *Minnesota Symposium on Child Psychology* (Vol. 18, pp. 189–212). Mahwah, NJ: Erlbaum.

Bjorkqvist, K., Lagerspetz, M. J., & Kaukiainen, A. (1992). Do girls manipulate and boys fight? Developmental trends in regard to direct and indirect aggression. *Aggressive Behavior, 18,* 117–127.

Cairns, R. B., Cairns, B. D., Neckerman, H. J., Ferguson, L. L., & Gariepy, J. L. (1989). Growth and aggression: 1. Childhood to early adolescence. *Developmental Psychology, 25,* 320–330.

Coie, J. D., & Dodge, K. A. (1998). Aggression and antisocial behavior. In W. Damon & N. Eisenberg (Eds.), *Handbook of child psychology: Vol. 3. Social, emotional, and personality development*(5th ed., pp. 779–862). New York: Wiley.

Coie, J. D., & Kupersmidt, J. B. (1983). A behavioral analysis of emerging social status in boys' groups. *Child Development, 54,* 1400–1416.

Crick, N. R. (1995). Relational aggression: The role of intent attributions, feelings of distress, and provocation type. *Development and Psychopathology, 7,* 313–322.

Crick, N. R. (1996). The role of overt aggression, relational aggression, and prosocial behavior in the prediction of children's future adjustment. *Child Development, 67,* 2317–2327.

Crick, N. R., Bigbee, M. A., & Howe, C. (1996). Gender differences in children's normative beliefs about aggression: How do I hurt thee? Let me count the ways. *Child Development, 67,* 1003–1014.

Crick, N. R., & Grotpeter, J. K. (1995). Relational aggression, gender and social-psychological adjustment. *Child Development, 66,* 710–722.

Crick, N. R., & Grotpeter, J. K. (1996). Children's treatment by peers: Victims of relational and overt aggression. *Development and Psychopathology, 8,* 367–380.

Crick, N. R., Werner, N. E., Casas, J. F., O'Brien, K. M., Nelson, D. A., Grotpeter, J. K., & Markon, K. (1999). Childhood aggression and gender: A new look at an old problem. In D. Bernstein (Ed.), *Nebraska Symposium on Motivation* (pp. 75–140). Lincoln: University of Nebraska Press.

Eder, D., & Hallinan, M. T. (1978). Sex differences in children's friendships. *American Sociological Review, 43,* 237–250.

Galen, B. R., & Underwood, M. K. (1997). A developmental investigation of social aggression among girls. *Developmental Psychology, 33,* 589–600.

Gottman, J. M., & Mettetal, G. (1986). The world of coordinated play: Same- and cross-sex friendship in young children. In J. M. Gottman & J. G. Parker (Eds.), *Conversations with friends: Speculations about affective development* (pp. 139–191). New York: Cambridge University Press.

Gottman, J. M., & Mettetal, G. (1986). The world of coordinated play: Same- and cross-sex friendship in young children. In J. M. Gottman & J. G. Parker (Eds.), *Conversations with friends: Speculations about affective development* (pp. 139–191). New York: Cambridge University Press.

Hart, C. H., Nelson, D. A., Robinson, C. C., Olsen, S. F., & McNeilly-Choque, M. K. (1998). Overt and relational aggression in Russian nursery-school-age children: Parenting style and marital linkages. *Developmental Psychology, 34,* 687–697.

Hughes, J. N., Cavell, T. A., & Thompson, B. (1998). The role of relational aggression in identifying aggressive boys and girls. *Journal of School Psychology, 36,* 457–477.

Kupersmidt, J. B., Putallaz, M., Coie, J. D., & Grimes, C. L. (2001, June). *Behavioral analysis of aggressive behavior in play groups of girls as a function of peer sociometric status.* Paper presented at the annual meeting of the International Society for Research in Child and Adolescent Psychopathology, Vancouver.

Lagerspetz, K. M., Björkqvist, K., & Peltonen, T. (1988). Is indirect aggression typical of females? Gender differences in aggressiveness in 11- to 12-year-old children. *Aggressive Behavior, 14,* 403–414.

Maccoby, E. E. (1990). Gender and relationships: A developmental account. *American Psychologist, 45,* 513–520.

Maccoby, E. E. (1998). *The two sexes: Growing up apart, coming together.* Cambridge, MA: Harvard University Press.

McKnight, K., Mariaskin, A. R., Putallaz, M., Grimes, C. L., Kupersmidt, J. B., & Coie, J. D. (2003, April). *A microanalytic look at the process of aggression in girls.* Paper presented at the biennial meeting of the Society for Research in Child Development, symposium on "Observational Studies of Aggression among Girls," Tampa, FL.

McNeilly-Choque, M. K., Hart, C. H., Robinson, C. C., Nelson, L. J., & Olsen, S. F. (1996). Overt and relational aggression on the playground: Correspondence among different informants. *Journal of Research in Childhood Education, 11*, 47–67.

Osterman, K., Bjorkqvist, K., Lagerspetz, K. M. J., Kaukiainen, A., Landau, S. F., Fraczek, A., & Caprara, G. (1998). Cross-cultural evidence of female indirect aggression. *Aggressive Behavior, 24*, 1–8.

Paley, V. G. (1992). *You can't say you can't play.* Cambridge, MA: Harvard University Press.

Paquette, J. A., & Underwood, M. K. (1999). Gender differences in young adolescents' experiences of peer victimization: Social and physical aggression. *Merrill-Palmer Quarterly, 45*, 242–265.

Parke, R. D., & Slaby, R. G. (1983). The development of aggression. In P. Mussen (Series Ed.) & E. M. Hetherington (Vol. Ed.), *Handbook of child psychology: Vol. 4. Socialization, personality, and social development* (pp. 547–641). New York: Wiley.

Putallaz, M., Kupersmidt, J., Grimes, C. L., DeNero, K., & Coie, J. D. (1999, April). *Overt and relational aggression: Aggressors, victims, and gender.* Paper presented at the biennial meeting of the Society for Research in Child Development, symposium on "Social Relationships and Two Forms of Aggression: Gender Considerations," Albuquerque, NM.

Putallaz, M., Rhule, D., Kupersmidt, J., Grimes, C. L., & McKnight, K. (2001, June). *Overt and relational aggression: Victims, aggressors and gender.* Paper presented at the annual meeting of the American Psychological Society, Toronto.

Rose, A. J., Lockerd, E., & Swenson, L. (2002, April). *Disliked and "popular" relationally aggressive youth: Differences in adjustment and manifestations of relational aggression.* Paper presented at the biennial meeting of the Society for Research on Adolescence, New Orleans, LA.

Rumors? About me? How readers handle bad gossip. (2002, September). *Parade* (News and Observer), p. 11.

Rys, G. S., & Bear, G. G. (1997). Relational aggression and peer relations: Gender and development issues. *Merrill-Palmer Quarterly, 43*, 87–106.

Simmons, R. (2002). *Odd girl out: The hidden culture of aggression in girls.* New York: Harcourt.

Thompson, M., Cohen, L. J., & Grace, C. O. (2002). *Mom, they're teasing me.* New York: Ballantine Books.

Thompson, M., & Grace, C. O. (2001). *Best friends, worst enemies: Understanding the social lives of children.* New York: Ballantine Books.

Tomada, G., & Schneider, B. H. (1997). Relational aggression, gender, and peer acceptance: Invariance across culture, stability over time, and concordance among informants. *Developmental Psychology, 33*, 601–609.

Underwood, M. K. (2003). *Social aggression among girls.* New York: Guilford Press.

Underwood, M. K., Galen, B. R., & Paquette, J. A. (2001). Top ten challenges for understanding aggression and gender: Why can't we all just get along? *Social Development, 10*, 248–266.

Waldrop, M. F., & Halverson, C. F. (1975). Intensive and extensive peer behavior: Longitudinal and cross-sectional analysis. *Child Development, 46,* 19–26.

Wiseman, R. (2002). *Queen bees and wannabes: Helping your daughter survive cliques, gossip, boyfriends, & other realities of adolescence.* New York: Crown.

Xie, H., Cairns, R. B., & Cairns, B. D. (2002). The development of social and physical aggression: A narrative analysis of interpersonal conflicts. *Aggressive Behavior, 28,* 341–355.

Xie, H., Swift, D. J., Cairns, B. D., & Cairns, R. B. (2002). Aggressive behaviors in social interaction and developmental adaptation: A narrative analysis of interpersonal conflicts during early adolescence. *Social Development, 28,* 341–355.

# PART III

# UNDERSTANDING ANTISOCIAL AND RELATED PROBLEM BEHAVIORS IN ADOLESCENT GIRLS

# CHAPTER 7

# Early Disruptive Behaviors Associated with Emerging Antisocial Behavior among Girls

Karen L. Bierman, Carole Bruschi, Celene Domitrovich,
Grace Yan Fang, Shari Miller-Johnson,
*and* the Conduct Problems Prevention Research Group

In recent years, researchers, practitioners, and policymakers alike have lamented the lack of good empirical data describing the developmental course of disruptive behavior problems and the emergence of antisocial behaviors among girls. Most of the available longitudinal research linking early disruptive behavior problems with adolescent antisocial activity focuses on developmental progressions in boys, due to prevalence rates that are typically 3–4 times higher in boys than girls during elementary school (American Psychiatric Association, 1994; Robins, 1986; Zoccolillo, 1993). Research on boys reveals that disruptive behavior problems are fairly stable, with year-to-year correlations typically in the .5 range. They predict serious social and academic adjustment difficulties, as well as later adolescent antisocial behavior, school dropout, and substance use (Dishion, French, & Patterson, 1995). Fifty percent of the children with moderate-to-severe levels of disruptive behaviors during the preschool years continue on during the school-age years, many developing clinically significant conduct and related disorders by late childhood and early adolescence (Campbell, 2002). Hence, these are significant problems that warrant early identification and intervention. Although prior research has focused primarily on boys, issues of early identification and intervention may be equally important for girls.

Despite being less prevalent among girls than boys, disruptive behavior problems represent a major mental health problem for girls with highly adverse consequences. By adolescence, antisocial activity and associated conduct disorder emerges as the second most common psychiatric disorder among girls (American Psychiatric Association, 1994). Like boys, girls with disruptive behavior problems who initiate antisocial activity in adolescence appear at high risk for associated adolescent mental health difficulties (particularly depression), as well as alcohol and substance abuse (Kovacs, Krol, & Voti, 1994; Zoccolillo, 1993). In addition, theorists have speculated that these girls represent a key link in the intergenerational transmission of male criminality, as they often associate romantically with antisocial men, become teen mothers, and show poor parenting abilities that increase the risk for disruptive behavioral development among their offspring (Capaldi, Kim, & Shortt, Chapter 11, this volume; Dishion, French, & Patterson, 1995; Serbin et al., Chapter 13, this volume; Zoccolillo, Paquette, Azar, Côté, & Tremblay, Chapter 12, this volume).

Recent studies suggest that there may be important gender differences in the development of disruptive behavior problems, leading investigators to argue that better attempts are needed to understand the early nature and course of these problems among girls (Silverthorn & Frick, 1999). In particular, questions exist concerning the use of early aggressive behaviors as indicators of at-risk status for later antisocial behavior. Whereas a near-consensus model has been reached regarding basic developmental progressions and mechanisms underlying the development of "early starting" patterns of antisocial behavior among boys, the degree to which this model fits girls remains open to question (Silverthorn & Frick, 1999). Researchers have suggested that screening strategies that focus on early aggression, which may be quite effective for identifying boys at risk for later antisocial activity, may result in the underidentification of at-risk girls (Zahn-Waxler, 1993; Zoccolillo, 1993). This chapter reviews literature relevant to this question and explores longitudinal data from the Fast Track Project (Conduct Problems Prevention Research Group [CPPRG], 1992) to compare the effectiveness of screening strategies that emphasize aggressive behaviors to a greater or lesser degree in identifying children as "at risk" for later antisocial behavior and related school adjustment difficulties.

## DEVELOPMENTAL MODEL OF THE "EARLY-STARTING" ANTISOCIAL PATHWAY

Based primarily on longitudinal studies of boys, developmental models suggest that "early-starting" or "life-course persistent" patterns of antisocial behavior begin to emerge during the preschool years. The initial behavior problems typically involve high rates of active, impulsive, and noncompliant behaviors that challenge the socialization efforts of parents, and escalate during early childhood to include the hostile aggressive behaviors that predict later antisocial activity (Campbell, 2002; Keenan & Shaw, 1994). Researchers have speculated that the temperamental characteristics (e.g., negative emotionality, high activity level) and/or neuropsychological deficits in executive functioning that contribute to attention deficits and hyperactivity increase socialization difficulties and create child vulnerability to the development of aggression (Lynam, 1996; Moffitt, 1993). Particularly in highly stressed family situations (e.g., families pressured with socioeconomic disadvantage, single parenting or marital discord, maternal depression, or low levels of social support), the parental response often involves inconsistent, harsh, and punitive control attempts, which serve to escalate child misbehavior through mechanisms of modeling of aggressive responding and intermittent negative reinforcement of child aggression in coercive interactions. In this early-starting pattern, negative transactions between parents and biologically vulnerable children contribute to social learning that involves the escalation from less severe noncompliant and argumentative and/or hyperactive–impulsive behaviors to more severe aggressive and antisocial behaviors (Patterson, 1986). By entry into grade school, the problem patterns shown by these children include salient levels of overt aggression, typically with high rates of concurrent oppositional defiant and inattentive–hyperactive behaviors (Moffitt, 1993; Stormshak, Bierman, & CPPRG, 1998).

Although inappropriate behavior is often their most salient problem, children with disruptive behaviors also experience significant social and academic adjustment problems during grade school, which contribute to their risk for antisocial activity and related maladaptation in adolescence (Conduct Problems Prevention Research Group, 1992; Patterson, Reid, & Dishion, 1992.) Perhaps in part a function of low levels of parental stimulation and support for the development of emotion control and social and cognitive skills (Greenberg, Kusche, & Speltz, 1991), children with disruptive behavior problems often enter school with deficiencies in critical social-cognitive skills, low levels of academic readiness, and low levels of social competence (Conduct Problems Prevention Research Group, 1992; Dodge, Bates, & Pettit, 1990). Children with disruptive behavior problems are rejected by their peers and develop conflictual relations with their teachers (Campbell, 2002; Coie, 1990). Consequently, these students often become disengaged from school and drift into deviant peer groups. Consistent with this developmental research, high rates of aggressive behavior at school entry serve as an effective "red flag" for boys, indicating significant risk for later psychosocial and academic adjustment problems in grade school and deviant group affiliation and antisocial activity in early adolescence (Coie, Lochman, Terry, & Hyman, 1992; Dishion, Andrews, & Crosby, 1995).

However, based upon evidence of gender differences in the display of aggressive behaviors, researchers have speculated that overt aggression may provide a less effective basis for early screening and identification of girls at risk for similar grade school adjustment problems and adolescent antisocial activity. Indeed, researchers have speculated that an emphasis on overt aggression as a basis for the early identification of at-risk children results in a significant underidentification of at-risk girls (Zahn-Waxler, 1993; Zoccolillo, 1993). The basis for concerns regarding gender differences in the utility of overt aggression as a marker of risk stems from evidence that rates of overt aggression show greater gender differences across childhood and adolescence than do other types of disruptive behavior problems.

## GENDER DIFFERENCES IN THE DISPLAY OF DISRUPTIVE BEHAVIORS

Of central importance to characterizing gender differences in disruptive behaviors is the concept, represented in the developmental model described in the preceding section, that aggressive behaviors are part of a broader-band spectrum of externalizing behavior problems that violate social expectations and norms, are aversive or harmful to others, and occur at levels high enough to impair the individual's developmental adaptation. In addition to aggressive behaviors, which involve hostile verbal and physical acts intended to cause harm to another, this spectrum also includes oppositional behaviors (e.g., negativistic, disobedient, moody, and angry reactive behaviors) and inattentive–hyperactive behaviors (e.g., impulsive, disorganized, disruptive, distractable, and off-task behaviors). From a developmental standpoint, oppositional behaviors and inattentive–hyperactive behaviors often predate and set the stage for child escalation to more aggressive and violent behaviors (Stormshak et al., 1998). Consistent with this developmental model, research on clinical populations suggest that oppositional defiant disorder (ODD), which is characterized by moody, oppositional, and noncompliant behaviors, is often a precursor to conduct disorder (CD), which is characterized by more severe aggressive and antisocial behaviors. Although the developmental progression of clinically significant disruptive behaviors ends with ODD for some children, most of the children who eventually develop CD also qualify for a diagnosis of ODD (77–96% across studies;

Loeber, Lahey, & Thomas, 1991), suggesting a developmental progression along a spectrum of disruptive behaviors.

Of the behaviors that comprise the spectrum of disruptive problems, rates of overt aggression show the strongest gender differences across childhood and adolescence. Boys are rated as more aggressive than girls by teachers and parents, and display a greater number of aggressive acts in observational studies (Hyde, 1984, 1986; Maccoby & Jacklin, 1980). The gender gap begins around age 4 (Keenan & Shaw, 1994) and remains fairly robust through middle childhood, decreasing in late adolescence and adulthood (Hyde, 1984). In their meta-analysis, Eagly and Steffen (1986) reported significant gender differences in aggression continuing in adulthood, although the presence and size of these differences varied across studies.

In contrast to rates of overt aggression, which show robust gender differences across childhood and adolescence, rates of oppositional behavior show only limited or nonsignificant gender differences across studies (Keenan & Shaw, 1994; Zahn-Waxler, Ianotti, Cummings, & Denham, 1990). Indeed, based on home observations of parent–child interactions conducted with children referred for treatment due to high rates of disruptive behavior problems, Webster-Stratton (1996) concluded that the behavioral symptoms of early-onset conduct problems for boys and girls show more similarities than differences. Specifically, she found equivalent levels of noncompliant, oppositional, defiant, and disruptive behaviors displayed by boys and girls; only physical aggression and physically destructive behaviors were more common in boys than girls. Apparently, disruptive boys more often hit, push, and destroy things than disruptive girls, but disruptive children of either gender have temper tantrums, argue, talk back, whine, break rules, and refuse to comply with parental requests.

Interestingly, boys who are inattentive and impulsive are more likely to become aggressive than are girls with equally severe attention deficits, suggesting that even among children with cognitive risk factors that increase vulnerability for aggressive behavior problems, boys are more vulnerable to the development of physical aggression that are girls (Berry, Shaywitz, & Shaywitz, 1985; deHaas & Young, 1984). Similarly, among children with diagnosed attention-deficit/hyperactivity disorder, boys are more likely to show comorbid aggression than are girls (Berry et al., 1985; deHaas, 1986).

Although some investigators have noted that gender differences in CD decrease markedly by adolescence (Zoccolillo, 1993), the gap closes primarily because of increases in girl's nonaggressive antisocial behavior; boys continue to predominate in aggressive crimes (McGee, Feehan, Williams, & Anderson, 1992; Offord, Boyle, & Racine, 1991). Indeed, in the Dunedin study (McGee et al., 1992) almost half of the boys with CD at age 15 had aggressive CD (defined largely by violent criminal acts), whereas all of the girls with CD exhibited nonaggressive patterns, involving truancy, running away, serious lying, substance use, and non-confrontational stealing. Similarly, in a large epidemiological study in Canada, Offord and colleagues (1991) found that by early adolescence (ages 12–16), rates of nonaggressive CD symptoms were almost equal between boys and girls, whereas boys continued to show significantly higher rates of aggressive CD symptoms. Hence, across studies and age, gender differences seem most pronounced for aggressive and less marked for the nonaggressive disruptive behaviors.

## ALTERNATIVE DEVELOPMENTAL MODELS

Perhaps as a function both of the limited research and the mixed findings that characterize the available research, theorists have come to different conclusions regarding the developmental implications of gender differences in the display of aggressive behaviors during the grade school years. Some researchers have suggested that girls do not follow the early-onset pathway to antisocial behaviors that has been documented among boys, but rather follow a delayed-onset developmental trajectory (see Silverthorn & Frick, 1999). There are two key findings that provide the foundation for the delayed-onset model. First, Silverthorn and Frick (1999) note that girls rarely show high rates of aggression in elementary school. Second, they review research describing the "closing of the gender gap" in antisocial activity in adolescence, as girls begin to display antisocial activity, and note that most of the girls initiating antisocial activity do not have a history of grade school aggression. Following the logic of Zoccolillo (1993), they suggest that the reduced gender differences in the prevalence of CD in adolescence reflects the fact that this disorder commonly begins later in females than males. Silverthorn and Frick contrast the early-starting pathway documented for boys with this "delayed-onset" pathway for girls, suggesting that their antisocial behavior problems usually emerge first in early adolescence. Based upon their longitudinal study of Swedish children, Stattin and Magnusson (1984) likewise argued that, for girls, aggressive behavior was not predictive of adult criminality until age 13, and suggested that aggressive behavior does not typically become predictive for girls until after they reach puberty.

Contrary to this viewpoint is one that suggests that girls, like boys, do experience early-starting patterns of disruptive behavior problems, but that their early hostility and dysregulation are expressed in nonaggressive ways that are missed by research focusing on overt aggression. The argument here is that the focus on overt aggression as a key marker of risk for disruptive behavior problems and associated psychosocial maladjustment in many studies has led to overestimations of gender differences (Cohen, 1991; Hyde, 1986) and underestimations and inadequate identification of at-risk girls (Zahn-Waxler, 1993; Zoccolillo, 1993). Whereas for boys, early aggression is the "red flag" of choice for identifying the early-starting pathway to antisocial behavior and related adolescent behavior problems, girls are less likely to show overt aggression. Hence, overt aggression may be a less powerful predictor of later conduct problems for girls compared with boys. In middle childhood, girls appear more likely to exhibit oppositional and disruptive behavior than overt aggression, and appear more likely to express interpersonal hostility with indirect or relational behaviors than physical acts of aggression against others (Cairns, Cairns, Neckerman, Ferguson, & Gariepy, 1989; Crick & Grotpeter, 1995).

It may be that there are both gender similarities and differences in the early predictors of antisocial behavior problems. Developmental models of conduct problems suggest that nonaggressive disruptive behaviors often indicate "first-stage" or entry-level socialization difficulties. Due to the stress they place on socializing agents (teachers and parents), as well as the negative impact they have on psychosocial adaptation (school learning and peer relations), nonaggressive disruptive behavior problems (e.g., oppositional–defiant and inattentive–hyperactive behaviors) may disturb socialization in ways that enhance coercive processes and interpersonal rejection, promoting escalation to the second stage or more advanced socialization problems indicated by aggressive disruptive behaviors (Stormshak et al., 1998).

Following the logic of this developmental model, the girls who do develop overt aggression may, like overtly aggressive boys, be at particularly high risk for later antisocial outcomes. Indeed, Kupersmidt and Coie (1990) found that high levels of aggression in grade school predicted high school police and juvenile court contacts for both boys and girls. Looking at a separate sample, Kupersmidt and Patterson (1991) found grade school teacher ratings of acting-out behaviors to be a significant predictor of later delinquency for both boys and girls. Similarly, in their longitudinal study of the Dunedin sample, Moffitt, Caspi, Rutter, and Silva (2001) found that girls who showed high rates of aggressive behavior in the early grade school years were, like boys, at high risk for antisocial outcomes in adolescence. However, the rate of overt aggression was so low among girls, Moffit and colleagues argued that overt aggression was unlikely to provide an effective screen for later antisocial activity among girls.

The question that remains is whether a screening strategy that focuses on nonaggressive behaviors in the disruptive behavior spectrum (e.g., oppositional and inattentive–hyperactive behaviors) as well as aggressive behaviors might provide a more effective method of identifying at-risk girls in comparison to a screening strategy focused primarily on overt aggression. As indicated in the prior review, gender differences are less marked for the nonaggressive (oppositional, inattentive–hyperactive) behaviors that comprise the spectrum of disruptive behaviors than they are for aggressive behaviors. Hence, including nonaggressive disruptive behaviors as indicators of early risk should increase the number of girls identified as "at risk" and, depending upon the predictability of those nonaggressive disruptive behaviors, may result in a more effective screening for girls likely to develop adolescent antisocial problems. Available research suggests that nonaggressive disruptive behaviors (oppositional and inattentive–hyperactive behaviors) disturb psychosocial adjustment in ways that are similar to aggressive behaviors, predicting problematic peer relations and poor academic performance (August & Stewart, 1982; Pope, Bierman, & Mumma, 1991). Evidence concerning their efficacy as indices of early risk for emerging antisocial behavior is lacking, but worth pursuing. Screening strategies that focus on nonaggressive as well as aggressive disruptive behaviors might provide a more comprehensive identification of girls as well as boys who are at risk for the development of later antisocial problem behaviors.

## THE PRESENT STUDY

The present study utilized data from the Fast Track longitudinal study of high-risk youth to compare gender differences in the efficacy of a narrow screening strategy (emphasizing overt aggression) compared with a broader screening strategy (including nonaggressive oppositional and inattentive–hyperactive behaviors along with overt aggression) applied at school entry to identify children at risk for psychosocial adjustment problems and antisocial behavior. Kindergarten teacher ratings on the Child Behavior Checklist (Achenbach & Edelbrock, 1983) were scored to represent aggressive and nonaggressive (oppositional and inattentive–hyperactive) disruptive behaviors. Using these assessments of risk at school entry, we tested the effectiveness of a screen that emphasized aggressive/disruptive behaviors only compared with a screen that included a broader spectrum of aggressive plus nonaggressive–disruptive behaviors to identify boys and girls who experienced later psychosocial adjustment difficulties (in grade school) and evidenced emerging antisocial behavior problems (in early adolescence). We hypothesized that, particularly for girls, using the broader screening strategy that included both aggressive and nonaggressive disruptive behaviors would result in greater sensitivity than a more narrow screen focused on aggressive/disruptive behaviors alone, thereby identifying more of the girls who would have adjustment difficulties in grade school and show antisocial behaviors in early adolescence.

## Methods

### Participants

Participants were 649 children representing the high-risk control and normative samples participating in a multisite investigation of the development and prevention of conduct problems (Fast Track; Conduct Problems Prevention Research Group, 1992). Participants were drawn from four demographically diverse sites: Durham, North Carolina; Nashville, Tennessee; Seattle, Washington; and rural areas of central Pennsylvania.

In the first step of the sampling process, kindergarten teachers in 55 participating schools completed the Authority Acceptance scale of the TOCA-R (Teacher Observation of Child Adaptation—Revised; Werthamer-Larsson, Kellam, & Wheeler, 1991), providing ratings of the disruptive behaviors shown by each student. To create the normative sample, approximately 100 participants (87 in Seattle) were randomly selected to represent the population at each site according to race, sex, and decile of problem behaviors on the kindergarten TOCA-R. To select a high-risk sample, parent ratings of disruptive behaviors were collected for children with the highest TOCA-R scores (those in the upper 40%). The teacher and parent ratings of child disruptive behaviors were standardized within site and summed, and children with the highest summed scores at each site (top 10–15%) were selected for the high-risk sample (see Lochman & CPPRG, 1995, for more details on the screening process). This study includes children who attended control schools and did not receive preventive intervention. By combining children from the normative and high-risk samples, the participants include an overrepresentation of children with disruptive behavior problems at school entry, enabling a focused study of gender differences in the pattern and predictability of those problems.

Of the 275 girls and 374 boys included, most were either African American ($n$ = 295; 45%) or European American ($n$ = 332; 51%). The mean age of children at the start of the study was 6.45 years ($SD$ = .50, range = 2.81 years). Socioeconomic levels for families, using the Hollingshead classification, showed 39% of the sample in the lowest level, and 26% of the sample in the next lowest level of socioeconomic status.

*Measures of Disruptive Behaviors at School Entry*

At the end of the kindergarten year, teachers rated child behavior problems using the Child Behavior Checklist—Teacher Report Form (CBCL-TRF; Achenbach & Edelbrock, 1983). Based upon a confirmatory factor analysis completed in a prior study (Stormshak et al., 1998), items were summed to create three narrow-band disruptive behavior subscales: (1) overt aggression ("gets in many fights," "physically attacks people," "threatens people"), (2) oppositional ("argues," "stubborn," "temper tantrums"), and (3) inattentive–hyperactive ("can't sit still," "impulsive, acts without thinking," "can't concentrate").

Using these kindergarten ratings, two profiles of disruptive behavior problems were identified. Children with aggression scores greater than .75 *SD* above the mean of the normative sample on these teacher ratings were identified with *aggressive disruptive behaviors.* Almost all of these children also had elevated scores on either or both of the other disruptive behavior scales (oppositional and inattentive–hyperactive). Children who had oppositional or inattentive–hyperactive scores greater than .75 *SD* above the mean of the normative sample but aggression scores lower than .75 *SD* above the mean were identified with *nonaggressive disruptive behaviors.* Given the focus of the study on screening children at-risk for the development of adolescent problems, a relatively liberal cutoff was used to designate children with elevated disruptive behaviors in kindergarten (e.g., symptoms elevated to .75 *SD* or more above the mean by teacher report). The goal was to include children with subclinical but elevated levels of problem behaviors to determine whether such elevations could be used as a screen to detect children who would later develop psychosocial adjustment and antisocial behavior problems.

*Measures of Psychosocial Adjustment in Grade School*

Three aspects of grade 4 school adjustment were assessed—classroom behavior, peer relations, and academic grades. Classroom behavioral adjustment was assessed using the 10-item Authority Acceptance scale of the TOCA-R, completed by classroom teachers at the end of the grade 4 year. This scale includes 10 disruptive and aggressive behaviors, which are rated along a 6-point scale (0 = almost never, to 5 = almost always). Prior studies reveal internal consistency (alpha = .85), and concurrent validity (Werthamer-Larsson et al., 1991). Children were considered to have problematic behavior outcomes if their score on this measure fell above .75 *SD* above the mean of the normative sample (placing them approximately in the highest 20%).

Peer relations were assessed using sociometric peer nominations. In interviews conducted individually with children in each classroom (on average, 75% participation), children were presented with a roster of all classmates and asked to identify the classmates they liked the best ("like most" nominations) and the classmates they liked the least ("like least" nominations). Unlimited nominations were accepted. Scores were standardized within class, and social preference scores were calculated by subtracting the standardized "like least" scores from the standardized "like most" scores. Children were considered to have problematic social outcomes if their social preference score fell below .75 SD beneath the mean of the normative sample (placing them approximately in the lowest 20%).

Grade 4 academic adjustment was assessed via examination of child grades in language arts and math derived from their school records. Grades were rated on a 13-point scale (1 = F, 4 = D, 7 = C, 10 = B, 13 = A), and children were considered to have problematic academic outcomes if their language arts and math grades combined were below .75 SD beneath the mean of the normative sample (placing them approximately in the lowest 20%).

### Measures of Adolescent Antisocial Behavior

In the summer following their seventh grade year (when most participating youth were 13–14 years old), they completed audio-assisted questionnaires on a laptop computer during a home interview (a procedure designed to enhance confidentiality and produce valid self-reports of antisocial behavior.) To assess involvement in antisocial activity, youth completed the 22-item Self-Reported Delinquency measure (Elliot, Huizinga, & Morse, 1986). For the purposes of this screening study, a dichotomous score was created to differentiate youth who did or did not report elevated levels of antisocial activity (e.g., using .75 SD above the mean of the normative sample as the cutoff).

## Results

### Kindergarten Problem Profiles

The distribution of aggressive and nonaggressive disruptive problem profiles by gender at school entry is shown in Table 7.1 (for a more complete exploration of gender differences in kindergarten problem profiles, see Bierman, Domitrovich, Fang, & CPPRG, 2003). In the Fast Track sample, a total of 122 girls showed elevated disruptive behaviors in kindergarten, and of those girls, 48% showed aggressive/disruptive profiles and 52% showed nonaggressive–disruptive profiles. In contrast, of the

TABLE 7.1. Proportion of Disruptive Boys and Girls
Exhibiting Aggressive and Nonaggressive Problems

|  | Boys |  | Girls |
| --- | --- | --- | --- |
| Aggressive disruptive | 65% (147) | > | 48% (59) |
| Nonaggressive disruptive | 35% (80) | < | 52% (63) |

*Note.* Percentages represent proportions of boys or girls with disruptive
problems who do or do not show concurrent aggression. Numbers of children
are in parentheses. Chi-square of 8.82 is significant at $p < .01$.

227 boys with disruptive behaviors, 65% exhibited aggressive/disruptive
profiles and 35% exhibited nonaggressive–disruptive profiles. The gender difference is statistically significant, chi-square (1) = 8.82, $p < .01$,
with disruptive boys much more likely to show concurrent aggression
than disruptive girls.

## Screening Strategies

Researchers have suggested that, by ignoring nonaggressive–disruptive
behaviors and emphasizing aggressive/disruptive behaviors in the screening of children at risk for later antisocial behavior problems, girls may
be underidentified. The alternative is to use a broader definition of disruptive behaviors (including nonaggressive as well as aggressive disruptive behaviors) in the screening process, which may provide a more sensitive identification of girls at risk for later psychosocial adjustment
problems and antisocial behaviors. To test this hypothesis, we compared
two screening strategies: (1) one that identified risk based upon elevated
aggression status (teacher ratings of aggression in kindergarten that exceeded .75 *SD* relative to the normative sample), labeled the *narrow aggression screen*, and (2) one that identified risk based on elevated scores
on any one of the disruptive behavior subscales (teacher ratings of aggressive, oppositional, or inattentive–hyperactive behaviors in kindergarten, any one of which exceeded .75 *SD* relative to the normative sample), labeled the *broad disruptive screen*. Outcomes included three
domains of psychosocial adjustment in fourth grade (classroom behavior
problems, academic difficulties, poor peer relations) and self-reported
antisocial behaviors in seventh grade.

The effectiveness of each screening model was evaluated by examining their sensitivity, specificity, odds-ratio, and Wald's statistic. Logistic
models were fit to predict each dependent variable, dichotomized to indicate problem versus nonproblem outcomes. Sensitivity represents the
proportion of children who were designated to be "at risk" by the kindergarten screening model and who were later known to experience a

given problem outcome. Specificity represents the proportion of children who were designated to be "nonrisk" by the kindergarten screening model and who were later known not to experience a given problem outcome. Thus, sensitivity indicates how effective the screening model was at correctly identifying "at risk" children, whereas specificity indicates how effective the screening model was at detecting low-risk children. Screening strategies that improve sensitivity often simultaneously decrease specificity. In this study, we were particularly interested in determining whether using oppositional and inattentive–hyperactive behaviors (rather than aggressive behaviors alone) would increase the sensitivity of the screening strategy for girls, increasing the identification of at-risk girls who might benefit from preventive intervention. The Wald statistic provides an overall test for the statistical significance of the screen, measuring the degree to which the kindergarten risk status impacts the later negative outcomes. It is calculated by dividing each estimate by its standard error and squaring the result. Odds ratios represent the odds of experiencing a negative outcome among children designated "at risk" by the kindergarten screening model relative to the odds of experiencing a negative outcome among children designated as "nonrisk" by the kindergarten screening model. Thus, when the odds ratio is 1, there is no association between kindergarten risk status and later negative outcomes; odds ratios larger than 1 reflect stronger associations between kindergarten risk status and later negative outcomes.

## Predicting Grade School Psychosocial Adjustment

Statistics reflecting the effectiveness of the narrow aggression kindergarten screen and the broad disruptive kindergarten screen in detecting girls and boys who experienced negative grade 4 psychosocial outcomes are shown in Table 7.2. Across the grade 4 outcome domains, the broad screening strategy (which includes elevated levels of oppositional and/or inattentive–hyperactive behaviors as indices of risk) resulted in an additional 5–9% of the sample (boys and girls) being correctly identified as "at risk" in kindergarten, relative to the narrow screening strategy that focused on aggression alone as the indicator of risk. The impact of the narrow versus broad screening strategies on sensitivity by gender is illustrated in Table 7.2. In each grade 4 outcome domain, the sensitivity of the broad screening strategy (e.g., the percentage of children designated as "at risk" who developed problematic outcomes) was notably higher than the sensitivity of the narrow screening strategy for girls (.65 vs. .37 for behavior problems, .64 vs. .27 for academic problems, .63 versus .30 for social problems). The broad screening strategy also increased the sensitivity of the screen for boys relative to the narrow screen, but the

TABLE 7.2. Grade 4 Psychosocial Adjustment Using Narrow versus Broad Screening Strategies

| Screening strategies by gender | n at risk | Indices of screening efficacy | | | |
|---|---|---|---|---|---|
| | | Wald statistic | Odds ratio | Sensitivity | Specificity |
| Grade 4 behavior problems | | | | | |
| Girls narrow screening | 17 ( 7%) | 9.26** | 3.00 | .37 | .84 |
| Girls broad screening | 30 (12%) | 13.91*** | 3.61 | .65 | .66 |
| Boys narrow screening | 66 (20%) | 23.20*** | 3.17 | .56 | .71 |
| Boys broad screening | 95 (29%) | 29.39*** | 4.40 | .81 | .51 |
| Grade 4 academic problems | | | | | |
| Girls narrow screening | 12 ( 5%) | 1.98 | 1.72 | .27 | .82 |
| Girls broad screening | 28 (11%) | 10.90*** | 3.14 | .64 | .64 |
| Boys narrow screening | 51 (15%) | 12.53*** | 2.41 | .55 | .67 |
| Boys broad screening | 78 (23%) | 24.99*** | 4.71 | .84 | .48 |
| Grade 4 social problems | | | | | |
| Girls narrow screening | 13 ( 7%) | 2.46 | 1.87 | .30 | .81 |
| Girls broad screening | 27 (15%) | 8.56** | 2.89 | .63 | .63 |
| Boys narrow screening | 37 (16%) | 3.36 | 1.67 | .44 | .68 |
| Boys broad screening | 59 (25%) | 9.30** | 2.39 | .69 | .51 |

Note. Numbers in parentheses indicate the percentage of the total sample that was correctly identified as at risk by the screening model for that outcome.
* $p < .05$; ** $p < .01$; *** $p < .001$.

gains in sensitivity were not as great as they were for girls, due in part to the higher sensitivity of the narrow aggression screen for boys compared to girls (.81 vs. .56 for behavior problems, .84 vs. .55 for academic problems, .69 vs. .44 for social problems.) Due to the lower prevalence of aggressive problems among girls compared to boys, the proportion of girls correctly identified as "at risk" was increased by about .28–.37 in accuracy when the broader screening strategy was used, whereas the proportion of boys correctly identified was increased by .15–.29. There was a corresponding loss in specificity in all cases when the broad screen strategy was used, but the overall efficacy of the model remained stronger for the broader compared to the narrow screening model, with the difference particularly notable for girls. For example, the Wald statistic for the narrow screening model was not significant for girls when predicting the academic or social outcomes, whereas this statistic was significant ($p < .01$) for all outcomes when using the broader screening strategy. An examination of the odds ratio likewise demonstrates the relatively stronger effectiveness of the broad compared with the narrow screening model, for both boys and girls.

## Predicting Early Adolescent Antisocial Behaviors

Table 7.3 shows the statistics evaluating the efficacy of the narrow versus broad screening model in identifying children at risk for emerging antisocial behavior in adolescence. When girls are considered, both the narrow and broad strategies provide statistically significant predictive accuracy. However, the narrow model results in an unacceptably low level of sensitivity (.35), indicating that the use of kindergarten teacher ratings of aggressive/disruptive behaviors alone as an early screen will underidentify girls at risk for later antisocial activity. Expanding the screening to include nonaggressive–disruptive behaviors (oppositional and/or inattentive–hyperactive behaviors) results in improved sensitivity, with specificity that is still in an acceptable range.

In contrast to the girls, the narrow screening model did not produce a statistically significant predictive screen for boys, whereas the broad screening model did. For boys, the broader screening model showed higher sensitivity than the narrow screen, but resulted in undesirably low specificity.

## Discussion

Over the past decade, it has become evident that more research is needed to understand the development of antisocial behavior among girls. Driven primarily by evidence that the gender gap in prevalence rates of antisocial behavior closes during adolescence, despite fairly robust gender differences in aggressive behavior during grade school, investigators have argued that developmental studies may need to look beyond early aggressive behaviors to understand risk factors that predispose girls to

TABLE 7.3. Predicting Adolescent Risky Outcomes Using Narrow versus Broad Screening Strategies

| Screening strategies by gender | Indices of screening efficacy | | | | |
| --- | --- | --- | --- | --- | --- |
| | $n$ at risk | Wald statistic | Odds ratio | Sensitivity | Specificity |
| Grade 8 antisocial behavior | | | | | |
| Girls narrow screening | 15 ( 7%) | 5.95* | 2.49 | .35 | .82 |
| Girls broad screening | 26 (12%) | 8.31** | 2.73 | .61 | .64 |
| Boys narrow screening | 45 (15%) | 2.10 | 1.44 | .47 | .62 |
| Boys broad screening | 68 (23%) | 4.17* | 1.72 | .71 | .42 |

*Note* Numbers in parentheses indicate the percentage of the total sample that was correctly identified as at risk by the screening model for that outcome.
* $p < .05$; ** $p < .01$.

becoming antisocial adolescents (Silverthorn & Frick, 1999; Zahn-Waxler, 1993; Zoccolillo, 1993). Some researchers have suggested that girls show a delayed-onset rather than early-onset pattern, in which their emerging antisocial behavior is not precipitated by early aggressive behavior (Silverthorn & Frick, 1999). Others have suggested that some girls exhibit early aggressive behavior and are, like boys, at high risk for antisocial outcomes, but that the prevalence rates of early overt aggression are so low among girls that aggressive girls represent only a very small, nearly insignificant proportion of the girls who become antisocial (Moffitt et al., 2001).

An alternative explored in this chapter is that girls do show early-starting patterns of disruptive behavior which can provide a basis for the identification of those at risk for later antisocial behavior, but their early-starting patterns are often characterized by nonaggressive–disruptive behaviors (rather than aggression). We hypothesized that nonaggressive–disruptive behaviors (e.g., oppositional and inattentive–hyperactive behaviors), which are a part of the broader spectrum of disruptive behaviors associated with the early-starting pathway progression of conduct problems for boys, might likewise be associated with early-starting problems for girls. Because many boys who show nonaggressive–disruptive behaviors also develop aggressive/disruptive behaviors, the "later stage" aggressive behaviors which may be more proximal indicators of antisocial activity provide a good index of early risk. Girls are much less likely to show aggressive behaviors than boys, and hence, relying on aggressive behavior to index their early-starting patterns of conduct problems may lead to the conclusion that girls are much less likely than boys to show early-starting difficulties. Hence, it may be particularly important to include nonaggressive–disruptive behaviors as "first-stage" indices of dysregulation and socialization difficulties in developmental models designed to detect early-starting patterns of disruptive behaviors that predict later antisocial outcomes among girls.

The present study tested the specific hypothesis that a screening strategy that included both nonaggressive and aggressive/disruptive behaviors as early risk indices would prove more effective at identifying girls who would develop grade school psychosocial adjustment difficulties and adolescent antisocial activity than a narrow screen that focused only on aggressive behavior problems. This hypothesis was supported for all three of the grade school outcomes examined—classroom behavior, social preference, and academic grades. In each case, the broad screening strategy, which included nonaggressive–disruptive as well as aggressive/disruptive behaviors as indices of risk, demonstrated superior sensitivity and higher odds ratios than the narrow screen that focused on aggression alone. The improvements in screening sensitivity were particularly marked for girls when elevations in oppositional and inattentive–

hyperactive behaviors were used as indices of early risk for later grade school academic and psychosocial adjustment problems, due to the very poor sensitivity of aggressive behaviors alone as early screen indicators for girls.

The broad screening strategy also proved more effective than the narrow screening strategy in identifying girls who would exhibit elevated levels of antisocial activity in early adolescence. Early aggression was strongly related to antisocial activity among girls, reflected in the high odds ratio produced by the narrow screening model, but given the low base rates of aggressive behaviors among girls, the use of aggression alone resulted in unacceptably low levels of screening sensitivity. Using the broader screening model, the number of antisocial girls correctly identified increased by 42% (from 15 to 26 girls) when elevated oppositional and inattentive–hyperactive behaviors, along with aggressive behaviors, were used for screening. Apparently, early aggression indicates high risk for later antisocial activity among girls, but there are a number of girls who become antisocial without showing early aggression. By including a focus on nonaggressive–disruptive behaviors (oppositional and inattentive–hyperactive), the number of antisocial girls correctly identified increased markedly. Including nonaggressive–disruptive as well as aggressive/disruptive behaviors in the screen for boys also improved the sensitivity of the model, but resulted in unacceptably low specificity. Additional screening analyses conducted on the Fast Track sample suggest that screening accuracy for boys is enhanced by the inclusion of parent as well as teacher ratings in kindergarten or by the use of first-grade rather than kindergarten teacher ratings (Hill, Lochman, Coie, Greenberg, & CPPRG, in press).

The clear implication from these findings is that programs designed to identify at-risk girls for early preventive intervention should utilize broad screening strategies, which include both nonaggressive–disruptive and aggressive/disruptive behaviors as early risk indices. Due to the relatively low base rates of overt aggression among girls, a screening strategy that recognizes the risk associated with oppositional and inattentive–hyperactive behaviors, even when these are not accompanied by aggressive behaviors is particularly important in order to avoid the under-identification of at-risk girls.

## DEVELOPMENTAL PROCESSES AND GENDER DIFFERENCES IN DISRUPTIVE PROBLEM PROFILES

In addition to the practical implications for prevention programs, the findings of this study also have implications for developmental theory. Interestingly, gender differences in aggressive behavior appear to emerge during the preschool years. For both boys and girls, rates of aggressive behavior increase as they begin to interact with others, and peak around age 3 as they begin to develop the language, self-regulation, and social skills that allow them to use alternative behaviors in social conflict situations (Keenan & Shaw, 1994). It is around 4 years of age that gender differences emerge, as girls show a greater responsivity to socialization pressures and a more marked decline in aggressive behaviors, whereas among boys rates of aggression decline more slowly (Keenan & Shaw, 1994). As reflected in the review provided by Susman and Pajer (Chapter 2, this volume), biological vulnerabilities may account for base rate differences in the prevalence of aggressive/disruptive behaviors among boys, and may contribute to gender differences in responsivity to socialization pressures. Interacting with these biological variables, Zahn-Waxler (1993; Zahn-Waxler & Polanicka, Chapter 3, this volume), among others, has speculated that differential socialization pressures may exacerbate gender differences in emotion regulation and behavioral display skills associated with anger and aggression.

Zahn-Waxler's model, including the interaction of socialization practices with biological vulnerabilities, is consistent with the findings of the present study, in which gender differences were less marked for disruptive behaviors (e.g., noncompliant and impulsive behaviors, temper tantrums) and more marked for aggressive/disruptive behaviors. Developmental models of aggressive behavior suggest that disruptive behaviors typically emerge first, and act as stressors to parents and teachers in their socializing efforts. Research suggests that adult responses to child disruptive behavior play a central role in promoting the escalation of problem behaviors from noncompliance to aggression (Campbell, 2002; Patterson, 1986; Patterson et al., 1992). Hence, it follows that, if parents and teachers respond differentially to the disruptive problem behaviors of girls and boys, these differential socialization pressures may contribute to the greater likelihood that boys (compared to girls) will escalate from disruptive to aggressive behaviors.

Indeed, researchers have documented gender differences in parental discipline strategies that may contribute to higher rates of aggression among boys. For example, in a large and diverse sample of school-age children, Deater-Deckard, Dodge, Bates, and Pettit (1998) found that boys were more likely to have received harsh discipline (55% of boys vs. 45% of girls) and to have mothers who valued aggression (8% of boys vs. 4% of girls). Similarly, Webster-Stratton (1996) found that mothers of disruptive boys showed higher rates of physically negative discipline (i.e., hitting, spanking, restraining) in response to their children's misbehaviors than did mothers of disruptive girls. This finding is consistent with research on normative samples, which suggests that, in general, mothers use more physical punishment with boys than girls (Lytton & Romney, 1991).

Parents also appear to respond differently to the angry emotional displays of girls compared with boys, in ways that might support more self-regulation among girls (Keenan & Shaw, 1994). For example, Smetana (1989) found that mothers more often gave explanations and inductions, explaining the harmful consequences of aggressive acts more often to their young girls than to young boys. Similarly, parents more often explicitly encourage girls to share toys in disputes, and impose consequences when they do not (Keenan & Shaw, 1994; Ross, Tesla, Kenyon, & Lollis, 1990). In these ways, parents may give girls more support and greater pressure to regulate their anger and inhibit aggressive behavior, while providing less support and more harsh discipline to boys—a combination associated with coercive escalations of aggressive behavior (Patterson, 1986; Zahn-Waxler & Polanichka, Chapter 2, this volume). Differential socialization patterns may account for social-cognitive differences found between adult men and women related to their evaluation of aggressive behavior. That is, women, more than men, tend to perceive aggression as a behavior that would produce harm to the target, evoke guilt and anxiety in oneself, and lead to retribution in a way that might put oneself in danger (Eagly & Steffan, 1986).

Gender similarities are evident in children's responses to socialization contexts, and girls who exhibit aggression are similar in many ways to aggressive boys. Studies of incarcerated juvenile delinquents suggest that antisocial girls experience many of the same risk factors as delinquent boys, including severe physical punishment (Lewis et al., 1991; Rosenbaum, 1989; Widom, 2000), and low levels of family cohesion and support (Rosenbaum, 1989). Similarly, developmental studies suggest that boys and girls respond in similar ways to family and community risk factors associated with aggressive development (Deater-Deckard et al., 1998; Webster-Stratton, 1996).

## GENDER DIFFERENCES IN THE STABILITY OF AGGRESSION AND PREDICTABILITY OF ANTISOCIAL BEHAVIOR

A major area of debate is the degree to which gender influences the stability and predictability of aggressive and nonaggressive disruptive behaviors. Some research suggests that teacher-rated overt aggression, which occurs less often among girls than boys, is actually more stable for girls when it does occur (Kohn & Rossman, 1972; Verhulst & Van der Ende, 1991). Other research shows no gender differences in the stability of aggression. For example, in a longitudinal study of aggressive grade school children (Lyons, Serbin, & Marchessault, 1988; Moskowitz, Schwartzman, & Ledingham, 1985), girls who exhibited elevated aggression displayed playground behavior that was equivalent to similarly identified boys, and their aggression proved equally stable over a 3-year follow-up period. Yet a third set of studies suggests that aggression may be more stable for boys than girls. For example, McGee and colleagues (1992) found that externalizing disorders at age 11 predicted externalizing disorders at age 15 for boys but not girls.

A similar set of mixed findings exist in data linking early aggressive behaviors to later antisocial activity. Some studies have found that grade school aggression is more predictive of adolescent delinquency for boys than girls (Lefkowitz, Eron, Walder, & Huesmann, 1977). Others, in contrast, have found that elementary school teacher ratings of aggression and acting-out behavior predict later police contact equally well for boys and girls (Kupersmidt & Coie, 1990) and self-reported delinquency (Kupersmidt & Patterson, 1991).

In the present study, a comparison of the odds ratios suggest that early aggression and associated disruptive behaviors may be more predictive of some outcomes for boys than girls (e.g., later disruptive behavior and antisocial activity), but equally predictive of other outcomes (e.g., social adjustment problems). Importantly, however, the predictability is significant for girls as well as boys, when the broad spectrum of disruptive behaviors is used to indicate early risk.

## FUTURE DIRECTIONS

The present findings validate concerns that the disruptive behavior problems of girls may be underidentified by measures that emphasize aggressive behavior, and suggest that nonaggressive–disruptive as well as aggressive/disruptive behaviors warrant concern as early indicators of risk for later antisocial activity. In this study, self-reported antisocial activity at ages 13–14 served as the indicator of antisocial outcomes, and further study is needed to validate these screening strategies and predictive links to additional measures of antisocial activity (e.g., police and court records) in later adolescence.

In addition, future studies are needed to examine developmental mechanisms that may link the early risk factors of nonaggressive– and aggressive/disruptive behaviors with later antisocial outcomes. The potential contributions to gender differences in antisocial development of early neuropsychological deficits (Moffitt, 1993) and academic difficulties and social maladjustment (Lewin, Davis, & Hops, 1999) warrant further consideration

Recent years have witnessed a growing interest in the study of indirect and relational aggression among girls (Underwood, 2003). Research suggests that, rather than displaying overt aggression, girls often express interpersonal hostility in other ways, such as excluding children from play, or spreading rumors about them (Crick & Grotpeter, 1995). Although relational aggression warrants study, the present findings suggest that high-risk girls also exhibit overt disruptive behavior, including moody, noncompliant, stubborn, inattentive, and impulsive acting-out, and that these overt, dysregulated behaviors are predictive of poor school adjustment and later antisocial activity. Hence, it is important to continue the study of overt behaviors among girls, including both aggressive/disruptive and nonaggressive–disruptive behaviors, which may have a lower prevalence among girls than boys, yet nonetheless be important indices of risk for maladjustment and antisocial activities.

Investigators have noted that the development of antisocial behavior in girls is important, not only from the perspective of the girls themselves, but also because of the link between antisocial girls and the intergenerational transmission of behavior problems (Dishion et al., 1995; Zoccolillo, Paquette, Azar, Côté, & Tremblay, Chapter 12, this volume). The possibility that nonaggressive–disruptive behaviors (as well as aggressive/disruptive behaviors) may increase risk rates for early sexual activity and pregnancy as well as dysfunctional parenting is worth pursuing empirically.

## AUTHOR NOTE

Members of the CPPRG in alphabetical order include Karen L. Bierman (Pennsylvania State University), John D. Coie (Duke University), Kenneth A. Dodge (Duke University), E. Michael Foster (Pennsylvania State University), Mark T. Greenberg (Pennsylvania State University), John E. Lochman (University of Alabama), Robert J. McMahon (University of Washington), and Ellen Pinderhughes (Vanderbilt University)

Support for this project came from the National Institute of Mental Health (Grant Nos. R18MH48083, R18MH50951, R18MH50952, and R18MH50953). Additional support was provided by the National Institute of Drug Abuse and the Center for Substance Abuse Prevention (through memorandums of agreement with the NIMH). This work was also supported in part by the Department of Education (Grant No. S184430002) and NIMH (Grant Nos. K05MH00797 and K05MH01027).

## REFERENCES

Achenbach, T. M., & Edelbrock, C. (1983). *Manual for the Child Behavior Checklist and Revised Child Behavior Profile*. Burlington, VT: University Associates in Psychiatry.

American Psychiatric Association. (1994). *Diagnostic and statistical manual of mental disorders* (4th ed.). Washington, DC: Author.

August, G. J., & Stewart, M. A. (1982). Is there a syndrome of pure hyperactivity? *British Journal of Psychiatry, 140,* 305–311.

Berry, C. A., Shaywitz, S. E., & Shaywitz, B. A. (1985). Girls with attention deficit disorder: A silent minority? A report on behavioral and cognitive characteristics. *Pediatrics, 76,* 801–809.

Bierman, K. L., Domitrovich, C., Fang, G. Y., & CPPRG. (2003). *Patterns of disruptive behaviors in girls and boys and their developmental consequences.* Unpublished manuscript, The Pennsylvania State University.

Cairns, R. B., Cairns, B., Neckerman, H., Ferguson, L., & Gariepy, J. L. (1989). Growth and aggression: 1. Childhood to early adolescence. *Developmental Psychology, 25,* 320–330.

Campbell, S. (2002). *Behavior problems in preschool children: Clinical and developmental issues* (2nd ed.). New York: Guilford Press.

Cohen, L. D. (1991). Sex differences in the course of personality development: A meta analysis. *Psychological Bulletin, 109,* 252–266.

Coie, J. D. (1990). Toward a theory of peer rejection. In S. R. Asher & J. D. Coie (Eds.), *Peer rejection in childhood* (pp. 365–401). Cambridge, UK: Cambridge University Press.

Coie, J. D., Lochman, J. E., Terry, R., & Hyman, C. (1992). Predicting early adolescent disorder from childhood aggression and peer rejection. *Journal of Consulting and Clinical Psychology, 60,* 783–792.

Conduct Problems Prevention Research Group. (1992). A developmental and clinical model for the prevention of conduct disorders: The Fast Track Program. *Development and Psychopathology, 4,* 509–527.

Crick, N. R., & Grotpeter, J. K. (1995). Relational aggression, gender, and social-psychological adjustment. *Child Development, 66,* 710–722.

Deater-Deckard, K., Dodge, K. A., Bates, J. E., & Pettit, G. S. (1998). Multiple risk factors in the development of externalizing behavior problems: Group and individual differences. *Development and Psychopathology, 10,* 469–493.

deHaas, P. A. (1986). Attention styles and peer relationships of hyperactive and normal boys and girls. *Journal of Abnormal Child Psychology, 14,* 457–467.

deHaas, P. A., & Young, R. D. (1984). Attention styles of hyperactive and normal girls. *Journal of Abnormal Child Psychology, 12,* 531–546.

Dishion, T. J., Andrews, D. W., & Crosby, L. (1995). Antisocial boys and their friends in early adolescence: Relationship characteristics, quality and interactional process. *Child Development, 66,* 139–151.

Dishion, T., French, D., & Patterson, G. (1995). The development and ecology of antisocial behavior. In D. Cicchetti & D. J. Cohen (Eds.), *Developmental psychopathology, Vol. 2: Risk, disorder, and adaptation* (pp. 421–471). Oxford, UK: Wiley.

Dodge, K. A., Bates, J. E., & Pettit, G. S. (1990). Mechanisms in the cycle of violence. *Science, 250* 1678–1683.

Eagly, A. H., & Steffan, V. J. (1986). Gender and aggressive behavior: A meta-analytic review of the social psychological literature. *Psychological Bulletin, 100,* 309–330.

Elliot, D. S., Huizinga, D., & Morse, B. (1986). Self-reported violent offending: A descriptive analysis of juvenile violent offenders and their offending careers. *Journal of Interpersonal Violence, 1*, 472–514.

Greenberg, M. T., Kusche, C. A., & Speltz, M. (1991). Emotional regulation, self control, and psychopathology: The role of relationships in early childhood. In D. Cicchetti & S. L. Toth (Eds.), *Internalizing and externalizing expressions of dysfunction: Rochester symposium on developmental psychopathology* (Vol. 2, pp. 21–66). Hillsdale, NJ: Erlbaum.

Hill, L. G., Lochman, J. E., Coie, J. D., Greenberg, M. T., & CPPRG. (in press). Effectiveness of early screening for externalizing problems: Issues of screening accuracy and utility. *Journal of Consulting and Clinical Psychology.*

Hyde, J. S. (1984). How large are gender differences in aggression? A developmental meta-analysis. *Developmental Psychology, 20*, 722–736.

Hyde, J. S. (1986). Gender differences in aggression. In J. S. Hyde & M. C. Linn (Eds.), *The psychology of gender: Advances through meta-analysis* (pp. 51–66). Baltimore: Johns Hopkins University Press.

Keenan, K., & Shaw, D. S. (1994). The development of aggression in toddlers: A study of low-income families. *Journal of Abnormal Child Psychology, 22*, 53–77.

Kohn, M., & Rossman, B. L. (1972). A social competence scale and symptom checklist for the preschool child: Factor dimensions, their cross-instrument generality and longitudinal persistence. *Developmental Psychology, 6*, 430–444.

Kovacs, M., Krol, R., & Voti, L. (1994). Early onset psychopathology and the risk for teenage pregnancy among clinically referred girls. *Journal of the American Academy of Child Adolescent Psychiatry, 33*, 106–113.

Kupersmidt, J., & Coie, J. (1990). Preadolescent peer status, aggression and school adjustment as predictors of externalizing problems in adolescence. *Child Development, 61*, 1350–1362.

Kupersmidt, J., & Patterson, C. (1991). Childhood peer rejection, aggression, withdrawal, and perceived competence as predictors of self-reported behavior problems in adolescence. *Journal of Abnormal Child Psychology, 19*, 427–449.

Lefkowitz, M. M., Eron, L. D., Walder, L. O., & Huesmann, L. R. (1977). *Growing up to be violent: A longitudinal study of the development of aggression.* Oxford, UK: Pergamon Press.

Lewin, L. M., Davis, B., & Hops, H. (1999). Childhood social predictors of adolescent antisocial behavior: Gender differences in predictive accuracy and efficacy. *Journal of Abnormal Child Psychology, 27*, 277–292.

Lewis, D. O., Yeager, C. A., Cobham-Portorreal, C. S., Klein, N., Showalter, C., & Anthony, A. (1991). A follow-up of female delinquents: Maternal contributions to the perpetuation of deviance. *Journal of the American Academy of Child and Adolescent Psychiatry, 30*, 197–201.

Lochman, J. E., & CPPRG. (1995). Screening of child behavior problems for prevention programs at school entry. *Journal of Consulting and Clinical Psychology, 6*, 549–559.

Loeber, R., Lahey, B. B., & Thomas, C. (1991). Diagnostic conundrum of oppositional defiant disorder and conduct disorder. *Journal of Abnormal Psychology, 100*, 379–390.

Lynam, D. R. (1996). Early identification of chronic offenders: Who is the fledgling psychopath? *Psychological Bulletin, 120*, 209–234.

Lyons, J., Serbin, L. A., & Marchessault, K. (1988). The social behavior of peer-identified aggressive, withdrawn, and aggressive/withdrawn children. *Journal of Abnormal Child Psychology, 16*, 539–552.

Lytton, H., & Romney, D. (1991). Parents' differential socialization of boys and girls: A meta-analysis. *Psychological Bulletin, 109*, 267–296.

Maccoby, E. E., & Jacklin, C. N. (1980). Sex differences in aggression: A rejoinder and reprise. *Child Development, 51*, 964–980.

McGee, R., Feehan, M., Williams, S., & Anderson, J. (1992). DSM-III disorders from age 11 to age 15 years. *Journal of the American Academy of Child and Adolescent Psychiatry, 31*, 50–59.

Moffit, T. E. (1993). The neuropsychology of conduct disorder. *Development and Psychopathology, 5*, 135–152.

Moffitt, T. E., Caspi, A., Rutter, M., & Silva, P. (2001). *Sex differences in antisocial behavior.* Cambridge, UK: Cambridge University Press.

Moskowitz, D. S., Schwartzman, A. E., & Ledingham, J. E. (1985). Stability and change in aggression and withdrawal in middle childhood and early adolescence. *Journal of Abnormal Psychology, 94*, 30–41.

Offord, D. R., Boyle, M. H., & Racine, Y. A. (1991). The epidemiology of antisocial behavior in childhood and adolescence. In D. J. Pepler & R. H. Rubin (Eds.), *The development and treatment of childhood aggression* (pp. 31–54). Hillsdale, NJ: Erlbaum.

Patterson, G. R. (1986). Performance models for antisocial boys. *American Psychologist, 41*, 432–444.

Patterson, G. R., Reid, J. B., & Dishion, T. J. (1992). *A social learning approach: Vol. 4. Antisocial boys.* Eugene, OR: Castalia.

Pope, A. W., Bierman, K. L., & Mumma, G. H. (1991). Aggression, hyperactivity, and inattention-immaturity: Behavior dimensions associated with peer rejection in elementary school boys. *Developmental Psychology, 27*, 663–671.

Robins, L. N. (1986). The consequences of conduct disorder in girls. In D. Olweus, J. Block, & M. Radke-Yarrow (Eds.), *Development of antisocial and prosocial behavior* (pp. 385–414). New York: Academic Press.

Rosenbaum, J. L. (1989). Family dysfunction and female delinquency. *Crime and Delinquency, 35*, 31–44.

Ross, H., Tesla, C., Kenyon, B., & Lollis, S. (1990). Maternal intervention in toddler peer conflict: The socialization of principles of justice. *Developmental Psychology, 26*, 994–1003.

Silverthorn, P., & Frick, P. J. (1999). Developmental pathways to antisocial behavior: The delayed-onset pathway in girls. *Development and Psychopathology, 11*, 101–126.

Smetana, J. G. (1989). Adolescents' and parents' reasoning about actual family conflict. *Child Development, 60*, 1052–1067.

Stattin, H., & Magnusson, D. (1984). *The role of early aggressive behavior for the frequency, the seriousness, and the types of later criminal offences.* Sweden: University of Stockholm.

Stormshak, E. A., Bierman, K. L., & the Conduct Problems Prevention Research Group. (1998). The implications of different developmental patterns of disruptive behavior problems for school adjustment. *Development and Psychopathology, 10,* 451–467.

Underwood, M. K. (2003). *Social aggression among girls.* New York: Guilford Press.

Verhulst, F. C., & Van der Ende, J. (1991). Four year follow-up of teacher-reported problem behaviours. *Psychological Medicine, 21,* 965–977.

Webster-Stratton, C. (1996). Early-onset conduct problems: Does gender make a difference? *Journal of Consulting and Clinical Psychology, 64,* 540–551.

Werthamer-Larsson, L., Kellam, S. G., & Wheeler, L. (1991). Effects of first-grade classroom environment on shy behavior, aggressive behavior, and concentration problems. *American Journal of Community Psychology, 19,* 585–602.

Widom, C. S. (2000). Motivation and mechanisms in the "cycle of violence." In D. J. Hansen (Ed.), *Nebraska Symposium on Motivation: Vol. 46. Motivation and child maltreatment* (pp. 1–37). Lincoln: University of Nebraska Press.

Zahn-Waxler, C. (1993). Warriors and worriers: Gender and psychopathology. *Development and Psychopathology, 5,* 79–89.

Zahn-Waxler, C., Ianotti, R. J., Cummings, M. E., & Denham, S. ( 1990). Antecedents of problem behaviors in children of depressed mothers. *Development and Psychopathology, 2,* 271–291.

Zoccolillo, M. (1993). Gender and the development of conduct disorder. *Development and Psychopathology, 5,* 65–78.

# CHAPTER 8

# Aggression and Antisocial Behavior in Sexually Abused Females

Penelope K. Trickett *and* Elana B. Gordis

Over the last two decades or so, as our understanding of the high prevalence of sexual abuse of females has increased, so has the number of research studies examining adverse developmental outcomes (Trickett, Kurtz, & Noll, in press). The emphasis of the majority of these studies has been on internalizing outcomes such as depression, anxiety, posttraumatic stress disorder, and dissociation (for reviews, see Beitchman, Zucker, Hood, daCosta, & Akman, 1991; Beitchman et al., 1992; Kendall-Tackett, Williams, & Finkelhor, 1993; Trickett et al., in press; Trickett & McBride-Chang, 1995; Trickett & Putnam, 1998). However, a number of studies have been concerned with such developmental outcomes as physical aggression, delinquency, and other antisocial behavior in sexually abused females. Some of this research has focused on more "sex-typed" forms of delinquency and antisocial behavior (e.g., running away or other status offenses, or sexual acting out). Other research has focused on other forms of delinquency and physical aggression usually associated more with male adolescents.

Table 8.1 presents a summary of findings of nine studies that examine how child sexual abuse relates to female aggression or other antisocial behavior. (This table does not include this research team's findings, which are to be described in more detail later in this chapter.) The list of studies included in Table 8.1 is not exhaustive. Rather, we have included only studies that met certain criteria. First, we included only studies that had an appropriate comparison group. Appropriate comparison groups

**TABLE 8.1. Studies Examining Links between Sexual Abuse and Aggression in Females**

| | Sample and comparisons | Definition of abuse/ characteristics of abused sample | Aggression measure | Findings |
|---|---|---|---|---|
| **Child** | | | | |
| Cosentino et al. (1992) | Girls ages 6–12, 20 sexually abused, 20 nonpsychiatric controls, and 20 psychiatric controls. | Females who had (1) at least one sexually abusive experience involving oral, anal, or vaginal intercourse or genital fondling with a person at least 5 years older, (2) had been referred to treatment within the past 48 months because of documented sexual abuse, and (3) were between ages 6 and 12 at the time of the study. | Gender Role Assessment Schedule—Child (GRAS-C): Child self-report measure assessing gender role behavior and preferences.<br><br>Child Game Participation Questionnaire (CGP): 64-item parent-report measure of gender-typical and atypical play patterns. | On GRAS-C, girls' self-report of aggression was higher in sexually abused group than in both comparison groups.<br><br>By parents report on CGP, sexually abused girls did more rough-and-tumble play than did both control groups and expressed more interest in body contact sports than did the nonpsychiatric controls. |
| Einbender & Friedrich (1989) | Comparison of 46 sexually abused to 46 matched comparison 6- to 14-year-old girls; comparison group matched on age, race, family income, family constellation variables, and presence of siblings. Some demographic differences in mothers' education and status of living with natural mother. | Sexually abused group had been abused within the previous 4 years. Abuse involved physical sexual contact between perpetrator and child. Perpetrator was 5 or more years older than child. Abuse was substantiated by state agency. Child was not living in same residence as perpetrator at time of study.<br><br>Eleven sexually abused girls living out of home had had an average of 2.4 out-of-home placements and had lived an average of 44.6 months out of the home. Forty-three of the abused girls had had therapy for problems related to sexual abuse. Only two comparison girls had had therapy. | Parent report on Child Behavior Checklist (CBCL). | By parents' reports, sexually abused girls higher than comparison girls on CBCL aggressiveness/bullying, delinquent/misbehavior, and cruel scales. |

*(continued)*

163

**TABLE 8.1.** (*continued*)

| | Sample and comparisons | Definition of abuse/ characteristics of abused sample | Aggression measure | Findings |
|---|---|---|---|---|
| Mannarino et al. (1989) | Females, ages 6–12, 94 referred from rape crisis centers within the previous 6 months, compared to 89 psychiatric controls who had been referred to outpatient child psychiatric clinics (excluding those who had been sexually abused) and 75 nonclinic controls recruited from schools. The sexually abused group had lower socioeconomic status (SES), which may be a confound. | Sexual abuse defined as "sexual contact of an exploitive nature between the perpetrator and the victim" and included genital, anal, and/or breast contact (oral kissing alone not included). Abuse required power difference due to age, size, and/or relationship. For all participants, abuse had been reported to child protection services prior to referral to the study. The most recent episode of abuse had to have occurred within the last 6 months prior to referral. Most often it was within several weeks. All were recruited within 2 weeks of disclosure of abuse, and participants were excluded if they had been to the rape crisis center more than two times. Frequency of abuse: 25 girls (25%) were abused 1 time, 27% abused 2–5 times, 11% abused 6–10 times. Most common type of abuse: genital fondling—51 girls (54%) reported this as the only type of abuse. Forty cases involved vaginal, anal, or oral intercourse. Ten girls were abused by more than one perpetrator. All perpetrators were male except one. Twenty-one percent were abused by father or stepfather; 13%, mother's boyfriend; 16%, extended family; 45%, familiar adult or adolescent; 4%, stranger. Fifty-six cases (60%) involved some type of force. | CBCL parent report | Sexually abused and psychiatric controls higher than normal controls but not different from each other on CBCL aggression and cruelty scales. Narrow-band CBCL scales: On delinquent, cruel scales: Sexually abused and psychiatric comparison groups higher than normal comparison children but not different from each other. No effects in analyses for characteristics of abuse (family member as perpetrator, abuse type, number of episodes, physical force). Authors suggest that low SES of sexually abused group may make them more problematic, contrasting with studies that found them not to have higher than normal behavior problems (Cohen & Mannarino, 1988; Friedrich et al., 1987). Conducted the following subgroup analyses: Table Text+3ab = Intrafamilial (father, mother, stepparent, older sibling; $n = 31$) versus extrafamilial ($n = 63$); fondling versus intercourse ($n = 51$ vs. 40); five or fewer versus six or more episodes (50 vs. 42); force (56). Conducted MANOVAs on CBCL scales versus groups, with no significant results. |

164

| Mannarino et al. (1991) | 6- and 12-month follow-up of preceding study. | Same sample, but only 79 sexually abused girls assessed at 6-month follow-up and 73 at 12-month follow-up. | CBCL Parent Report | At both 6- and 12-month follow-up: Sexually abused and psychiatric controls higher than normal controls on CBCL aggressive and cruel scales but not different from each other. Repeated measures: Sexually abused girls improved only on the cruel subscale of narrow-band CBCL scores. |
| | | | | At both 6- and 12-month follow-up, sexually abused and psychiatric comparisons scored higher than normal comparisons on delinquent, cruel scales of CBCL but not differently from each other. Sexually abused improved only on cruel subscale of narrow band. Normal controls improved on delinquent scale. |
| | | | | Conducted similar subgroup analyses as in original study for 6- and 12-month data. Significant findings for type of abuse (intercourse vs. fondling) on ANOVAs for CBCL Externalizing, Total Behavior Problems, Total Social Competence scale. Intercourse was related to less competence and more problems. ANOVAs on narrow-band scales were nonsignificant (comparison was 40 fondled vs. 32 intercourse in total sample). |

(continued)

165

**TABLE 8.1.** (*continued*)

| | Sample and comparisons | Definition of abuse/ characteristics of abused sample | Aggression measure | Findings |
|---|---|---|---|---|
| **Adolescent** | | | | |
| Garnefski & Diekstra (1997) | 1,490 adolescents ages 12–19, 80% female, with separate analyses within gender. Compared group reporting sexual abuse (*n* = 745) with comparison group matched on age and gender. | Sexual abuse assessed through self-report responses to the question: Have you ever been sexually abused, for example, been forced to perform sexual acts, assaulted, or raped? Also assessed whether the sexual abuse was accompanied by physical abuse. | Aggressive/criminal behavior measured through self-report items measuring 10 emotional/behavioral problem areas. Principal components analysis resulted in four dimensions, one of which was aggressive/criminal behavior, defined as at least one of the following behaviors: felony assault, criminal behavior (destruction of property; stolen items worth more than 50 Dutch guilders; involved with police because of doing something on two or more occasions during the previous year). Behavior was treated as dichotomous variable. | Sexually abused (SA) girls were more likely to indicate aggressive criminal behavior than were nonabused girls (NSA). (SA girls: 25.3%; NSA girls: 10.1%.) Nonabused boys were higher than SA girls. The combination of suicidality and aggressive/ criminal behavior reported 13.3 times more by SA girls than by NSA girls. Physical abuse increased likelihood of problems, especially aggressive/criminal and suicidality in both boys and girls. |

| Harrison et al. (1989). | Male and female adolescent sample drawn from 1,824 adolescents entering inpatient treatment for substance abuse between 1984 and 1986 who gave consent to be interviewed. Final sample include 444 girls (210 of whom reported sexual abuse) and 971 boys (81 of whom reported sexual abuse). Comparisons within sex for effect of sexual abuse. | Assessment with two questions from semistructured interview: Has anyone in your family ever been sexual with you? Has anyone else ever sexually abused you? Interviewers probed to clarify answers and decided what constituted abuse at their own discretion. Of 597 girls, 43 reported both intrafamilial and extrafamilial sexual abuse, 47 intrafamilial abuse only, and 120 extrafamilial abuse only. | Semistructured interview administered during the second week of treatment. | More sexually abused girls reported any arrest, an arrest before age 14, out-of-home placement, detention in a detention center, and time spent in a juvenile correction facility than did nonabused girls. |
|---|---|---|---|---|
| Runtz & Briere (1986) | Retrospective report of 150 female 17- to 40-year-olds comparing those reporting sexual abuse (sexual contact with someone at least 5 years older) versus those not reporting abuse on whether they engaged in outcome behaviors during "teenage years." | Finkelhor items used to identify sexually abused females, defined as having had sexual contact with a person at least 5 years older than themselves before the age of 15 (41 of 278 identified; final sample was 39 abused and 111 nonabused). | Single-item retrospective self-report measures. | Sexually abused were more likely to have skipped school, gotten in trouble with the law. No differences on stealing or providing sex for money. |
| Widom & Kuhns (1996) | Included 908 physically and/or sexually abused and neglected males and females processed through courts from 1967–1971. Control group was matched on age, sex, race, and SES. Abused and neglected youth were under 11 at time of maltreatment, followed through adolescence. Separate analyses conducted within gender. Other groups were almost equally male and female, but sexually abused group was more than 80% female. | Sexual abuse ranged from "assault and battery with intent to gratify sexual desires" to fondling, touching in an obscene manner, sodomy, incest "and so forth." | Single items assessing teenage pregnancy, promiscuity (having had sex with 10 or more people in a single year), and prostitution (ever having been paid for having sex with someone). | Bivariate analyses: All types of maltreatment increased likelihood of female subjects endorsing prostitution question, compared to controls. For male subjects, not significant. No effect emerged for promiscuity and teenage pregnancy. Sexual abuse and neglect remained significant predictors of prostitution for women even after controlling for age, race, gender, and SES indicator (receiving welfare as a child). Null results for other outcomes. |

*(continued)*

**TABLE 8.1.** (*continued*)

| | Sample and comparisons | Definition of abuse/ characteristics of abused sample | Aggression measure | Findings |
|---|---|---|---|---|
| **Wider age span/adult** | | | | |
| Rimsza et al. (1988) | 72 girls ages 2–17 from sexual abuse clinic compared to matched controls using chart review and follow-up phone calls. Physically abused girls excluded. | Abuse defined as forced sexual activity or sexual activity between an adult and a child or adolescent.<br><br>Most common type of abuse (*n* = 44) was intercourse. Other types included genital fondling (including nonpenile vaginal penetration; *n* = 20), sodomy (*n* = 9), and oral–genital contact (*n* = 14).<br><br>Perpetrators included strangers (*n* = 11); relatives (*n* = 26, 17 of whom were fathers or stepfathers); mothers' boyfriends (*n* = 6); family friends, acquaintances, and neighbors (*n* = 19).<br><br>Duration ranged from under 6 months (*n* = 31) to greater than 6 months (41 cases).<br><br>Mean duration of follow-up was 24 months, range of 9–48 months. | Chart review and follow-up phone call to caretaker asking six questions, including one about behavior problems. "Does the child have any behavior problems? If so, What?" | Sexually abused girls were more likely than were comparison girls to run away from home (6 vs. 0) and have other behavior problems. No group differences emerged on school problems and early pregnancy.<br><br>Analyses specifically on duration of abuse were significant, such that those who had been abused longer were more likely to report at least one symptom (not specifically running away). No other characteristics of abuse were significant, though age of victim approached it for some behaviors (not running away). |
| Stein et al. (1988) | 3,132 adults age 18 or over from two Los Angeles mental health catchment areas. Forty-four women had reported child sexual abuse. Separate analyses within gender. | Sexual abuse assessed by the question: "In your lifetime, has anyone ever tried to pressure or force you to have sexual contact? By sexual contact, I mean their touching your sexual parts, your touching their sexual parts, or sexual intercourse." If yes (*n* = 447), participants were asked if they had ever been forced or pressured for sexual contact before age 16 and their age at first incident. | NIMH Diagnostic Interview Schedule, antisocial personality disorder | No significant difference between women reporting versus not reporting childhood sexual abuse. |

168

are crucial because of the clear evidence that demographic variables such as poverty and social class adversely influence many of the outcome measures of interest in child abuse research, and that most child abuse samples tend to be of lower socioeconomic status. Thus without an appropriate comparison group, one cannot distinguish between abuse effects and poverty effects. Second, because our interest was on female development, we included only research with all-female samples or research that analyzed for gender effects in samples that included males and females. (A number of studies have predominantly female samples [e.g., 70–80%] but do not contain analyses for gender differences or separate analyses by gender. These are not included here.)

Of the nine studies included in Table 8.1, five have all-female samples and four have samples with males and females. Three of the studies focus on middle childhood to early adolescence (with ages ranging from 6–10 to 6–14; Cosentino, Meyer-Bahlburg, Albert, & Gaines, 1992; Einbender & Friedrich, 1989; Mannarino, Cohen, & Gregor, 1989; Mannarino, Cohen, Smith, & Moore-Motily, 1991). One has a sample that ranges from early childhood to adolescence (ages 2–17; Rimsza, Berg, & Locke, 1988). Three studies have all-adolescent samples (Garnefski & Diekstra, 1997; Harrison, Hoffman, & Edwall, 1989; Widom & Kuhns, 1996) and one has an adult sample but measures, retrospectively, adolescent adjustment (Runtz & Briere, 1986). Only one study reports on adult functioning (Stein, Golding, Siegel, Burnam, & Sorenson, 1988). In brief, these studies indicate that mothers of school-age sexually abused girls consistently rate their daughters higher in aggressive behavior (including physical and verbal aggression, and rough-and-tumble play) than do mothers of nonabused girls (Cosentino et al., 1992; Einbender & Friedrich, 1989), although one of these (Mannarino et al., 1989, 1991) found that sexually abused girls were more aggressive than the nonclinical comparison groups but were not different from the psychiatric comparison group. As can be seen from Table 8.1, findings from the studies of adolescent samples are less clear. Some studies find sexually abused girls to be more aggressive and more delinquent than nonabused peers (Garnefski & Diekstra, 1997; Harrison et al., 1989; Widom & Kuhns, 1996). Others have clearly mixed findings (Rimsza et al., 1988; Runtz & Briere, 1986). The one study of adult females reports no difference in rates of antisocial personality disorder among those who had experienced child sexual abuse versus those who had not.

Although at first glance considerable research appears to exist on aggression and antisocial behavior in sexually abused females, a closer examination reveals that knowledge is limited, in part due to limitations of these studies. Researchers often define aggression, antisocial behavior, and delinquency inconsistently and with insufficient clarity. The same label, for example, delinquency, sometimes refers to aggressive or violent behavior, whereas other times refers to status offenses such as truancy, running away, or sexual acting out. The studies in Table 8.1 have other limitations as well. With one exception (Mannarino et al., 1989, 1991), these studies are one-time cross-sectional studies. Whereas these studies may in fact be measuring acute reactions to sexual abuse, in most of them we know little about when the sexual abuse occurred in relation to the time of measurement. Variability in the time between the abuse and the data collection could account for variability in findings. Similarly, most of the studies provide little information about other characteristics of the sexual abuse that may relate to developmental outcomes (Trickett et al., in press), including the identity of the perpetrator, chronicity, and co-occurrence of violence or other forms of child maltreatment. Variability in these factors may account for variability in the findings.

What follows is a summary of findings concerning aggression and antisocial behavior in sexually abused females from a longitudinal study that has addressed some of these limitations and problems. This study has been concerned with many domains of adjustment and adaptation, most of which are outside the scope of this chapter. We focus here specifically on aggression and delinquency, and not on behavior that falls into a more general "acting-out" or "externalizing" category, for example, sexual activity and early pregnancy or self-harm. (The reader is referred to Noll, Horowitz, Bonnano, Trickett, & Putnam, 2003; Noll, Trickett, & Putnam, 2003.) Thus, this summary focuses on findings concerning conventionally defined physical and verbal aggression and delinquency.

## THE RESEARCH PROGRAM

The findings we describe come from a program of research on the psychobiological impact of familial sexual abuse on female development begun by Putnam and Trickett in 1987 (see, e.g., Putnam & Trickett, 1993; Trickett & Putnam, 1993). Figure 8.1 illustrates the basic conceptualization of this research. The tenets of this research are, first, that sexual abuse experienced during childhood is generally very stressful and appropriately considered traumatic, although the degree of trauma varies depending upon certain characteristics of the abuse, as listed at the far left of Figure 8.1. Second, this abuse produces both psychological distress and physiological stress, both of which affect the adjustment and adaptation of abused girls as indexed by the compromised development of competencies and emergence of behavior problems or psychiatric symptoms (see the far right of Figure 8.1). Third, these outcomes are mediated (1) by other experiences, especially the provision of support by

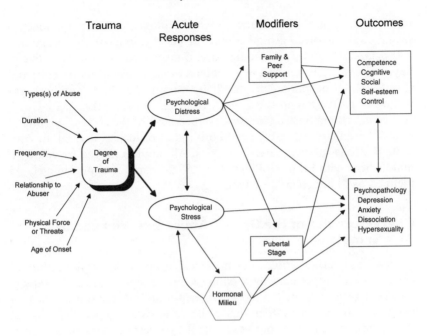

**FIGURE 8.1.** Conceptual model of impact of sexual abuse on female development.

the mother and other family members, peers, and professionals (e.g., in the form of psychotherapy), and (2) by developmental factors, especially the passage through puberty and the transition into and through adolescence. The most distinctive features of this research program are its longitudinal design, which involves a longer time frame than any prior study, its explicitly developmental focus emphasizing puberty and transition into adolescence, and its focus on not only psychological but also physiological variables, especially those related to pubertal maturation and to stress.

## Participants in the Study

Initially, 166 families participated in this research. Approximately half of these families consisted of sexually abused female children and adolescents and their mothers (or other nonabusing caretaker), and the other half were a demographically similar comparison group. Abused females were referred by protective service agencies in the greater Washington, DC, metropolitan area. Eligibility criteria for inclusion in the study were (1) the victim was female, age 6–16 years of age; (2) disclosure of referring abuse occurred within 6 months of participation; (3) sexual abuse involved genital contact or penetration; (4) the perpetrator was a family member, including parent, stepparent, or mother's live-in boyfriend, or other relative (e.g., older sibling, uncle, grandparent); and (5) a nonabusing parent or guardian (usually the child's mother) was willing to participate in the project. A group of comparison females recruited via community advertising were similar to the abused subjects in terms of ethnicity, age, SES, neighborhood of residence, and family constellation (one- or two-parent families). All families ranged from low to middle SES, with mean Hollingshead (1975) scores of approximately 35 (defined as "blue collar," or working class).

## Characteristics of the Sexual Abuse Experienced by This Sample

As described earlier, criteria for inclusion in the sexual abuse group included abuse perpetrated by a family member. For 23% of the sample the perpetrator was the biological father; for 36% of the sample the perpetrator was another father figure (i.e., stepfather or mother's live-in boyfriend), and for 41% of the sample the perpetrator was another relative (including grandfather, uncle, older brother, or stepbrother). The average age of onset of the abuse was about 8 years, and the average duration was about 2 years. Almost 50% of the sample experienced physical violence or threats of physical violence associated with the sexual abuse, and/or physical abuse (not associated with the sexual abuse). For 70% of the sample, the abuse included penetration of some sort (vaginal, anal, or digital), and in 42% of the sample, other instances of sexual abuse involving a different perpetrator had also occurred.

These summary characteristics indicate first that the abuse experienced by this sample overall is quite severe, and second that despite somewhat restrictive inclusion criteria, considerable variability regarding the abuse experience exists in this sample. Because, as noted in the discussion of Figure 8.1, we hypothesized that variation in the degree of trauma would relate to the degree of psychological distress and physiological stress, some of our analyses examine differences in abuse experiences. We have done this in two ways. In some analyses, we have used the characteristics described earlier and shown in Figure 8.1 (e.g., age of onset of abuse, duration of abuse, identity of perpetrator) as predictor variables in multiple regressions to examine associations among these variables and developmental outcomes (see, e.g., Trickett, Horowitz, Reiffman, & Putnam, 1997). In other analyses, we have developed what we call "profile groups," based on cluster analysis, that subdivide the abuse group into three subgroups based on the dimensions of abuse characteristics. This procedure is described in detail in Trickett, Noll, Reiffman, and Putnam (2001). In brief, the profile 1 subgroup included girls whose abuse involved multiple perpetrators, none of whom was the biological father; the duration of abuse extended over a relatively short period of time but often occurred with physical violence. Abuse by a single perpetrator who was not the biological father characterized the girls of the profile 2 subgroup. Duration of the abuse for this profile was relatively short, and violence was not frequent. The third profile subgroup was characterized by abuse by the primary father (in all but three cases the biological father) over a long period, beginning at a relatively young age. In 45% of these cases, there was also sexual abuse by another perpetrator. The amount of violence for profile 3 was intermediate to that of the other two profile subgroups.

As this chapter was being written, this research was conducting its sixth round of data collection, having assessed the sample of sexually abused girls and the comparison group at median ages 11, 12, 13, 18, and 20 (time 1–time 5). The retention rate from time 1 to time 4 or 5 is about 95% (see, e.g., Trickett et al., 2001, for details). The findings summarized herein come from analyses of time 1 and times 4 and 5.

## Measurement of Aggressive and Antisocial Behaviors

At the inception of the study (time 1), we assessed many domains of psychological and physical development. Measures of aggression or antisocial behavior included the following:

1. Aggressiveness/bullying and delinquent/misbehavior factors were derived from the Child Behavior Checklist (CBCL; Achenbach, 1991a). This parent report measure consists of 120 items covering many types of problem behaviors. Invariance analyses within a sample of 944 maltreated children indicated five factors, two of which concerned aggressive or antisocial behavior (Noll, Trickett, Horn, Long, & Putnam, 2004). The first, aggressiveness/bullying, consists of 21 items and includes behaviors such as "gets in many fights," "destroys things," "physically attacks people," "argues a lot," and "swearing and obscene language." For this sample this factor has an internal consistency reliability of .90. The second, delinquent/misbehavior has 13 items and, in this sample, an internal consistency reliability of .76. Items in this factor include, for example, "steals outside the home," "disobedient at school," "vandalism," "lying or cheating." It should be noted that although these factors are psychometrically independent, in this sample they are very highly related ($r = .81$).

2. *Diagnostic and Statistical Manual of Mental Disorders*, third

edition, revised (DSM-III-R; American Psychiatric Asociation, 1987) diagnoses of oppositional defiant disorder, conduct disorder, and attention-deficit/hyperactivity disorder were derived from the child's self-report on the Diagnostic Interview for Children and Adolescents (DICA; Reich & Welner, 1988). Note that these diagnoses are based on DSM-III-R criteria rather than DSM-IV (fourth edition) criteria. Conduct disorder (CD) represents a pattern of violating others' rights and violating social norms and rules, and includes several types of behaviors: aggression toward people and animals (e.g., bullying others, initiating physical fights, using a weapon, etc.), destruction of property (e.g., by fire setting or other means), deceitfulness or theft (e.g., breaking into buildings, stealing items of nontrivial value), and rule violations (e.g., staying out past curfews, running away, truancy from school). To earn this diagnosis, at least three of these behaviors must occur at around the same time for at least 6 months. Oppositional defiant disorder (ODD) represents aggressive, irritating, and/or oppositional behavior that often is less extreme than CD and includes such behaviors as arguing, losing temper, deliberately irritating others, being spiteful and vindictive, and blaming others for things. At least five of these behaviors must occur for at least 6 months. Attention-deficit/hyperactivity disorder (ADHD) includes symptoms of inattention and hyperactivity, such as fidgeting, being easily distracted, talking excessively, failing to complete activities, losing things, and having difficulty following through with things. A diagnosis requires eight of these behaviors occurring at around the same time for at least 6 months, with an age of onset before age 7.

3. Acting-out behavior in the classroom is a subscale of the Teacher Child Rating Scale (Hightower, Spinell, & Lotyczewski, 1986). It has six items (e.g., "disruptive in class," "defiant, obstinate, stubborn," "overly aggressive to peers"), and good internal consistency reliability, and is based on teacher report.

At times 4 and 5, somewhat different measures of aggression and antisocial behavior were assessed:

1. The self-report version of the CBCL, the Youth Self Report (YSR; Achenbach, 1991b) contains the same items and the same factors were derived: Aggressiveness/bullying (with internal consistency reliability of .86) and delinquent/misbehavior (with internal consistency of .68). These two factors had a correlation of .63.

2. Three indices of delinquent behavior were derived from the Adolescent Delinquency Questionnaire (ADQ; Huizinga & Elliott, 1986). These were, first, person offenses with 7 items and an internal consistency reliability of .71. Sample items include "attack with weapon," "hit to hurt," "get into fights." Second, property offenses, with 14 items and an internal consistency reliability of .81. Examples of items include "de-

stroy property," "break in to steal," "steal car." And, third, drug/alcohol offenses, with 3 items and an internal consistency reliability of .72. Items on this scale concerned alcohol use and abuse and marijuana use. (Use of other drugs was assessed, but reported so infrequently that inclusion in this scale reduced the internal consistency notably.)

## Group Differences in Aggression and Antisocial Behavior

Several sets of analyses (Gordis, Trickett, & Susman, 2003; Trickett et al., 2001; Trickett, McBride-Chang, & Putnam, 1994) have indicated consistently higher levels for the abuse group as compared to the comparison group on all measures of antisocial behavior at entry into the study (i.e., our time 1 assessment). These group effects emerged for mother, teacher, and child self-report variables. Thus, analysis of mother-reported CBCL factors of aggressiveness/bullying and delinquent misbehavior revealed overall group differences at time 1 (Trickett et al., 2001). Similarly, on the Teacher Child Rating Scale at time 1, teachers reported higher levels of acting-out behavior in the classroom for the sexually abused girls as compared with the comparison girls (Trickett et al., 1994). For the child-reported DSM diagnoses, all three "disruptive disorders," namely ODD, CD, and ADHD, were more prevalent among the sexually abused girls than among the comparison group girls (Gordis et al., 2003). Thus one can clearly say that in the period shortly following the disclosure of sexual abuse, the girls in this study were exhibiting more aggressive and antisocial behavior.

This finding of overall group differences does not hold for our time 4–5 analyses. Thus no group differences emerged for the self-reported YSR factors of aggressiveness/bullying or delinquent misbehavior (Trickett et al., 2001; Trickett, Kurtz, & Putnam, 2003), nor for any of the delinquency subscales, person offenses, property offenses, or alcohol/drug use (Trickett et al., 2003). Thus, 7 or 8 years later, the consistent differences in levels of aggressive or antisocial behavior found in sexually abused girls as compared with the nonabused comparison group are no longer discernable.

### Subgroup Differences

As described earlier, one of our interests has been in determining the salience of the variability in the sexual abuse experienced by the participants in the study. At time 1, we have examined how the three profile subgroups compared with one another and with the comparison group on levels of aggressiveness/bullying and delinquent misbehavior. These analyses indicated that for aggressiveness/bullying the profile 3 subgroup (biological father perpetrator) showed the most elevated scores, which were significantly higher than the other profile subgroups and than the comparison group. Profile subgroups 1 (multiple perpetrator/nonbiological father) and 2 (single perpetrator/nonbiological father) were also elevated significantly as compared with the comparison group, but did not differ from one another. For delinquent misbehavior the pattern was similar in that the profile 3 subgroup showed the most elevated scores, which were significantly higher than the profile 1 subgroup. In this instance, both of these subgroups were significantly higher than profile 2 and than the comparison group, which did not differ from one another. Thus, these analyses indicate that in this sample soon after the disclosure of abuse, the subset of sexual abuse victims who were abused by their biological father exhibited the highest levels of aggression and antisocial behavior—higher than victims abused by nonbiological father perpetrator(s), who for the most part, exhibit higher levels of aggression and antisocial behavior than nonabused comparison group members. These findings are supported by multiple regression analyses, which indicated that at time 1, of all the characteristics of the abuse considered, abuse by the biological father was the strongest predictor of aggression, acting-out behaviors, and disruptive disorders (Trickett, Reiffman, Horowitz, & Putnam, 1997).

Although, at time 4–5, no overall group difference emerged on the YSR factors of aggressiveness/bullying and delinquent misbehavior, significant differences did emerge when comparing the profile subgroups on these dimensions to the comparison group. However, the pattern of differences changed somewhat from those found at time 1. In these time 4–5 analyses, profile 3 and profile 2 subgroup members showed significantly elevated scores on both aggressiveness/bullying and delinquent misbehavior as compared with the comparison group, but did not differ from one another. Profile 1 subgroup members had scores on these two dimensions that were similar to those of the comparison group. When the scores on the three delinquency scales were examined for the three profile subgroups and the comparison group, no significant differences were found.

Thus, for the delinquency measures, no overall abuse–comparison group differences were found, nor were there differences in mean levels of the three profile groups. For the YSR factors, on the other hand, the pattern at time 4–5 was somewhat different. Although there were no overall group differences, two of the profile subgroups showed elevated scores on both factors relative to the comparison group. One of these was profile 3 (biological father perpetrator), which is consistent with the time 1 findings. Girls abused by their biological father continued to show more aggressive and antisocial behavior 7 or more years after the disclosure of the abuse. However, now profile 2 subgroup members (abused by a single perpetrator who is not the biological father), who at the earlier time point showed the least aggressive and antisocial behavior as compared with the other abuse profile groups, now show levels comparable to those girls abused by the biological father.

## Summary of Group Differences

Table 8.2 summarizes the group differences found in the several analyses described. Clearly, in the period shortly after the disclosure of the sexual abuse, indices of aggression and delinquency, whether reported by the mother, teacher, or child herself and including a broad range of activities, including physical and verbal aggressiveness, argumentativeness, destructiveness, and stealing were elevated in sexually abused girls as compared with a demographically similar comparison group. It is also apparent that characteristics of the abuse have discernable effects over and above the overall group effects. Thus, abuse by a biological father is associated with the highest levels of aggressiveness, but abuse by (nonbiological father) multiple perpetrators is associated with worse outcomes than abuse by (nonbiological father) single perpetrators.

After approximately 7 years (time 4–5), the findings are quite different. No overall group effects are evident. The only subgroup effects are for aggressiveness/bullying and delinquent misbehavior, where those girls abused by their biological father and those abused by a (nonbiological father) single perpetrator have elevated scores as compared with those abused by (nonbiological father) multiple perpetrators who are similar to the comparison group. It is important to remember, however, that at time 1 measures included mother report, teacher report, and self-report, whereas at the later measurement points all measures were self-report. Also, although attrition was low, the $ns$ at time 4–5 were smaller than at time 1, and power was thus reduced somewhat.

## Moderating Effect of Abuse Status

In one set of analyses we have begun to examine maternal child-rearing approaches as possible predictors of aggression and delinquency, and abuse status as a possible moderator of these relationships (Trickett et al., 2003). The child-rearing indices in these analyses, assessed at time 1, are composite scores derived from the Child-Rearing Practices Q Sort (Block, 1981) that measure three key domains of child rearing: *enjoyment of child and parental role*, *authoritarian control*, and *encouragement of independence*. As might be expected from prior research on de-

TABLE 8.2. Summary of Group Differences on Measures of Aggression and Delinquency at Time 1 and Time 4–5

| Measure | Overall group effect | Subgroup effects |
|---|---|---|
| | Time 1 | |
| CBCL (Mother Report) | | |
| Aggressiveness/Bullying | A > C | 3 > 1 = 2 > C |
| Delinquent/Misbehavior | A > C | 3 > 1 = 2 > C |
| Teacher Child Rating Scale | | |
| Acting Out Behavior | A > C | Not examined |
| DSM-III-R Diagnoses (Self-Report) | | |
| CD, ODD, ADHD | A > C | Not examined |
| | Time 4–5 | |
| CBCL Youth Self-Report | | |
| Aggressiveness/Bullying | A = C | 3 = 2 > 1 = C |
| Delinquent/Misbehavior | A = C | 3 = 2 > 1 = C |
| Adolescent Delinquency Questionnaire | | |
| Person Offenses | A = C | 1 = 2 = 3 = C |
| Property Offenses | A = C | 1 = 2 = 3 = C |
| Drug/Alcohol Use | A = C | 1 = 2 = 3 = C |

Note. CBCL, Child Behavior Checklist; CD, conduct disorder; ODD, oppositional–defiant disorder; ADHD, attention-deficit/hyperactivity disorder. A, abuse group, C, comparison group. In subgroup analyses, 1, 2, and 3 indicate profile subgroups.

linquency in males (e.g., Farrington & Hawkins, 1991; McCord, 1991), mothers' espousal of support for authoritarian discipline and control techniques was found to be positively related to person offenses, property offenses, and drug/alcohol offenses, assessed approximately 7 years later (at time 4–5) for both the sexually abused girls and the comparison girls.

A moderating effect of abuse emerged for the relationship of this child-rearing domain and delinquent misbehavior. Here a positive association between authoritarian control and delinquent misbehavior was found for the sexual abuse group but not for the comparison group (for which the relationship was, in fact, negative but nonsignificant). Some other moderating effects have been found for the other child-rearing domains as well. First, high enjoyment of child and parental role was associated with low delinquent misbehavior and person offenses for the comparison group but with high scores on these indices for the sexually abused girls. A similar but nonsignificant pattern of results was found for property offenses and drug/alcohol offenses. Another similar pattern indicated that high espousal of encouraging independence was associated with higher delinquency (especially person offenses and property offenses) for the comparison group whereas, for the abuse group, no such association was found.

These latter results may indicate that maternal child-rearing perspectives, at least as assessed close to the disclosure of the abuse, have different meanings for the mothers of sexually abused girls than for mothers on girls who are not abused and, as a result, different implications for long-term development. So, for example, it could be that in the months following disclosure of a daughter's sexual abuse, a mother's views about the value of promoting independence in the preadolescent or adolescent daughter would be changed by the recent experience and/or be less frankly stated than for a mother with a daughter of a similar age but no recent disclosure of abuse.

In other analyses (Gordis et al., 2003) we are examining the relations among sexual abuse, reproductive hormones, and aggression and antisocial behavior, assessed shortly after the disclosure of abuse (time 1). Specifically, we are interested in whether sexual abuse is associated with the levels of estradiol, testosterone, and the gonadatrophins, luteinizing hormone (LH), and follicle-stimulating hormone (FSH), and whether sexual abuse affects the relationship between each of these hormones and behavior problems. In regression analyses, controlling for age and menstrual status, no main effects of abuse status emerged on serum levels of any of the hormones, although sexually abused girls had marginally higher levels of testosterone. Next, we examined the relationships of hormone levels, abuse status, and their interaction on aggressiveness/bullying and delinquent misbehavior and on the DICA diagnoses of ODD, CD, and ADHD. In each case, as noted earlier, the main effect of abuse status predicted the behavior problem. Hormone level was never a significant predictor of the behavior problems.

In several cases, however, the hormone by abuse status interaction was significant. Specifically, the interaction between FSH and abuse status significantly predicted aggressiveness/bullying, delinquent misbehavior, and a diagnosis of ODD, and the interaction between LH and abuse status significantly predicted delinquent misbehavior. The pattern of these interactions was always the same: For the sexual abuse group, but not the comparison group, level of FSH and LH was negatively related to levels of aggression and antisocial behavior; that is lower hormone levels were related to higher scores on the behavior problem measures. For the comparison group, this negative relationship between hormone level and behavior problem did not emerge.

Hormone–behavior relationships in normal and altered developmental trajectories are still being elucidated. Whereas some links have been established between estrogen and aggressive behavior in females, we still know little about how the gonadotropins FSH and LH relate to aggression and antisocial behavior in normal development. In our comparison group, the relation between these hormones and aggressive/delinquent behavior was null. However, in the abuse group, the relation was negative. Some evidence in the literature suggests that adverse life events can alter hormone behavior relations (Susman & Pajer, Chapter 2, this volume). Consistent with this idea, our data suggest that the experience of abuse may override whatever relationship FSH and LH have with aggressive and delinquent behavior in normal developmental trajectories.

## CONCLUSIONS

Our research program has expanded knowledge about the association between sexual abuse and the development of aggression and antisocial behavior in females in several ways. To reiterate, our results indicate, first, large, clear, elevated levels of aggression and antisocial behavior in sexually abused female children and adolescents in the period shortly after the disclosure of the abuse. These elevated levels are perceived and reported on by mothers or other caretakers, teachers, and the girls themselves. Second, overall differences between the abused and comparison females in aggression and antisocial behavior are less easily discernable 7–8 years later. Although overall group effects are not detectable, subgroup effects remain significant even 7–8 years after the abuse. The subgroup of abuse victims for whom the biological father was the perpetrator remained more aggressive and delinquent at this later assessment. In addition, the subgroup abused by a single perpetrator who was not the biological father (profile 2) showed elevated levels of aggression similar to the profile 1 subgroup. Even though no effect held at the longitudinal follow-up between all the abused girls versus the comparison girls, certain patterns of abuse did still predict elevated aggression and delinquency.

Thus, these findings do not suggest that the adverse impact of sexual abuse dissipates or disappears over time. Rather these findings as well as our (and other researchers') analyses of other outcome variables indicate, first, that there are likely different developmental trajectories that can follow childhood sexual abuse. That is, different individuals may develop differing levels or severity of problems in differing behavioral domains depending on the nature of the abuse, characteristics of the individual, characteristics of the family environment, and the supports and services provided to the victim after the abuse is disclosed. To examine the multiple variables requires a long-term perspective that considers the developing child in her family context. That the poorest long-term outcomes are for the girls abused by their biological fathers attests to this. Such abuse may well be more traumatic and damaging because of the nature of the primary father–daughter relationship, involving greater betrayal of trust and greater exploitation of love and dependency (Freyd, 1996; Russell, 1984).

It also cannot be discounted that, to the degree that there is a genetic component to antisocial behavior and that sexually abusive behavior is clearly antisocial, there may be a genetic component to the antisocial behavior of daughters of these men. Our research design does not allow us to examine this hypothesis. Neither this hypothesis nor our first hypothesis of the salience of greater betrayal by abusive biological fathers accounts for our finding that those girls in profile 2—abused by a single perpetrator who is not a biological father—also exhibit long-term adjustment problems involving aggression and antisocial behavior. At first glance this finding seems quite counterintuitive, since the abuse experienced by profile 2 subgroup members seems less severe than that of either profile 1 or 3 subgroups. We have, however, found similar results for other outcomes as well (Noll, Trickett, & Putnam, 2003; Trickett et al., 2001) and have posited that, perhaps because of the apparent lower severity of the abuse and the lower levels of acute distress symptoms at the time of disclosure, these individuals may receive less support and fewer mental health services (Horowitz, Putnam, Noll, & Trickett, 1997) over time, resulting in adverse outcomes.

This research has begun to elucidate some of the factors that may mediate or moderate the development of aggressive and antisocial behavior in this sample. First, the results underscore the need to include information about the characteristics of the sexual abuse in models of the effects of abuse on behavior. Our inclusion criteria—familial, contact sexual abuse, with recent disclosure—was more restrictive than much research, and resulted, one might predict, in a more homogeneous sample. Nonetheless, the sample represented considerable variability in experience, with different implications for both short and long term. Few of the studies summarized in Table 8.1 explicitly examined any characteristics of abuse. Those that did found worse outcomes associated with intercourse versus fondling (Mannarino et al., 1989, 1991), with sexual abuse combined with physical abuse (Garnefski & Diekstra, 1997), and with abuse of longer duration (Rimsza et al., 1988). However, as we have noted elsewhere (Trickett, Reiffman, et al., 1997), much inconsistency has been found in research that examined the impact of only one characteristic of sexual abuse, probably, at least in part, because of associations among characteristics (e.g., abuse by a biological father often begins at a young age and lasts a long time). None of the preceding studies examined relationships among the characteristics of abuse, and none examined the characteristic of abuse that we have found to be associated with the most serious problems—abuse by the biological father as compared with another father figure (e.g., stepfather, etc.). Combining into one category girls abused by biological fathers and other father figures may obscure the result that abuse by the biological father causes the most serious consequences on average.

We have begun examining other mediators and moderators as well. We have found that the espoused child rearing attitudes of mothers of sexually abused girls do not have the same relationship with later aggressiveness and delinquency as do the attitudes of comparison group mothers. And we find that the relationships between certain reproductive hormones which come "on line" in puberty and various indices of aggression and antisocial behavior also differ for sexually abused females as compared with nonabused females. Much more remains to be done if we are to understand the complex interactions among multiple variables that determine which victims of sexual abuse become aggressive or antisocial adults.

Our findings and the other research studies reviewed here also indicate the importance of carefully defining what behaviors are being used as indicators of antisocial behavior or delinquency and of carefully measuring these constructs. The context of sexual abuse changes the meaning of many acts that fall into the category of delinquent behavior, for example, running away or staying out late and sexual offenses. A girl who is being abused at home may need to function in a survival mode and may resort to running away from an unsafe home situation or stay out late at night to avoid abuse. Thus, in a sample of nonabused girls, this behavior may represent delinquency, but in an abused sample it may represent self-protection, and though it may be associated with negative outcomes over time, the meaning and trajectory may be different.

In addition, we need to consider the relationship manifestations of aggression, which may be especially relevant to girls' functioning and to the study of the effects of abuse on girls' development. In particular, research needs to attend to the effects of abuse on anger and hostility, and on clinical outcomes that are associated with anger and hostility, such as borderline personality disorder, which may be more typical expressions of the emotions and cognitions underlying aggressive and acting-out constructs affected by abuse. Hostility and anger may be major problems for at least subgroups of sexual abuse victims (e.g., Bonanno et al., 2002; Porter & Long, 1999; Trull, 2001). Problems with management of anger and hostility could have very serious consequences for developing romantic relationships and later family relationships, including parenting. As yet, this area remains understudied. Integrative research on the roles that negative emotions of anger and hostility, in addition to aggressive and antisocial behavior, play in female adolescent and young adult development is sorely needed.

## REFERENCES

Achenbach, T. M. (1991a). *Manual for the Child Behavior Checklist/4-18 and 1991 Profile*. Burlington: University of Vermont, Department of Psychiatry.

Achenbach, T. M. (1991b). *Manual for the Youth Self-Report and 1991 Profile*. Burlington: University of Vermont, Department of Psychiatry.

American Psychiatric Association. (1987). *Diagnostic and statistical manual of mental disorders* (3rd ed., rev.). Washington, DC: Author.

Beitchman, J. H., Zucker, K. J., Hood, J. E., daCosta, G. A., & Akman, D. (1991). A review of the short-term effects of child sexual abuse. *Child Abuse and Neglect, 15, 537–556.*

Beitchman, J. H., Zucker, K. J., Hood, J. E., daCosta, G. A., Akman, D., & Cassavia, E. (1992). A review of the long-term effects of child sexual abuse. *Child Abuse and Neglect, 16, 101–118.*

Block, J. H. (1981). *The child-rearing practices report (CRPR)*. Unpublished manuscript, University of California at Berkeley.

Bonanno, G., Keltner, D., Noll, J. G., Putnam, F. W., Trickett, P. K., LeJeune, J., & Anderson, C. (2002). When the face reveals what words do not: Facial expressions of emotion, smiling, and the willingness to disclose childhood sexual abuse. *Journal of Social and Personality Psychology, 83, 94–110.*

Cosentino, C. E., Meyer-Bahlburg, H. F. L., Albert, J. L., & Gaines, R. (1992). Cross-gender behavior and gender conflict in sexually abused girls. *Journal of the American Academy of Child and Adolescent Psychiatry, 32, 940–947.*

Einbender, A., & Friedrich, W. (1989). The psychological functioning and behavior of sexually abused girls. *Journal of Consulting and Clinical Psychology, 57, 155–157.*

Farrington, D. P., & Hawkins, J. D. (1991). Predicting participation, early onset and later persistence in officially recorded offending. *Criminal Behavior and Mental Health, 1, 1–33.*

Freyd, P. (1996). False memory syndrome. *British Journal of Psychiatry, 169, 794–795.*

Garnefski, N., & Diekstra, R. F. W. (1997). Child sexual abuse and emotional and behavioral problems in adolescence: Gender differences. *Journal of the American Academy of Child and Adolescent Psychiatry, 36, 323–329.*

Gordis, E. B., Trickett, P. K., & Susman, E. J. (2003). *Hormone-behavior relations among sexually abused and comparison girls*. Presented at the annual meeting of the American Psychological Association, Toronto.

Harrison, P. A., Hoffman, N. G., & Edwall, G. E. (1989). Sexual abuse correlates: Similarities between male and female adolescents in chemical dependency treatment. *Journal of Adolescent Research, 4, 385–399.*

Hightower, A. D., Spinell, A., & Lotyczewski, B. S. (1986). The Teacher–Child

Rating Scale: A brief objective measure of elementary children's school problem behaviors and competencies. *School Psychology Review, 15*, 383–409.

Hollingshead, A. F. (1975). *Four Factor Index of Social Status.* Unpublished manuscript, Yale University.

Horowitz, L. A., Putnam, F. W., Noll, J. G., & Trickett, P. K. (1997). Factors affecting utilization of treatment services by sexually abused girls. *Child Abuse and Neglect, 21*, 35–48.

Huizinga, D., & Elliott, D. S. (1986). Reassessing the reliability and validity of self report delinquency measures. *Journal of Quantitative Criminology*, 293–327.

Kendall-Tackett, K. A., Williams, L. M., & Finkelhor, D. (1993). Impact of sexual abuse on children: A review and synthesis of recent empirical studies. *Psychological Bulletin, 113*, 164–180.

Mannarino, A. P., Cohen, J. A., & Gregor, M. (1989). Emotional and behavioral difficulties in sexually abused girls. *Journal of Interpersonal Violence, 4*, 437–451.

Mannarino, A. P., Cohen, J. A., Smith, J. A., & Moore-Motily, S. (1991). Six- and twelve-month follow-up of sexually abused girls. *Journal of Interpersonal Violence, 6*, 494–511.

McCord, J. (1991). The cycle of crime and socialization practices. *Journal of Criminal Law and Criminology, 82*, 211–228.

Noll, J. G., Horowitz, L. A., Bonnano, G. A., Trickett, P. K., & Putnam, F. W. (2003). Revictimization and self-harm in females who experienced childhood sexual abuse: Results from a prospective study. *Journal of Interpersonal Violence, 18*, 1452–1471.

Noll, J. G., Trickett, P. K., Horn, J. L., Long, J., & Putnam, F. W. (2004). *Mega-factoring of CBCL items for maltreated children.* Manuscript in preparation.

Noll, J. G., Trickett, P. K., & Putnam, F. W. (2003). A prospective investigation of the impact of childhood sexual abuse on the development of sexuality. *Journal of Consulting and Clinical Psychology, 71*, 575–586.

Porter, C. A., & Long, P. J. (1999). Locus of control and adjustment in female adult survivors of childhood sexual abuse. *Journal of Child Sexual Abuse, 8*, 3–25.

Putnam, F. W., & Trickett, P. (1993). Child abuse, a model of chronic trauma. *Psychiatry, 56*, 84–92.

Reich, W., & Welner, Z. (1988). *Diagnostic interview for children and adolescents: DSM-III-R version.* St. Louis, MO: Washington University.

Rimsza, M. E., Berg, R. A., & Locke, C. (1988). Sexual abuse: Somatic and emotional reactions. *Child Abuse and Neglect, 12*, 201–208.

Runtz, M., & Briere, J. (1986). Adolescent "acting-out" and childhood history of sexual abuse. *Journal of Interpersonal Violence, 1*, 326–334.

Russell, D. E. (1984). The prevalence and seriousness of incestuous abuse: Stepfathers vs. biological fathers. *Child Abuse and Neglect, 8*, 15–22.

Stein, J. A., Golding, J. M., Siegel, J. M., Burnam, M. A., & Sorenson, S. B. (1988). Long-term psychological sequelae of child sexual abuse: The Los Angeles Epidemiologic Catchment Area Study. In G. E. Wyatt & G. J. Powell (Eds.), *Lasting effects of child sexual abuse* (pp. 135–154). Newbury Park, CA: Sage.

Trickett, P. K., Kurtz, D. A., & Noll, J. G. (in press). The consequences of child sexual abuse for female development. In D. Bell-Dolan, S. Foster, & E. Mash (Eds.), *Handbook of behavioral and emotional disorders in girls.* New York: Kluwer Academic/Plenum Press.

Trickett, P. K., Kurtz, D. A., & Putnam, F. W. (2003). *Patterns of aggressive and antisocial behavior in sexually abused females.* Poster presented at the biennial conference of the Society for Research in Child Development, Tampa, FL.

Trickett, P. K., & McBride-Chang, C. (1995). The developmental impact of different forms of child abuse and neglect. *Developmental Review, 15,* 311–337.

Trickett, P. K., McBride-Chang, C., & Putnam, F. W. (1994). The classroom performance and behavior of sexually abused females. *Development and Psychopathology, 6,* 183–194.

Trickett, P. K., Noll, J. G., Reiffman, A., & Putnam, F. W. (2001). Variants of intrafamilial sexual abuse experience: Implications for short- and long-term development. *Developmental Psychopathology, 13,* 1001–1019.

Trickett, P. K., & Putnam, F. W. (1993). Impact of child sexual abuse on females: Toward a developmental, psychobiological integration. *Psychological Science, 4*(2), 81–87.

Trickett, P. K., & Putnam, F. W. (1998). Developmental consequences of child sexual abuse. In P. K. Trickett & C. D. Schellenbach (Eds.), *Violence against children in the family and the community* (pp. 39–56). Washington, DC: American Psychological Association.

Trickett, P. K., Reiffman, A., Horowitz, L. A., & Putnam, F. W. (1997). Characteristics of sexual abuse trauma and the prediction of developmental outcomes. In D. Cicchetti & S. L. Toth (Eds.), *Developmental perspectives on trauma: Theory, research and intervention* (Vol. 8, pp. 289–314). Rochester, NY: University of Rochester Press.

Trull, T. J. (2001). Structural relations between borderline personality disorder features and putative etiological correlates. *Journal of Abnormal Psychology, 110,* 471–481.

Widom, C. S., & Kuhns, J. B. (1996). Childhood victimization and subsequent risk for promiscuity, prostitution, and teenage pregnancy: A prospective study. *American Journal of Public Health, 86,* 1607–1612.

# CHAPTER 9

# A Long-Term Follow-Up of Serious Adolescent Female Offenders

Peggy C. Giordano, Stephen A. Cernkovich,
*and* Allen R. Lowery

Males are more likely than their female counterparts to commit serious acts of antisocial and violent behavior (Cernkovich & Giordano, 1979; Chesney-Lind & Shelden, 1992; Renzetti & Goodstein, 2001; Robins, Tipp, & Pryzbeck, 1991). This basic difference in rates of involvement has a continuing impact on research emphases, theory development, and the kinds of sampling/measurement strategies that dominate the study of these behaviors. In the individual case, a greater emphasis on the male offender seems warranted, but the cumulative effect is that we still do not know very much about female offense patterns. Cross-sectional studies have provided useful data, particularly as they have dispelled a number of myths/stereotypes about the characteristics and correlates of female delinquency. But we are in agreement with Warren and Rosenbaum (1986), who emphasized that little is known about "female offender behavior over time" (p. 393). Although longitudinal designs are now a preferred methodological strategy, many of the most important contributions to our knowledge either exclude girls or have focused most research attention on boys' development (Laub & Sampson, 2003; Loeber, Stouthamer-Loeber, Van Kammen, & Farrington, 1991; McCord, 1983; Patterson, 1982; Sampson & Laub, 1993; Wolfgang, Thornberry, & Figlio, 1987).

Another problem is that unselected cohort or school designs, even if quite large, will not often capture a sufficiently large number of serious female offenders to allow for meaningful analysis. For example, Stattin and Magnusson (1990) found in a follow-up of 1,393 pupils in Sweden that only 15 girls had an official crime record as juveniles, while 165 boys were convicted of at least one offense prior to age 18. Wolfgang and colleagues (1987) reported that 1.9% of the girls in his large cohort study had committed a violent offense resulting in injury to a victim. When examining youth who offended at a high rate for more than a year of the study, only two girls in the National Youth Survey qualified as serious violent offenders (Huizinga, Morse, & Elliott, 1992). Cairns and colleagues (Cairns, Cairns, Neckerman, Ferguson, & Gariepy, 1989; Schlossman & Cairns, 1991) found that 6% of their female sample had at least one serious arrest charge by age 18. Moffitt, Caspi, Rutter, and Silva (2001) recently analyzed female as well as male patterns of behavior, but classified only six females in their long-term study as "life-course persistent" offenders.

This reliable disparity in rates of involvement influences topic choices (e.g., the literature contains more studies of adolescent female depression than of female delinquency), and researchers interested in gender have also frequently redefined what it is that constitutes antisocial behavior (e.g., an increased focus on relational or social aggression among girls). However, a small number of adolescent girls do commit traditional acts of delinquency and/or exhibit violent behaviors. Yet we know little about them, and less about their long-term prospects. Recent statistics document that "the relative growth in juvenile arrests involving females was more than double the growth for males" (Poe-Yamagata & Butts, 1996, p. 5). These statistics also reveal a higher percentage increase in female arrests for violent crime index offenses, also underscoring the need for more research.

The criminological literature does reflect increased interest in the female offender, but many works are essentially reviews of the literature, where no original data have been collected (Heidensohn, 1985; Leonard, 1982; Ross & Fabiano, 1986; Schur, 1984; Smart, 1976; Weisheit & Mahan, 1988). Several important qualitative studies, such as Campbell's (1981, 1984, 1990) observational analyses of female gang members in New York and Miller's (1986) study of female prostitutes in Milwaukee, are extremely useful sources for theory building, but it is difficult to generalize from these studies because of their reliance on small samples and lack of a longitudinal design. Carlen (1985) did conduct a follow-up of a small sample of women in England, and found that all of the women she studied "have now rejected lawbreaking. No longer do they see it as being either a satisfying mode of self expression or a satisfactory way of making a living" (p. 12). But because of the small sample size (only four women were followed up), we cannot be certain that this pattern of movement away from antisocial behavior would be characteristic of a larger, more heterogeneous sample of serious adolescent female offenders.

Warren and Rosenbaum (1986) examined adult arrest records of 159 females incarcerated as adolescents, and found that a high percentage of these women continued to have problems as adults. Robins's (1966, 1986) research included follow-ups with women as well as men seen at a psychiatric clinic for antisocial behavior either in childhood or adolescence. This study, like that of Warren and Rosenbaum, documented elements of continuity in the antisocial behavior patterns of the females. In addition, Robins underscored the importance of examining outcomes such as mental health in addition to antisocial behavior, as rates of internalizing problems were high among the adult women. The Ohio Serious Offender study we recently completed focuses on a more contemporary sample of young female offenders, all of whom had committed serious and/or repeated offenses (see Cernkovich, Giordano, & Pugh, 1985, for a more complete description of the delinquent behavior profiles of this sample, compared with a sample derived from a household survey of youth we also conducted). In this chapter, we describe how the young women we followed up have fared as adults, when compared with their male counterparts.

Although our primary objective is to examine the adult criminal involvement of these women, a comprehensive assessment of adult outcomes requires attention to other aspects of their lives. Thus, we also review the women's marital and employment circumstances, as well as their levels of educational and occupational achievement. It is also important to focus on areas of life that may be of special interest given the focus on women offenders. Thus, we present basic comparisons of levels of psychological distress and parenting difficulties of the male and female respondents who participated in the Ohio Serious Offender Study. Finally, we describe similarities and differences in the causal processes linked to *variations* in the success of women and men's adult transitions, and throughout the discussion highlight the unique challenges facing minority women and men with an early history of conduct problems.

## DIFFERENT VIEWS ABOUT WOMEN'S ADULT PROSPECTS

While longitudinal research in this area is limited, several contrasting hypotheses about gender and long-term outcomes are quite plausible. Some have suggested that serious adolescent female offenders will tend to evidence more favorable adult outcomes than male serious offenders. Even though delinquent girls may have some antisocial tendencies, it has been suggested that the continuing force of gender socialization, including the weight of "nurturant role obligations" (Robbins, 1989, p. 119) and stronger pressures toward conformity confronting all women (Scarr-Salapatek & Salapatek, 1973; Schur, 1984), could result in a greater likelihood that these young women more often than their male counterparts would mature out of deviant roles, behaviors, and lifestyles. This notion is also consistent with some research on gang youth. For example, Moore and Hagedorn (1999) found that the female Hispanic gang members they studied infrequently went on to be arrested as adults. These researchers also focused on the importance of having children as a factor that was associated with movement away from criminal and gang involvement. Similarly, Graham and Bowling (1995), in a study of British offenders, found that women more often than men ended their criminal involvement abruptly, and movement away from crime was often linked to the birth of a child.

Other work in this area foreshadows more problematic adult circumstances, however. As Robins (1986) has pointed out, the generally low base rate of occurrence of girls' conduct problems somehow implies that there may be more "serious" implications when it *does* occur. The conception of seriousness may encompass several related areas. The behavior itself may be more firmly entrenched/chronic, or it may be seen as more symptomatic of psychological disturbance, or as more likely to co-occur with psychological disorders (Crites, 1976; Ross & Fabiano, 1986; Widom, 1984). In addition, the greater social stigma attached to female in contrast to male involvement in antisocial behavior may be more limiting to life chances/opportunities for a return to conventional roles (Schur, 1984). According to this logic, then, we might expect that adolescent female offenders will tend to evidence more problematic outcomes, including continued involvement in antisocial behavior, greater psychological distress, lower academic/occupational attainment, and difficulty adapting to prosocial adult roles such as that of parent or spouse.

Yet another possibility is that few differences will be found in the long-term prospects of male and female delinquents, or in the processes linked to variations in the success of their adult transitions. Some researchers have emphasized that while fewer girls than boys become involved in criminal behavior, the processes leading to delinquency are actually quite similar across gender (Dornfeld & Kruttschnitt, 1991; Giordano & Cernkovich, 1997; Matseuda & Jeglum-Bartusch, 1991; Moffitt et al., 2001; Smith & Paternoster, 1987). By extension, then, similarly aged men and women with an early history of conduct problems might experience similar adult trajectories and a fairly equal likelihood of making an exit from a criminal lifestyle. For example, Baskin and Sommers (1998) interviewed a sample of women who had desisted from crime and found the reasons women gave for "maturing out" were quite similar to those found in studies of male offenders (see also Uggen & Kruttschnitt, 1998).

A final complication is suggested by the work of feminist theorists, who have increasingly highlighted the ways in which gender may be linked with and influenced by experiences deriving from other important characteristics, notably minority status (Collins, 2000; Hill & Sprague, 1999; King, 1988). This work connects to a much larger literature documenting that minority individuals face continuing social and economic disadvantages in general and in their criminal justice system contacts (Flowers, 1990). Thus, while the study we describe focuses on the central contrast between male and female offenders, it is important to highlight variations in the nature of the adult experiences of white and African American respondents as these women and men have navigated the transition to adulthood.

## THE OHIO SERIOUS OFFENDER STUDY

In 1982 we conducted interviews ($n$ = 127) with the entire population of the only state-level institution for delinquent girls in Ohio; a comparable sample was drawn from the populations of three institutions for boys ($n$ = 127). We conducted the follow up in 1995–1996, and were eventually able to locate and interview 85% of the original group of respondents (109 women, 101 men) who had participated in the adolescent interviews. It was necessary to conduct interviews within 25 different prison settings, where a total of 44 interviews took place. The final sample was 48% white and 37% African American, and averaged approximately 29 years of age. An analysis of self-reported delinquency data collected in 1982 indicated that the female and male respondents in this sample were not only more delinquent in comparison to the average youth who participated in the related household survey described in the next section, but also when compared to the most delinquent youth in the household survey (Cernkovich et al., 1985). The study included structured interviews with each respondent, and open-ended life history narratives elicited from a majority of those who completed the structured protocol.

## THE TOLEDO HOUSEHOLD STUDY

Although the primary focus of our review is on the preceding sample of formerly institutionalized youth, for some purposes it is useful to compare this group to a more random sample of youths who completed the identical structured interviews as adolescents and again as young adults. The household study was based on interviews with 942 youth, 12–19 years of age, living in private households in the Toledo, Ohio, metropolitan area. A multistage modified probability sampling procedure was employed, and respondents were equally divided among males and females and African American and white youths. An effort was made in 1992 to locate and reinterview all of the original 942 household respondents. The overall completion rate for the adult follow-up was 77% of the original sample (adjusting the base rate for 10 confirmed deaths); of these, 82% completed personal interviews. Of the 721 respondents interviewed at time 2, 45% were male and 47% were white.

## KEY FINDINGS OF THE SERIOUS OFFENDER FOLLOW-UP STUDY

A fundamental but important question is the degree to which these women and men had persisted or desisted in criminal involvement, as reflected by their behavior profiles at the time of the adult follow-up. Figure 9.1 presents the percentages of respondents in each race/gender category who could be classified as desisters using three independent raters and multiple sources of information (self-reported crime, arrest data, and information contained within the life history narratives). The raters used information contained within the arrest histories, self-reports, and

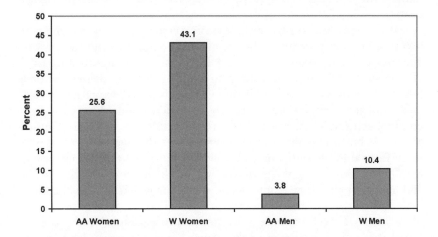

**FIGURE 9.1.** Serious offenders who had desisted at the adult follow-up. (AA, African American; W, white.)

qualitative life history data to classify respondents as desisters, persisters, or belonging to a less clear-cut middle category. A desister classification resulted if the individual did not have an arrest within a 2-year window prior to the interview, and if the self-report and narrative data did not include more than minor reported criminal activity in the past year. We note that although a high rate of interrater reliability was achieved, these data nevertheless reflect a somewhat subjective evaluation process and should thus be interpreted with caution. Our use of several sources of data clearly decreases the number of desisters when compared with the more typical strategy of relying solely on arrest records. However, we believe this offers a more accurate portrait of the actual levels of involvement in criminal activity we encountered at the time of the adult follow-up.

Data described in Figure 9.1 document that female respondents were significantly more likely to have desisted than male respondents, and within gender categories being African American was associated with a greater likelihood of persistence. Although these data thus indicate that being female is somewhat "advantageous" or protective, it is important to underscore that 74% of the African American women and 57% of their white counterparts could not be clearly categorized as having desisted from criminal activity. Figure 9.2 presents data on self-reported criminal involvement for each of the race/gender categories. Consistent with the profile represented in Figure 9.1, white female respondents report the lowest levels of criminal involvement, and black males report the highest levels. However, in this comparison the self-reported involvement of African American women is slightly higher than that of white males, although this difference is not statistically significant.

It is important to situate these basic outcome data within the context of a broader portrait of the social and economic circumstances of a majority of those who participated in the study. Sampson and Laub (1993), in their analyses derived from a large sample of delinquent boys followed up by Glueck and Glueck (1968), found that marital attachment and job stability were strongly related to adult desistance from criminal activity. These researchers argued that it was not marriage or a job per se but the quality of those experiences that was associated with more favorable life outcomes. However, it appeared that a majority of the Glueck men were, at the time of the adult follow-up, both married and had stable full-time employment. Our view is that the social control potential of these circumstances is greatly enhanced when both are in place as a relatively complete "respectability package." However, we found that only 8.1 percent of the young adults we interviewed in connection with the Ohio Serious Offender Study could be characterized as

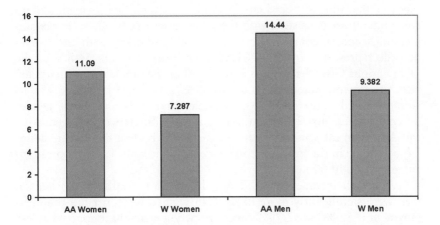

**FIGURE 9.2.** Self-reported criminal involvement of serious offenders. (AA, African American; W, white.)

having access to this high-quality package (which we defined as an average or better report of marital attachment and a job earning wages above the 1995 poverty line.) The men and women in the sample appeared relatively equally disadvantaged in these basic respects (7.7% of the women and 8.6% of the men had achieved the total "respectability" package). Furthermore, the follow-up data indicate that African American respondents were particularly unlikely to be both married and fully employed. Only 5.1% of the African American women and no African American males were so positioned (see Giordano, Cernkovich, & Rudolph, 2002).

Our view is that declines in the likelihood and permanence of marriage and reduction in the type of manufacturing jobs available to many of the Glueck men are important underpinnings of the differences in findings across these two studies. The data described in Figure 9.3 add to the overall portrait. Figure 9.3 depicts the percentage of respondents in the Ohio Serious Offender Study who had graduated from high school. A comparison of male and female percentages indicates no differences by gender. Overall, 83.2% of the women and 82.7 % of males failed to graduate from high school. Only 6% had educational experience beyond high school, and the majority of these were either associate degrees (4%) or other technical training (1.5%). These educational levels stand in sharp contrast to the academic achievement levels reported by the respondents who had participated in the Toledo Household Study, and it is important to note that even most household "offenders" reported that they had graduated from high school. Employment and income figures are consistent with these low levels of education. For example, household incomes were divided into quartiles, with the lowest quartile represented by the 0-$14,000 category. Overall, 54.8% of the Ohio Serious Offender women and 52.7% of their male counterparts fell into this lowest category, and only 7.6% (8.6% of men, 6.7% of women) listed household incomes higher than $40,000. These gender differences were not significant, but again race differences emerged. African American men and women were more likely than their white counterparts to be in the lowest income category, and only 1.5% reported incomes over $40,000.

Although income data did not differ dramatically across gender, men were significantly more likely than women to report full-time employment (65.6% vs. 32.7%). Since women in general are somewhat less likely to be employed full time we also compared this group to the neighborhood women, and found that the latter were significantly more likely than the Serious Offender women to be fully employed. The life history narratives reveal that whether male or female, the Serious Offender respondents rarely garnered "above the table" wages. Men were more likely to describe construction or roofing work, while women frequently listed service sector jobs such as nurse's aide or waitress. Clearly, for those who were classified as belonging to the "persister" category, selling drugs and prostitution often added to the meager wages earned legitimately. Housing circumstances encountered by the interviewers (government housing, living with friends or relatives, basement of

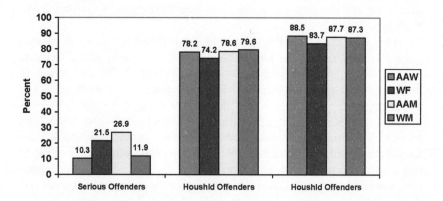

FIGURE 9.3. Educational achievement (percent graduated from high school). (AAW, African American women; WF, white females; AAM, African American men; WM, white males.)

crackhouse, dilapidated trailer in rural Kentucky) are consistent with the low reported incomes, and only a handful of respondents were home-owners. One woman interviewed in a shelter for battered women admit-ted that she was not currently in an abusive relationship, but was desper-ate for some sort of housing ("I've been trying for 3 months to get in the regular homeless shelters . . . ").

Given the array of legal and social difficulties experienced by many respondents, it is perhaps not surprising that reports of psychological distress are very high. Consistent with the findings of Robins's (1966) classic follow-up; the women in our sample report higher levels of psy-chological distress (see Figure 9.4) at the adult follow-up when com-pared with male respondents (3.53 vs. 3.08). Since women often score higher on measures of depression, we also compared these women to their counterparts in the household sample and found that the offender women on average report significantly higher levels of distress (3.53 vs. 2.92). Men within the offender group also reported higher levels of dis-tress than their neighborhood counterparts (3.08 vs. 2.80).

Figure 9.5 depicts parenting experiences of the offender and house-hold sample groups. Among offenders, being female can again be con-sidered advantageous or protective, in that Serious Offender women were more likely than their male counterparts to have physical custody of all of their children. However, in this instance it is also important to note the contrast with the household sample of women, including those who were classified as delinquent as adolescents. Only 9.5% of the Afri-can American women identified in the neighborhood study as delinquent

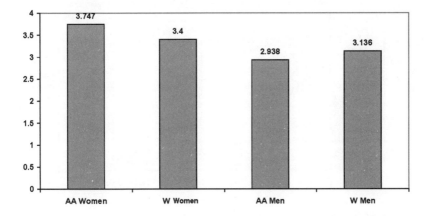

**FIGURE 9.4.** Self-reported psychological distress at adult follow-up. (AA, African American; W, white.)

lost or never had custody of one or more of their children, but 61.8% of
African American women in the Serious Offender group reported loss of
custody of at least one child. And while 17.1% of the white female delinquents identified in the neighborhood study reported that they did not
currently have physical custody of one of their biological children, this
situation characterized 41% of the family situations of white female Serious Offenders.

## FACTORS ASSOCIATED WITH VARIATIONS IN THE SUCCESS OF THE TRANSITIONS OF THE OHIO SERIOUS OFFENDER SAMPLE

Although the preceding descriptive portrait depicts multiple layers of
disadvantage encountered at the time of the follow-up, the sample is
nevertheless characterized by significant variations in adult functioning
and well-being. Thus, we have also examined factors that appear to be
associated with these patterns of variation and explored the degree to
which movement away from crime connects to generic or distinctly
gendered processes.

We began with the factors highlighted by Sampson and Laub's influential analysis of male delinquents who had participated in the Gluecks'
follow-up study (Laub, Nagin, & Sampson, 1998; Sampson & Laub,

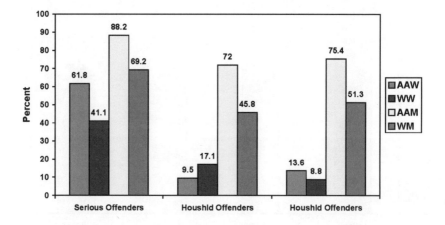

**FIGURE 9.5.** Percent who have lost/never had physical custody of one or more biological children. (AAW, African American women; WW, white women; AAM, African
American men; WM, white men.)

1993). We found that marital attachment and job stability were not significantly related to levels of desistance from crime for either the female or male respondents in the Ohio Serious Offender Study (Giordano et al., 2002). It is likely that the low base rates of marriage, high rates of marital instability, and dismal economic circumstances described earlier influenced this pattern of results. Nevertheless, in our analysis of the detailed qualitative life history data we found that a subset of the respondents indicated that they had indeed benefited from a "good marriage effect." The qualitative data are thus especially useful as they have suggested the presence of subtypes within the larger group of women. Some of the domestic arrangements described appeared to be quite traditional in character ("he don't trust me around men . . . he don't want me being around men . . . he don't like me to work at all . . . ") and reports of marital happiness varied considerably. Yet these women linked their movement away from crime to a conventional family life that included their husband and children. Our analyses of the life history narratives suggested a more conditional effect of marriage that takes into account the important role played by the individual's motivation to change as well as the social control potential of the spouse or romantic partner.

It is also important to consider the spouse's own attitudes and behavioral repertoire. While Sampson and Laub (1993) have argued that the spouse's prosocial or antisocial tendencies are not as important as the character or quality of the marital bond itself, we found that the partner's level of involvement in crime is a very significant predictor of the respondent's own self-reported criminal activity (Giordano, Cernkovich, & Holland, 2003). We also found that while the spouse's crime level was a strong predictor for both male and female respondents, a gender by partner crime interaction also was significant. That is, analyses revealed that spouse's crime level was a stronger predictor of *male* than of female self-reported criminality.

This finding seems to contradict the perspective offered by researchers who have emphasized how many offenses of women tie either directly or indirectly to the influence of marital partners (see, e.g., Richie, 1996). Evidence for this idea can certainly be found within our data, but the findings described here may also reflect the difficulties women such as the Serious Offender respondents have in locating a traditional prosocial spouse. While some of the women's problems do appear to relate to their romantic entanglements, our longitudinal perspective documents that many problems predate them; the findings also illustrate that some women have apparently been able to break away from crime and drug use even as their partners continue to participate in this type of lifestyle. This suggests the importance of continuing to include attention to cognitive and motivational variables (the slippery but important concept of human agency) as well as to interpersonal and economic factors that have previously been found to influence desistance processes (see also Maruna, 2001).

Other women within the sample who described an increasing disenchantment with the street/criminal lifestyle described how they had been able to "hook" onto other sources of change, such as a deepening religious faith or involvement with their children's lives. Indeed, these particular "hooks for change" were mentioned more frequently by female than male respondents (Giordano et al., 2002). However, in this sample, it is clear that such changes are far from automatic (the high rates of custody loss described earlier underscore this point). Virtually all women in the sample expressed love for their children, but some continued to dissociate their experiences as a good parent from their criminal or addictive behaviors. For example, one woman noted that she is a good, strict parent, even though "I might be a drug addict, and I may not get up but even if I'm not up, they will get up for school, dress proper for school . . . " (p. 1039). Those who had made more drastic lifestyle changes had apparently experienced a number of important and interrelated cognitive transformations. Such women frequently described the parent role as fundamentally incompatible with continued deviation. As one particularly successful respondent put it, "I couldn't imagine . . . even spending the night in jail and having him know about it" (p. 1040). In addition, such women more often moved their social contacts into alignment with these more prosocial identities (e.g., they made friends with other church members, or other mothers they met through their children's' activities).

## CONCLUSION

These data indicate that an accurate portrait of long-term consequences of early female delinquency necessitates gathering data not only from neighborhood or school samples, but from truly "high-risk" offenders such as those we followed up in this study. These offenders are extremely marginal educationally and socially, and the low percentage who had completely desisted from crime reflects the multiple, overlapping layers of disadvantage we encountered at the time of the adult follow-up. High levels of psychological distress reflect and undoubtedly directly inhibit attempts to move away from a criminal lifestyle, obtain decent employment and housing, and adequately parent the next generation.

The data reviewed herein suggest some gender similarities and differences. In spite of similarly low educational levels and low incomes, women more often than men could be placed in the desister category. Because of the higher levels of stigma and social sanctions associated with being a deviant or criminal woman, these women may be much more highly motivated to latch onto almost any opportunities/resources/ socially supportive network members available that will facilitate an exit from a criminal lifestyle. However, a minimum level of cultural and social capital is required to successfully effect these types of lifestyle changes. Some of the women we encountered could be considered as almost fully encapsulated within deviant worlds that provide few prospects for any type of escape to a different way of life. As one young woman explained it, referring to her involvement in prostitution, "It's all I know. . . . "

The findings with regard to parenting experiences also reflect gendered processes. While there is now much greater attention to the father's role in child development, the reality is that much close-in caregiving is provided by mothers. It is highly unusual for children to live in households without their biological mother (census data reveal that 92% of U.S. children live with their biological mothers). Thus, our findings about high rates of custody loss in this sample have practical implications, and underline the need to add considerations of parenting and child protection/development in treatment settings for both women and men. We are currently interviewing the adolescent children born to these respondents, with the goal of adding knowledge about those factors that can best serve to interrupt what appears to be a strong cultural press toward intergenerational continuity in antisocial problems experienced by this next generation.

The data also indicate that minority women and men in our sample are, on average, even more disadvantaged than white respondents. The higher levels of adult criminal involvement and greater psychological distress undoubtedly reflect specific challenges of discrimination and social and economic disadvantage. They also underscore the need to develop culturally sensitive programs for minority youth, along with gender-specific prevention and intervention programs.

## ACKNOWLEDGMENT

This research was supported by Grants Nos. MH29095 and MH46410 from the National Institute of Mental Health.

## REFERENCES

Baskin, D. R., & Sommers, I. B. (1998). *Casualities of community disorder: Women's careers in violent crime*. Boulder, CO: Westview Press.
Cairns, R. B., Cairns, B. D., Neckman, H. J., Ferguson, L. L., & Gariepy, J. L.

200 PROBLEM BEHAVIORS IN ADOLESCENT GIRLS

(1989). Growth and aggression: I. childhood to early adolescence. *Child Development, 25,* 320–330.

Campbell, A. (1981). *Girl delinquents.* New York: St. Martin's Press.

Campbell, A. (1984). *The girls in the gang: A report from New York City.* Oxford, UK: Blackwell.

Campbell, A. (1990). Female participation in gangs. In C. R. Huff (Ed.), *Gangs in America* (pp. 163–182). Newbury Park, CA: Sage.

Carlen, P. (Ed.). (1985). *Criminal women: Autobiographical accounts.* Cambridge, UK: Polity Press.

Cernkovich, S. A., & Giordano, P. C. (1979). A comparative analysis of male and female delinquency. *Sociological Quarterly, 20,* 131–145.

Cernkovich, S. A., Giordano, P. C., & Pugh, M. D. (1985). Chronic offenders: The missing cases in self-report delinquency research. *Journal of Criminal Law and Criminology, 76,* 705–732.

Chesney-Lind, M., & Shelden, R. G. (1992). *Girls, delinquency, and juvenile justice.* Pacific Grove, CA: Brooks/Cole.

Collins, T. H. (2000). *Black feminist thought: Knowledge, consciousness, and the politics of empowerment* (10th anniversary ed.). New York: Routledge.

Crites, L. (Ed.). (1976). *The female offender.* Lexington, MA: Lexington Books.

Dornfeld, M., & Kruttschnitt, C. (1991, November). *Is there a weaker sex? Mapping gender-specific outcomes and their risk factors.* Paper presented at the annual meeting of the American Society of Criminology, San Francisco.

Flowers, R. B. (1990). *Minorities and criminality.* New York: Praeger.

Giordano, P. C., & Cernkovich, S. A. (1997). Gender and antisocial behavior. In D. M. Stoff, J. Breiling, & J. D. Maser (Eds.), *The handbook of antisocial behavior* (pp. 496–510). New York: Wiley.

Giordano, P. C., Cernkovich, S. C., & Holland, D. (2003). Changes in friendship relations over the life course: Implications for desistance from crime. *Criminology, 41,* 293–328.

Giordano, P. C., Cernkovich, S. A., & Rudolph, J. L. (2002). Gender, crime, and desistance: Toward a theory of cognitive transformation. *American Journal of Sociology, 107,* 990–1064.

Glueck, S., & Glueck, E. (1968). *Delinquents and nondelinquents in perspective.* Cambridge, MA: Harvard University Press.

Graham, J., & Bowling, B. (1995). *Young people and crime.* London: Home Office Research Study 145.

Heidensohn, F. (1985). *Women and crime.* New York: New York University Press.

Hill, S. A., & Sprague J. (1999). The gendering of violent delinquency. *Criminology, 27*(2), 277–313.

Huizinga, D., Morse, B. J., & Elliott, D. S. (1992). *The National Youth Survey: An overview and description of recent findings* (National Youth Survey Project Report No. 55). Boulder: Institute of Behavioral Science, University of Colorado.

King, D. K. (1988). Multiple jeopardy, multiple consciousness: The contest of black feminist ideology. *Signs: Journal of Women in Culture and Society, 14,* 42–72.

Laub, J. H., Nagin, D. S., & Sampson, R. J. (1998). Trajectories of change in criminal offending: Good marriages and the desistance process. *American Sociological Review, 63,* 3–24.

Laub, J. H., & Sampson, R. J. (2003). *Shared beginnings, divergent lives: Delinquent boys to age 70!* Cambridge, MA: Harvard University Press.

Leonard, E. (1982). *Women, crime, and society: A critique of theoretical criminology.* New York: Longman.

Loeber, R., Stouthamer-Loeber, M., Van Kammen, W., & Farrington, D. P. (1991). Initiation, escalation, and desistance in juvenile offending and their correlates. *Journal of Criminal Law and Criminology, 82,* 36–82.

Maruna, S. (2001). *Making good: How ex-offenders reform and reclaim their lives.* Washington, DC: American Psychological Association.

Matsueda, R., & Jeglum-Bartusch, D. R. (1991). *Gender, reflected appraisals and labeling: A cross-population test of an interactionist theory.* Paper presented at the annual meeting of the American Society of Criminology, San Francisco.

McCord, J. (1983). A longitudinal study of aggression and antisocial behavior. In K. T. VanDusen & S. A. Mednick (Eds.), *Prospective studies of crime and delinquency* (pp. 269–276). Boston: Kluwer-Nijhoff.

Miller, E. (1986). *Street women.* Philadelphia: Temple University Press.

Moffitt, T. E., Caspi, A., Rutter, M., & Silva, P. A. (2001). *Sex differences in antisocial behavior: Conduct disorder, delinquency, and violence in the Dunedin Longitudinal Study.* Cambridge, UK: Cambridge University Press.

Moore, J. W., & Hagedorn, J. M. (1999). What happens to girls in the gang? In M. Chesney-Lind & J. M. Hagerdorn (Eds.), *Female gangs in America: Essays on girls, gangs, and gender* (pp. 177–186). Chicago: Lake View Press.

Patterson, G. R. (1982). *Coercive family process.* Eugene, OR: Castalia.

Poe-Yamagata, E., & Butts, J. A. (1996). *Female offenders in the juvenile justice system* (OFFDP Research Report). Washington, DC: Office of Juvenile Justice and Delinquency Prevention, U.S. Department of Justice.

Renzetti, C. M., & Goodstein, L. (2001). *Women, crime, and criminal justice: Original feminist readings.* Los Angeles: Roxbury.

Richie, B. (1996). *Compelled to crime: The gender entrapment of battered black women.* New York: Routledge.

Robbins, C. (1989). Sex differences in psychosocial consequences of alcohol and drug abuse. *Journal of Health and Social Behavior, 30,* 117–130.

Robins, L. N. (1966). *Deviant children grown up.* Baltimore: Williams & Wilkins.

Robins, L. N. (1986). The consequences of conduct disorder in girls. In D. Olweus, J. Block, & M. Radkey-Yarrow (Eds.), *Development of antisocial and prosocial behavior* (pp. 385-414). Orlando, FL: Academic Press.

Robins, L. N., Tipp, J., & Pryzbeck, T. (1991). Antisocial personality. In L. N. Robins & D. A. Regier (Eds.), *Psychiatric disorders in America: The epidemiologic catchment area study* (pp. 258–290). New York: Free Press.

Ross, R. R., & Fabiano, E. A. (1986). *Female offenders: Correctional afterthoughts.* Jefferson, NC: McFarland.

Sampson, R., & Laub, J. H. (1993). *Crime in the making: Pathways and turning points through life.* Cambridge, MA: Harvard University Press.

Scarr-Salapatek, S., & Salapatek, P. (Eds.). (1973). *Socialization.* Columbus, OH: Charles E. Merrill.

Schlossman, S., & Cairns, R. B. (1991). Problem girls: Observations on past and present. In G. H. Elder, Jr., R. D. Park, & J. Modell (Eds.), *Children in time and place: Relations between history and developmental psychology.* New York: Cambridge University Press.

Schur, E. (1984). *Labeling women deviant.* New York: Random House.

Smart, C. (1976). *Women, crime and criminology: A feminist critique.* London: Routledge & Kegan Paul.

Smith, D. A., & Paternoster, R. (1987). The gender gap in theories of deviance: Issues and evidence. *Journal of Research in Crime and Delinquency, 24,* 140–172.

Stattin H., & Magnusson, D. (1990). *Pubertal maturation in female development.* Hillsdale, NJ: Erlbaum.

Uggen, C., & Kruttschnitt, C. (1998). Crime in the breaking: Gender differences in desistance. *Law and Society Review, 32,* 339–366.

Warren, M. Q., & Rosenbaum, J. L. (1986). Criminal careers of female offenders. *Criminal Justice and Behavior, 13,* 393–418.

Weisheit, R., & Mahan, S. (1988). Women, crime and criminal justice. Cincinnati, OH: Anderson.

Widom, C. S. (1984). Sex roles, criminality and psychopathology. In C. Spatz Widom (Ed.), *Sex roles and psychopathology* (pp. 183–217). New York: Plenum Press.

Wolfgang, M. E., Thornberry, T. P., & Figlio, R. M. (1987). *From boy to man: From delinquency to crime.* Chicago: University of Chicago Press.

# CHAPTER 10

# Trends in Delinquent Girls' Aggression and Violent Behavior

## A Review of the Evidence

Meda Chesney-Lind *and* Joanne Belknap

Girls in the juvenile justice system were once "dubbed" the "forgotten few" (Bergsmann, 1989). That construction of female delinquency has rapidly faded as increases in girls' arrests have dramatically outstripped those of boys for most of the last decade. Girls now account for 28% of juvenile arrests, up from 23% at the beginning of the last decade (Federal Bureau of Investigation, 1991, 2001), and attention is being drawn to the fact that their arrests for nontraditional, even violent, offenses are among those showing the greatest increases. These shifts and changes all bring into sharp focus the need to better understand the dynamics involved in female delinquency and the need to tailor responses to the unique circumstances of girls growing up in the new millennium.

This chapter provides a critical examination of these trends in female juvenile delinquency with a specific focus on current research examining trends in girls' aggression and violence. We examine national trends, and then we take a closer look at self-report data, which amplify the trends seen in the more global arrest and incarceration data. The findings emphasize the importance of examining how girls' violence and aggression is measured and framed. The authors conclude that girls' violence and aggression has been misrepresented too often in both research forums and the media, whether by criminologists or journalists.

## PATTERNS IN GIRLS' DELINQUENCY: ARE GIRLS REALLY CLOSING THE GENDER GAP IN VIOLENCE?

Between 1991 and 2000 in the United States, girls' arrests increased 25.3%, while arrests of boys actually decreased by 3.2% (Federal Bureau of Investigation, 2001, p. 221). Concomitant with these arrest increases are increases in girls' referral to juvenile courts; between 1987 and 1996, the number of delinquency cases involving girls increased by 76%, compared to a 42% increase for males (Stahl, 1999). Arrests of girls for serious violent offenses increased by 27.9% between 1991 and 2000; arrests of girls for "other assaults" increased by even more: 77.9% (Federal Bureau of Investigation, 2001, p. 221). The Office of Juvenile Justice and Delinquency Prevention (1999) found that the female violent crime rate for 1997 was 103% above the 1981 rate, compared to 27% for males. This prompted them to assert that "increasing juvenile female arrests and the involvement of girls in at-risk and delinquent behavior has been a pervasive trend across the United States" (p. 2). Discussions of girls' gang behavior and, more recently, girls' violence have also been extremely prevalent in the media (see Chesney-Lind, 1999, for a review).

## TRENDS IN GIRLS' VIOLENCE

With reference to what might be called girls' "nontraditional" delinquency, it must be recognized that girls' capacity for aggression and violence has historically been ignored, trivialized or denied. For this reason, self-report data, particularly from the 1970s, showed higher involvement of girls in assaultive behavior than official statistics from that period would indicate.[1]

More recent self-report data of youthful involvement in violent offenses fail to show the dramatic changes found in official statistics during either the 1980s or the 1990s. Consider data collected by the Centers for Disease Control and Prevention (CDC) over the last decade (see Table 10.1). The CDC has been monitoring youthful behavior in a national sample of school-age youth in a number of domains (including violence) at regular intervals since 1991 in a biennial survey titled the Youth Risk Behavior Survey. A quick look at data collected over the 1990s reveals that while 34.4% of girls surveyed in 1991 said that they had been in a physical fight in the last year, by 1999 that figure had dropped to 27.3%, or a 21% decrease in girls' fighting; boys' violence also decreased during the same period but only slightly—from 44.0% to

TABLE 10.1. Trends in Girls' and Boys' Self-Reported Violence

|                    | 1991 | 1993 | 1995 | 1997 | 1999 |
|--------------------|------|------|------|------|------|
| Girls' behavior    |      |      |      |      |      |
| In a physical fight | 34.2 | 31.7 | 30.6 | 26.0 | 27.3 |
| Carried a weapon   | 10.9 | 9.2  | 8.3  | 7.0  | 6.0  |
| Carried a gun      |      | 1.8  | 2.5  | 1.4  | 0.8  |
| Boys' behavior     |      |      |      |      |      |
| In a physical fight | 50.2 | 51.2 | 46.1 | 45.5 | 44.0 |
| Carried a weapon   | 40.6 | 34.3 | 31.1 | 27.7 | 28.6 |
| Carried a gun      |      | 13.7 | 12.3 | 9.6  | 9.0  |

Note. Compiled by the authors from Youth Risk Surveillance data (Centers for Disease Control and Prevention, 1992, 1994, 1998, and 2000).

42.5% (a 3.4% drop) (Brener, Simon, Krug, & Lowry, 1999, p. 443; Centers for Disease Control and Prevention, 1992, 1994, 1996, 1998, 2000). Similarly, the rate of girls who reported carrying weapons and carrying guns also declined substantially. A logistic analysis of these trends (for the years 1991–1997) published in the *Journal of the American Medical Association* concluded that "while analyses revealed a significant linear decrease in physical fighting for both male and female students the β [beta] for females was larger, suggesting they had a steeper decline" (Brener et al., 1999, p. 444).

Earlier, a matched sample of "high-risk" youth (ages 13–17) surveyed in the 1977 National Youth Study and the more recent 1989 Denver Youth Survey also revealed significant *decreases* in girls' involvement in felony assaults, minor assaults, and hard drugs, and no change in a wide range of other delinquent behaviors—including felony theft, minor theft, and index delinquency (Huizinga, 1997). Finally, there are the trends in girls' lethal violence. While girls' arrests for all forms of assault have been skyrocketing in the 1990s, girls' arrests for robbery fell by 45.3% and murder by 1.4% between 1991 and 2000. If girls were in fact closing the gap between their behavior and that of boys, would not one expect to see the same effect across all the violent offenses (including the *most* violent offense)? That simply is not happening.

Further support of this notion comes from recent research on girls' violence in San Francisco (Males & Shorter, 2001). Scholars' analyses of vital statistics maintained by health officials (rather than arrest data) conclude that there has been a 63% drop in San Francisco teen-girl fatalities between the 1960s and the 1990s, and they also report that hospital injury data show that girls are dramatically underrepresented among those reporting injury (including assaults: Girls are 3.7% of the population but were only 0.9% of those seeking treatment for violent injuries) (Males & Shorter 2001, pp. 1–2).

They conclude: Compared to her counterpart of the Baby Boom generation growing up in the 1960s and 1970s, a San Francisco teenage girl today is 50% less likely to be murdered, 60% less likely to suffer a fatal accident, 75% less likely to commit suicide, 45% less likely to die by a gun, 55% less likely to become a mother, 60% less likely to commit murder, and 40% less likely to be arrested for property crimes (Males & Shorter 2001, p. 1).

Data from Canada indicate the same pattern. A recent report on delinquent girls incarcerated in British Columbia concludes that "despite isolated incidents of violence, the majority of offending by female youth in custody is relatively minor" (Corrado, Odgers, & Cohen, 2000). Even a study of girls tried and convicted as adults in the United States found the majority of the girls had relatively minor offenses (Gaarder & Belknap, 2002).

In short, other measures of girls' violent crime that are less susceptible to changes in policing practices fail to reflect the trends shown in the arrest data. Having said that, there is still a need to understand the gender dynamics in girls' and boys' aggression and violence, a topic the next section covers in more detail. Moreover, once these are fully understood, it is clear that they interface with the various societal changes in the framing of girl's aggression that have occurred in the past decades.

## WHAT'S IN A NAME?: ENFORCEMENT PRACTICES AND ARREST DATA

If the levels of girl's physical aggression, or violence, has not changed, what explains the dramatic increases in female arrest, particularly in arrests of girls for "other assaults"? Relabeling of behaviors that were once categorized as status offenses (noncriminal offenses like "runaway" and "person in need of supervision") into violent offenses cannot be ruled out in explanations of arrest rate shifts, nor can changes in police practices with reference to domestic violence. A review of the over 2,000 cases of girls referred to Maryland's juvenile justice system for "person-to-person" offenses revealed that virtually all of these offenses (97.9%) involved "assault." A further examination of these records revealed that about half were "family centered" and involved such activities as "a girl hitting her mother and her mother subsequently pressing charges" (Mayer, 1994).

More recently, Acoca's (1999) study of nearly 1,000 delinquent girls' files from four California counties found that while a "high per-centage" of these girls were charged with "person offenses," a majority of these involved assault. Furthermore, "a close reading of the case files of girls charged with assault revealed that most of these charges were the result of nonserious, mutual combat, situations with parents." Acoca de-tails cases that she regards as typical including: "father lunged at her while she was calling the police about a domestic dispute. She [girl] hit him." Finally, she reports that some cases were quite trivial in nature, in-cluding a girl arrested "for throwing cookies at her mother" (Acoca 1999, pp. 7–8). In a Colorado study, a girl reported that she was ar-rested for "assault" for throwing her Barbie doll at her mother (Belknap, Winter, & Cady, 2001).

In essence, when exploring the dramatic increases in the arrests of girls for "other assault," it is likely that changes in enforcement practices have dramatically narrowed the gender gap. As noted in the preceding examples, a clear contribution has come from increasing arrests of girls and women for domestic violence. A recent California study found that the female share of these arrests increased from 6% in 1988 to 16.5% in 1998 (Bureau of Criminal Information and Analysis, 1999). African American girls and women had arrest rates roughly 3 times that of white girls and women in 1998: 149.6 compared to 46.4 (Bureau of Criminal Information and Analysis, 1999).

Relabeling of girls' arguments with parents from status offenses (like "incorrigible" or "person in need of supervision") to assault is a form of "bootstrapping" that has been particularly pronounced in the official delinquency of African American girls (Bartollas, 1993; Robin-son, 1990). This practice also facilitates the incarceration of girls in de-tention facilities and training schools—something that would not be possible if the girl were arrested for noncriminal status offenses. Simi-larly, some parents admit to using detention as a "time out" from con-flict with their daughters, including some mothers who would rather have their daughters in detention than at home with the mothers and their boyfriends, when it is often the mothers' boyfriends who caused the girls' running away (Lederman & Brown, 2000).

"Up-criming" cannot be ruled out in terms of the increases seen in arrests of youth for schoolyard fights and other instances of bullying that formerly were ignored or handled internally by schools and parents. Such an explanation is particularly salient as increasing numbers of schools adopt "zero tolerance" policies for physical aggression and/or weapon carrying. It has long been known that arrests of youth for minor or "other" assaults can range from schoolyard tussles to relatively seri-ous, but not life-threatening, assaults (Steffensmeier & Steffensmeier, 1980). Currie (1998) adds to this the fact that these "simple assaults without injury" are often "attempted" or "threatened" or "not completed." At a time when official concern about youth violence is almost unparalleled and school principals are increasingly likely to call police onto their campuses, it should come as no surprise that youthful arrests in this area are up. It is noteworthy that this unparalleled police involvement on secondary school campuses is largely due to "Columbine" and other school shootings and "massacres" perpetrated almost exclusively by boys (see Steinem, 2001).

The possibility of up-criming of minor forms of youthful violence is supported by research on the dynamics of juvenile robbery in Honolulu (another violent offense where girls' arrests showed sharp increases in the mid-1990s). In the last decade, Hawaii, like the rest of the nation, had seen an increase in the arrests of youth for serious crimes of violence[2] coupled with a recent decline. In Hawaii, violent crime (murder, rape, robbery, and aggravated assault) arrests increased 60% from 1987 to 1996, coupled with an 8.6% decline between 1996 and 1997 (Crime Prevention and Justice Assistance Division, 1997, 1998). Most of the change can be attributed to increases in the number of youth arrested for two offenses: aggravated assault and robbery. Between 1994 and 1996, for example, the number of youth arrested for robbery doubled in Honolulu.

These increases prompted a study of the actual dimensions of juvenile robbery in Honolulu (see Chesney-Lind & Paramore, 2001). In this study, police files from two time periods (1991 and 1997) that focused on robbery incidents resulting in arrest were identified. According to these data, in 1991, the vast majority of those arrested for robbery in Honolulu were male—114 (95%) versus 6 (5%) female. However, a shift occurred in 1997—83.3% were males. Thus, the proportion of robbery arrests involving girls more than tripled between 1991 and 1997.

Taken alone, these numeric increases, along with anecdotal information, are precisely why the "surge" in girls' violence has been made. However, in this study we were able to carefully characterize of each of these "robberies" during the two time periods. Essentially, the data suggested that no major shift in the pattern of juvenile robbery occurred between 1991 and 1997 in Honolulu. Rather, it appears that less serious offenses, including a number committed by girls, are being swept up into the system, perhaps as a result of changes in school policy and parental attitudes (many of the robberies occurred as youth were going to and from school). Consistent with this explanation are the following observable patterns in our data: During the two time periods under review, the age of offenders shifts downward, as does the value of items taken. In 1991, the median value of the items stolen was $10.00; by 1997, the median value had dropped to $1.25. Most significantly, the proportion of adult victims declined sharply, while the number of juvenile victims increased. Finally, while more of the robberies involved weapons in 1997, those weapons were less likely to be firearms and the incidents were less likely to result in injury to the victim. In short, the data suggest that the problem of juvenile robbery in the City and County of Honolulu is largely characterized by slightly older youth bullying and "hijacking" younger youth for small amounts of cash and occasionally jewelry and that arrests of youth for these forms of robbery accounted for virtually all of the increase observed.

Major gender differences were found in another study of youthful violence, in which 444 incarcerated delinquent youth in Ohio were recently asked to report on an anonymous survey the offenses involved in their current incarceration (Holsinger, Belknap, & Sutherland, 1999). Although girls and boys reported similar rates for burglary as an offense (one-fifth of both), girls (one-third) were more likely than boys (one-fifth) to report an assault as an offense, and far more likely to report a property crime as an offense (53% of girls and 31% of boys). Boys (16%) were twice as likely as girls (8%) to be incarcerated for an offense involving drugs, almost 5 times as likely to be incarcerated for a sex offense (5% of girls, and 24% of boys), and more than twice as likely to report robbery as an offense that resulted in their current incarceration (7% of girls and 16% of boys). There were no significant gender differences in the youths' reports of whether they were in for a violent offense; about half of both sexes reported violent offenses as leading to their current incarceration (Holsinger et al., 1999).

An examination of these youths' self-reported offenses leading to their current incarcerations implies that the girls and boys are similar in the severity of their levels of offending overall. Yet the girls received significantly shorter sentences (mean = 12 months for girls, mean = 16 months for boys) (Holsinger et al., 1999). It is useful to examine some of the qualitative data in order to speculate why this may be the case. Focus groups with delinquent girls in this same state found reports of girls' attempts to protect themselves to be incriminating (Belknap, Dunn, & Holsinger, 1997). For example, when asked why she was incarcerated, one girl told a story of her otherwise "clean" delinquent record until she carried a knife to school. She had repeatedly told school authorities that an older boy in the school was following her as she walked to and from school and that she was afraid of him. The school refused to look into it, but when the girl put a knife in her sock in order to protect herself getting to and from school, the school's "no tolerance" code for weapons was triggered. This girl reported extreme frustration regarding the school's tolerance of the boy stalking and sexually harassing her, but no tolerance for her attempts to protect herself when the school failed to assure her safety.

## GENDER MATTERS IN GIRLS' AGGRESSION AND VIOLENCE

The psychological literature on aggression, which considers forms of aggression other than physical aggression (or violence), is also relevant here. Taken together, this literature generally reflects that, while boys and men are more likely to be physically aggressive, differences begin to even out when verbal aggression is considered (yelling, insulting, teasing; Bjorkqvist & Niemela, 1992). Furthermore, girls in adolescence may be more likely than boys to use "indirect aggression," such as gossip, telling bad or false stories, or telling secrets (Bjorkqvist, Osterman, & Kaukiainen, 1992). When this broad definition of "aggression" is utilized, only about 5% of the variance in aggression is explained by gender (Bjorkqvist & Niemela, 1992).

Does relational aggression occur more frequently with girls and boys? Research addressing this question has been mixed (see Okamoto & Chesney-Lind, 2002). Crick and Grotpeter (1995), consistent with Bjorkqvist and Niemla (1992), found that girls in their sample of third-through sixth-grade students were significantly more relationally aggressive than were boys. They found that these youth were significantly more disliked and lonelier than nonrelationally aggressive peers. Other research, however, has found no difference in the frequency of relational aggression between boys and girls (e.g., Gropper & Froschl, 2000; Tiet, Wasserman, Loeber, McReynolds, & Miller, 2001). In these studies, however, researchers coded observations of aggression, while in the Crick and Grotpeter study, peer nomination was used as the data collection procedure. This suggests that manifestations of relational aggression may be difficult to detect by adult observers, and may need to be identified by members of the youth peer group. Because of the relatively indirect nature of behaviors related to relational aggression, Crick and Gropeter state that "it might be difficult for those outside the peer group to reliably observe and evaluate [this form of aggression] in naturalistic settings" (p. 712).

Why is relational aggression important for those concerned about girls in the juvenile justice system? First, it is likely that girls in delinquency prevention and intervention programs have considerable problems with relational aggression, since it has been shown to be related to internalizing problems, peer rejection, and depression (Crick et. al, 1998, pp. 126–127). Second, while girls' aggressive behavior often remains relational in nature, overt manifestations of aggression are often preceded by relational aggression. This phenomenon is evident in both the school and group home settings for girls. Often the rationale for a physical fight is "She's talking behind my back" or "She's after my boyfriend." By addressing the relational aspect of aggression early and often, practitioners working with youth are in essence conducting overt violence prevention. The significance of this process extends to boys as well. The massacre at Columbine High School, for example, might have been prevented if the relational aggression associated with the ostracism and ridicule extended to Eric Harris and Dylan Klebold by their peers were addressed. In other words, relational aggression, while seemingly insignificant, can lead to serious consequences if left unaddressed by youth practitioners.

Finally, research suggests that relational aggression is one of the factors contributing to the stereotype that "girls are more difficult to work with" for practitioners. Using in-depth interviews, Freitas and Chesney-Lind (2001) described how difficult it is for practitioners to watch girls be "mean" to other girls and boys, and the challenges for practitioners associated with being targets of relational aggression themselves. Okamoto (2002) describes the unique challenges that male practitioners face in working with female youth clients. These findings suggest the importance of training practitioners on how to appropriately respond to relational aggression, and the need for ongoing practitioner support and supervision.

Those who study aggression in young children and young adults also note that girls' aggression is usually within the home or "intra-female" and, thus, likely to be less often reported to authorities (Bjork-qvist & Niemela, 1992). The fact that scholars as well as the general public have largely ignored these forms of aggression also means that there is substantial room for girls' aggression to be "discovered" at a time where concern about youthful violence is heightened.

Finally, girls' behavior, including violence, needs to be put in its patriarchal context. In her analysis of self-reported violence in girls in Canada, Artz (1998) has done precisely that, and the results were striking. First, she noted that violent girls reported significantly greater rates of victimization and abuse than their nonviolent counterparts, and that girls who were violent reported great fear of sexual assault, especially from their boyfriends. Specifically, 20% of violent girls stated they were physically abused at home, compared to 10% of violent males and 6.3% of nonviolent girls. Patterns for sexual abuse were even starker; roughly 1 out of 4 violent girls had been sexually abused, compared to 1 in 10 of nonviolent girls (Artz, 1998). Follow-up interviews with a small group of violent girls found that they had learned at home that "might makes right" and engaged in "horizontal violence" directed at other powerless girls (often with boys as the audience). Certainly, these findings provide little ammunition for those who would contend that the "new" violent girl is a product of any form of "emancipation."

Detailed comparisons drawn from supplemental homicide reports from unpublished FBI data also hint at the central, rather than peripheral, way in which gender has colored and differentiated even the most serious of girls' and boys' violence. In a study of these FBI data on the characteristics of girls' and boys' homicides between 1984 and 1993, Loper and Cornell (1996) found that girls accounted for "proportionately fewer homicides in 1993 (6%) than in 1984 (14%)" (p. 324). They found that, in comparison to boys' homicides, girls who killed were more likely to use a knife than a gun and to murder someone as a result of conflict (rather than in the commission of a crime). Girls were also more likely than boys to murder family members (32 %) and very young victims (24% of their victims were under the age of 3 compared to 1% of the boys' victims). When involved in a peer homicide, girls were more likely than boys to have killed as a result of an interpersonal conflict and were more likely to kill alone, while boys were more likely to kill with an accomplice. Loper and Cornell concluded that "the stereotype of girls becoming gun-toting robbers was not supported. The dramatic increase in gun-related homicides . . . applies to boys but not girls" (p. 332).

In conclusion, what needs to be understood about girls' delinquency, particularly from a programmatic and policy standpoint is that gender provides an important and complex context within which even violence is enacted. For girls who enter the juvenile justice system, including girls with a history of violence and aggression, there is a clear link between victimization, trauma, and delinquency. The other major theme that must be addressed is the fact that most often this trauma produces not violent offenses but rather what have long been regarded as "trivial" or unimportant offenses like running away from home.

Simply stated, the current trends in juvenile justice suggest that social control of girls is once again on the criminal justice agenda—this century it is justified by their purported "violence," just as in the past century it was justified by their sexuality. (See Corrado et al., 2000, for a similar pattern in Canada.)

## GIRLS' TROUBLES AND TRAUMA: NONAGGRESSIVE OFFENSES AND VIOLENT VICTIMZATIONS

While the media has focused attention on girls' violent, nontraditional delinquency, most of girls' delinquency is not of that sort at all. However, understanding these offenses is also important in exploring girl's aggression and violence, since these are the behaviors that are currently being relabeled as "person offenses."

Examining the types of offenses for which girls have historically been arrested, it is clear that most are arrested for the less serious criminal acts and status offenses (noncriminal offenses for which only youth can be taken into custody, such as "running away from home" or "curfew violation"). Even today, despite the increases in girl's arrests for violent offenses, roughly half of girls' arrests were for either larceny theft (21.5%) much of which, particularly for girls, is shoplifting (Shelden & Horvath, 1986) or status offenses (21.8%). Boys' arrests were far more dispersed (Federal Bureau of Investigation, 2001, p. 221).

## Status Offenses

Status offenses have long played a significant role among the offenses that bring girls into the juvenile justice system. They accounted for about a quarter all girls' arrests in 2000, but only 10% of boys' arrests—figures that remained relatively stable during the last decade. In 2000, over half (58.9%) of those arrested for one status offense—running away from home—were girls (Federal Bureau of Investigation, 2001, p. 221). Running away from home and prostitution remain the only two arrest categories where more girls than boys are arrested.

The passage of the Juvenile Justice and Delinquency Prevention Act in 1974, which, among other things, encouraged jurisdictions to divert and deinstitutionalize youth charged with status offenses, did result in a slight decrease in these arrests. As an example, the last decade did show a 16.3% drop in arrests of girls for runaway (although, ironically, the decrease for boys was sharper—20.2%). However, some of the leveling off of these arrest numbers is likely explained by the relabeling of these offenses as person offenses. Parents increasingly seek to do this, since police will often refuse to arrest and detain youth charged only with status offenses because of the deinstitutionalization mandates. Such is not the case with person offenses, particularly "domestic violence," which in some states, like Florida, *requires* detention.

Similarly, abolishing status offenses and the implementation of the fair-procedure 1982 *Young Offenders Act (YOA)* in Canada is reported by some to have not changed or improved the treatment of delinquent girls (Corrado et al., 2000; Duffy, 1996; Reitsma-Street, 1999). Specifically, since passage of the YOA, the use of custodial dispositions for young females did not decrease as expected, particularly for minor offenses (Corrado et al., 2000).

Why are girls more likely than boys to be arrested for running away from home? There are no simple answers to this question. Studies of actual delinquency (not simply arrests) show that girls and boys run away from home in about equal numbers. As an example, Canter (1982) found in a National Youth Survey that there was no evidence of greater female involvement, compared to males, in any category of delinquent behavior. Indeed, in this sample males were significantly more likely than females to report status offenses. There is some evidence to suggest that parents and police may be responding differently to the same behavior. Parents may be calling the police when their daughters do not come home, and police may be more likely to arrest a female than a male runaway youth.

Finally, research on the characteristics of girls in the California Youth Authority (CYA) system reveals that while these girls cannot be incarcerated in the Youth Authority for status offenses, nearly half (45%) had been charged with status offenses prior to their incarceration in the CYA for more serious offenses (Bloom & Campbell, 1998). Focus groups with program staff working in a variety of settings in California also indicated that these individuals felt that girls in that state were chiefly involved in the juvenile justice system for offenses such as "petty theft, shoplifting, assault and battery, drug violations, gang activity and truancy, lying to a police officer, and running away" (Bloom & Campbell, 1998).

## Sexual and Physical Abuse

Research illustrates the differences in the reasons that boys and girls have for running away. Girls are, for example, much more likely than boys to be the victims of child sexual abuse, with some experts estimating that roughly 70% of the victims of child sexual abuse are girls (Finkelhor & Baron, 1986). Not surprisingly, the evidence also suggests a link between this problem and girl's delinquency—particularly running away from home.

Studies of girls on the streets or in court populations depict high rates of both sexual and physical abuse. A study of a runaway shelter in Toronto found, for example, that 73% of the female runaways and 38% of the males had been sexually abused. This same study found that sexually abused female runaways were more likely than their nonabused counterparts to engage in delinquent or criminal activities such as substance abuse, petty theft, and prostitution. No such pattern was found among the male runaways (McCormack, Janus, & Burgess, 1986). A similar study of 372 homeless and runaway youth in Seattle living on the street and in shelters reported that girls (30%) were twice as likely as boys (15%) to report sexual abuse histories, and that "extreme violence" was higher among the girls' than the boys' sexual abuse reports (Tyler, Hoyt, Whitbeck, & Cauce, 2001). Girls were significantly more likely than boys to report being victimized in their homes as well as on the street after they ran away. Furthermore, the more sexual abuse the youth experienced at home, the more likely he or she was to run away at a younger age. This is particularly important given research that finds for both boys and girls that an early age of delinquency onset is related to more serious delinquency past age 14 (Piquero & Chung, 2001). The Seattle study also found that the runaway girls were more likely than the runaway boys to report both selling sex and being sexually victimized on the street (Tyler et al., 2001). This is consistent with Schaffner's (1998) contention that the "solutions" to girls' sexual victimization (such as running away from home to escape sexual abuse) are often sexually troubling situations.

Detailed studies of youth entering the juvenile justice system in Florida have compared the "constellations of problems" presented by girls and boys entering detention (Dembo, Schmeidler, Sue, Borden, & Manning, 1995; Dembo, Williams, & Schmeidler, 1993). These researchers have found that female youth were more likely than male youth to have abuse histories and contact with the juvenile justice system for status offenses, while male youth had higher rates of involvement with various delinquent offenses. Further research on a larger cohort of youth ($n$ = 2,104) admitted to an assessment center in Tampa concluded that "girls' problem behavior commonly relates to an abusive and traumatizing home life, whereas boys' law violating behavior reflects their involvement in a delinquent life style" (Dembo et al., 1995, p. 21).

More recent research confirms Dembo's insights; Cauffman, Feldman, Waterman, and Steiner (1998) studied the backgrounds of 96 girls in the custody of the CYA and compared these results with those garnered from a comparison sample of male youth ($n$ = 93) held by CYA. In this comparison, Cauffman and colleagues found that while boys were more likely to be traumatized as observers of violence, "girls were more likely to be traumatized as direct victims" (more than half the girls were the victims of either sexual or physical abuse). Perhaps as a result, girls were significantly more likely than boys to be currently suffering from posttraumatic stress disorder (PTSD); the levels of PTSD found in this population were "significantly higher than among the general adolescent female population" (11% compared to 65%; Cauffman et al., 1998). Interestingly, about two-thirds of the girls in this sample were serving time for a violent offense (murder, assault, robbery), and 43% of the girls identified as gang members (Cauffman et al., 1998).

A study of 444 incarcerated youth in Ohio found that for every measure of experienced or witnessed violence, girls reported significantly higher rates. Given that the boys' reported rates were still alarmingly high, this is particularly troubling. The most extreme gender differences were for sexual abuse, followed by physical abuse by non-family members. Two-thirds of the boys and three-fourths of the girls reported physical abuse from a family member, while two-thirds of girls and one-third of boys reported physical abuse by a non-family member. Three-fifths of girls and almost one-fifth of boys reported sexual abuse histories (Holsinger et al., 1999).

In short, while these offenses appear trivial, girls who exhibit these behaviors have problems (usually as a result of exposure to sexual and physical victimization) that are profound. All the more ironic is the fact that if current trends continue, more and more of these girls will find themselves arrested, detained, and labeled as "violent" themselves when they seek to escape violent situations.

## CONCLUSIONS

Girl's aggression and violence has long been ignored, trivialized, and minimized. This denial not only permits the occasional "discovery" of "bad girls," particularly by the media, but it also means that minor changes in enforcement practices can make it appear that girls' behavior has changed, when in actuality, that is not the case.

Specifically, we suggest that the "closing gender gap" in youthful violence and aggression is largely a myth. Rather, it appears that changes in arrest data over time are likely the product of changes in the behavior of parents, school officials, and law enforcement. One of these shifts is the relabeling of behaviors that were once subsumed under status offenses as crimes of violence (often so that the parent can get their daughter arrested and detained). For example, youth who hit a parent were once charged as CHINS (Children in Need of Supervision) or PINS (Persons in Need of Supervision). Today these girls are likely to be charged with "assault." In addition to this "relabeling," the popularity of "zero tolerance policies" on and around school campuses has meant the minor forms of youth-on-youth violence that were once handled internally are increasingly criminalized.

This chapter also emphasizes the need to avoid both denial and demonization of girl's violence, and to seek to understand the context which produces girl's aggressive behavior. How is it that girls and boys use aggression differently? How do those who label the behavior as criminal decide to do so? Finally, despite dramatic changes in girl's arrests for "violent" offenses, most girls are still arrested for non-aggressive and drug offenses. Even those girls arrested for "violent" offenses are likely quite different from their violent male counterparts and far more like the "traditional" girl delinquent than many assumed.

## NOTES

1. As an example, Canter (1982) reported a male versus female, self-reported delinquency ratio of 3.5:1 for serious assault and 3.4:1 for minor assault in a survey done in 1976. At that time, arrest statistics showed much greater male participation in aggravated assault (5.6:1) and simple assault (3.8:1) (Federal Bureau of Investigation, 1980). Currently, arrest statistics show a 3.3:1 ratio for "aggravated assault" and a 2.2:1 ratio for "other assaults" (Federal Bureau of Investigation, 1999).
2. In this report, "serious crimes of violence" will refer to the Federal Bureau of Investigation's index offenses which are used to measure violent crime: murder, forcible rape, aggravated assault, and robbery.

## REFERENCES

Acoca, L. (1999). Investing in girls: A 21st century challenge. *Juvenile Justice, 6*(1), 3–13.

Artz, S. (1998). *Sex, power and the violent school girl.* Toronto: Trifolium Books.

Bartollas, C. (1993). Little girls grown up: The perils of institutionalization. In C. Culliver (Ed.), *Female criminality: The state of the art* (pp. 469–482). New York: Garland Press.

Belknap, J., Dunn, M., & Holsinger, K. (1997, February). *Moving toward juvenile justice and youth-serving systems that address the distinct experience of the adolescent female* (Gender Specific Work Group Report to the Governor). Columbus, OH: Office of Criminal Justice Services.

Belknap, J., Winter, E., & Cady, B. (2001). *Assessing the needs of committed delinquent and pre-adjudicated girls in Colorado: A focus group study* [Report]. Denver: Colorado Division of Youth Corrections.

Bergsmann, I. R. (1989). The forgotten few: Juvenile female offenders. *Federal Probation, 53*(1), 73–78.

Bjorkqvist, K., & Niemela, P. (1992). New trends in the study of female aggression. In K. Bjorkqvist & P. Niemela (Eds.), *Of mice and women: Aspects of female aggression* (pp. 1–16). San Diego, CA: Academic Press.

Bjorkqvist K., Osterman K., & Kaukiainen, A. (1992). The development of direct and indirect aggressive strategies in males and females. In K. Bjorkqvist & P. Niemela (Eds.), *Of mice and women: Aspects of female aggression* (pp. 51–64). San Diego, CA: Academic Press.

Bloom, B., & Campbell, R. (1998). Literature and policy review. In B. Owen & B. Bloom (Eds.), *Modeling gender-specific services in juvenile justice: Policy and program recommendations* (pp. 1–96). Sacramento, CA: Office of Criminal Justice Planning.

Brener, N. D., Simon, T. R., Krug, E. G., & Lowry, R. (1999). Recent trends in violence-related behaviors among high school students in the United States. *Journal of the American Medical Association, 282,* 330–446.

Bureau of Criminal Information and Analysis. (1999). *Report on arrests for domestic violence in California, 1998.* Sacramento: State of California, Criminal Justice Statistics Center.

Canter, R. J. (1982). Sex differences in self-report delinquency. *Criminology, 20,* 373–393.

Cauffman, E., Feldman, S. S., Waterman, J., & Steiner, H. (1998). Posttraumatic stress disorder among female juvenile offenders. *Journal of the American Academy of Child and Adolescent Psychiatry, 31,* 1209–1216.

Centers for Disease Control and Prevention. (1992). *Youth Risk Behavior Surveillance—United States, 1991* (CDC Surveillance Summaries, U.S. Department of Health and Human Services). Atlanta, GA: Author.

Centers for Disease Control and Prevention. (1994). *Youth Risk Behavior Surveillance—United States, 1993* (CDC Surveillance Summaries U.S. Department of Health and Human Services). Atlanta, GA: Author.

Centers for Disease Control and Prevention. (1996). *Youth Risk Behavior Surveillance—United States, 1995* (CDC Surveillance Summaries, U.S. Department of Health and Human Services). Atlanta, GA: Author.

Centers for Disease Control and Prevention. (1998). *Youth Risk Behavior Surveillance—United States, 1998* (CDC Surveillance Summaries, U.S. Department of Health and Human Services). Atlanta, GA: Author.

Centers for Disease Control and Prevention. (2000). *Youth Risk Behavior Surveillance—United States, 1999* (CDC Surveillance Summaries, U.S. Department of Health and Human Services). Atlanta, GA: Author.

Chesney-Lind, M. (1999). Media misogyny: Demonizing "violent" girls and women. In J Ferrel & N. Websdale (Eds.), *Making trouble: Cultural representations of crime, deviance, and control* (pp. 115–141). New York: Aldine.

Chesney-Lind, M., & Paramore, V. (2001). Are girls getting more violent?: Exploring juvenile robbery trends. *Journal of Contemporary Criminal Justice, 17,* 142–166.

Corrado, R. R., Odgers, C., & Cohen, I. M. (2000). The incarceration of female young offenders: Protection for whom? *Canadian Journal of Criminology, 2,* 189–207.

Crick, N. R., & Grotpeter, J. K. (1995). Relational aggression, gender, and social-psychological adjustment. *Child Development, 66,* 710–722.

Crick, N. R., Werner, N. E., Casas, J. F., O'Brien, K. M., Nelson, D. A., Grotpeter, J. K., & Markon, K. (1998). Childhood aggression and gender: A new look at an old problem. In D. Bernstein (Ed.), *Gender and motivation* (pp. 75–141). Lincoln: University of Nebraska Press.

Crime Prevention and Justice Assistance Division. (1997). *Crime in Hawaii: 1998.* Honolulu: Department of the Attorney General.

Crime Prevention and Justice Assistance Division. (1998). *Crime in Hawaii: 1978.* Honolulu: Department of the Attorney General.

Currie, E. (1998). *Crime and punishment in America.* New York: Metropolitan Books.

Dembo, R., Schmeidler, J., Sue, S. C., Borden, P., & Manning, D. (1995). Gender differences in service needs among youths entering a juvenile assessment center: A replication study. *Journal of Correctional Health Care, 2,* 191–217.

Dembo, R., Williams, L., & Schmeidler, J. (1993). Gender differences in mental health service needs among youths entering a juvenile detention center. *Journal of Prison and Jail Health, 12,* 73–101.

Duffy, A. (1996). Bad girls in hard times: Canadian female juvenile offenders. In G. O'Bireck (Ed.), *Not a kid anymore* (pp. 203–220). Scarborough: Nelson Canada.

Federal Bureau of Investigation. (1980). *Crime in the United States 1979*. Washington, DC: U.S. Government Printing Office.

Federal Bureau of Investigation. (1991). *Crime in the United States 1990*. Washington, DC: U.S. Government Printing Office.

Federal Bureau of Investigation. (1999). *Crime in the United States 1998*. Washington, DC: U.S. Government Printing Office.

Federal Bureau of Investigation. (2001). *Crime in the United States 2000*. Washington, DC: U. S. Government Printing Office.

Finkelhor, D., & Baron, L. (1986). Risk factors for child sexual abuse. *Journal of Interpersonal Violence, 1*, 43–71.

Freitas, K., & Chesney-Lind, M. (2001, August/September). Difference doesn't mean difficult: Workers talk about working with girls. *Women, Girls, and Criminal Justice, 2*, 65–78.

Gaarder, E., & Belknap, J. (2002). Tenuous borders: Girls transferred to adult court. *Criminology, 40*, 481–517.

Gropper, N., & Froschl, M. (2000). The role of gender in young children's teasing and bullying behavior. *Equity and Excellence in Education, 33*(1), 48–56.

Holsinger, K., Belknap, J., & Sutherland, J. L. (1999). *Assessing the gender specific program and service needs for adolescent females in the juvenile justice system* (Report). Columbus, OH: Office of Criminal Justice Services.

Huizinga, D. (1997). *Over-time changes in delinquency and drug use: The 1970's to the 1990's* [Unpublished report]. Washington, DC: Office of Juvenile Justice and Delinquency Prevention.

Lederman, C. S., & Brown, E. N. (2000). Entangled in the shadows: Girls in the juvenile justice system. *Buffalo Law Review, 48*, 909–925.

Loper, A. B., & Cornell, D. G. (1996). Homicide by girls. *Journal of Child and Family Studies, 5*, 321–333.

Males, M., & Shorter, A. (2001). *To cage and serve*. Unpublished manuscript, Center for Juvenile Justice.

Mayer, J. (1994). *Girls in the Maryland juvenile justice system: Findings of the female population taskforce*. Presentation to the Gender Specific Services Training Group, Minneapolis, MN.

McCormack, A., Janus, M. D., & Burgess, A. W. (1986). Runaway youths and sexual victimization: Gender differences in an adolescent runaway population. *Child Abuse and Neglect, 10*, 387–395.

Office of Juvenile Justice and Delinquency Prevention. (1999). *What about girls? Females in the juvenile justice system* [Flyer]. Washington, DC: U.S. Department of Justice.

Okamoto, S., & Chesney-Lind, M. (2002, October/November). Girls and relational aggression: Beyond the "mean girl" hype. *Women, Girls, and Criminal Justice*, 81–90.

Okamoto, S. K. (2002). The challenges of male practitioners working with female youth clients. *Child and Youth Care Forum, 31*, 257–268.

Piquero, A. R., & Chung, H.L. (2001). On the relationships between gender, early onset, and the seriousness of offending. *Journal of Criminal Justice, 29*, 189–206.

Reitsma-Street, M. (1999). Justice for Canadian girls: A 1990's update. *Canadian Journal of Criminology, 41*, 335–364.

Robinson, R. (1990). *Violations of girlhood: A qualitative study of female delinquents and children in need of services in Massachusetts.* Unpublished doctoral dissertation, Brandeis University.

Schaffner, L. (1998). Female juvenile delinquency: Sexual solutions, gender bias, and juvenile justice. *Hastings Women's Law Journal, 9*, 1–25.

Shelden, R., & Horvath, J. (1986). *Processing offenders in a juvenile court: A comparison of male and female offenders.* Paper presented at the annual meeting of the Western Society of Criminology, Newport Beach, CA.

Stahl, A. L. (1999). *Delinquency cases in juvenile courts, 1996.* (OJJDP Publication No. 109). Washington, DC: U.S. Department of Justice.

Steffensmeier, D. J., & Steffensmeier, R. H. (1980). Trends in female delinquency: An examination of arrest, juvenile court, self-report, and field data. *Criminology, 18*, 62–85.

Steinem, G. (2001). Supremacy crimes. In L. Richardson, V. Taylor, & N. Whittier (Eds.), *Feminist frontiers* (pp. 462–464). Boston: McGraw-Hill.

Tiet, Q. Q., Wasserman, G. A., Loeber, R., McReynolds, L. S., & Miller, L. S. (2001). Developmental and sex differences in types of conduct problems. *Journal of Child and Family Studies, 10*(2), 181–197.

Tyler, K. A., Hoyt, D. R., Whitbeck, L. B., & Cauce, A. M. (2001). The impact of childhood sexual abuse or later sexual victimization among runaway youth. *Journal of Research on Adolescence, 11*, 151–176.

# PART IV

# GIRLS AS PERPETRATORS AND VICTIMS OF ABUSIVE AND CONFLICTUAL RELATIONSHIPS

*Adolescence and Adulthood*

# CHAPTER 11

# Women's Involvement in Aggression in Young Adult Romantic Relationships

## A Developmental Systems Model

Deborah M. Capaldi, Hyoun K. Kim, *and* Joann Wu Shortt

The image of physical aggression in romantic relationships that is commonly portrayed by the media is that of a man who is violent toward his female partner due to his desire to control her, or perhaps to his innate violent tendencies. Much research from a feminist perspective has utilized specialized samples such as agency populations (e.g., shelter samples) and concentrated on aggressive behaviors in men, the impact on women (e.g., injuries, depressive symptoms), and on women's responses to men's violence toward them, including coping behaviors. Studies based on this conceptualization typically focus on factors influencing men's violence, such as cultural and historical attitude, power, and resource imbalance between partners (e.g., Walker, 1984).

In this chapter, we begin with discussions of how leading theoretical perspectives in the area of partner violence view women's role in partner violence and point to the need to move beyond a primary focus on men only toward a view of partner violence as a dyadic process focusing on both partners within the dyad. We describe a developmental systems perspective that incorporates *both* partners' developmental characteristics, behaviors, and interactional processes to explain violence within these intimate dyads, and we present findings from our studies that have tested aspects of a developmental contextual or systems model of aggression toward a partner. Throughout the chapter, we emphasize the importance of examining women's role in the study of aggression in intimate relationships.

## BATTERER TYPOLOGIES: WOMEN AS VICTIMS, NOT AGENTS, OF AGGRESSION

Several recent research efforts have focused on defining typologies of men who are aggressive toward a partner—the batterer typologies (Gottman, 2001; Gottman et al., 1995; Holtzworth-Munroe & Stuart, 1994; Meehan, Holtzworth-Munroe, & Herron, 2001). Batterer typologies are driven largely by the goal of improving the outcomes of treatment programs for men by defining subtypes who may respond to different forms of treatment and intervention. Holtzworth-Munroe and Stuart (1994) identified three subtypes of batterers, namely generally violent/antisocial, dysphoric/borderline, and family only. Holtzworth-Munroe, Meehan, Herron, Rehman, and Stuart (2000) added a fourth subtype, namely low-level antisocial. However, the purpose of typology work has been extended to attempting to explain men's aggression toward women. Consistent with feminist theories, batterer typology work rests on the assumption that domestic violence is men's aggression toward women and can best be understood by focusing only on traits of the men. The typologies have largely been tested on samples recruited by flyers and newspaper advertising with respondents screened for men's violence toward women. The behavior of the women toward the men, including aggression, is generally not considered, or they are portrayed as victims and not agents of aggression.

## FAMILY VIOLENCE PERSPECTIVE: COUPLES AS MUTUALLY AGGRESSIVE

Contrary to the assumption that aggression within couples generally involves women being assaulted by men, almost one-half of the violent episodes reported in intimate relationships involve men and women being mutually aggressive (Brush, 1990; Stets & Straus, 1990). Findings across other studies have also indicated a similar or even a higher prevalence and frequency of physically aggressive acts toward partners by women, particularly during young adulthood (e.g., Harned, 2001; Straus, 1997; Straus & Gelles, 1986, 1990; Sugarman & Hotaling, 1989). In a cross-national comparison between the United States and New Zealand (National Family Violence Surveys—Straus & Gelles, 1986; National Youth Survey—Elliott, Huizinga, & Morse, 1985; and Dunedin Multidisciplinary Health and Development Study—Magdol, Moffitt, Caspi, & Silva, 1997) for young adults (under age 25 years), the perpetration rates reported by women ranged from 36 to 51%, whereas rates reported by men were from 22 to 43%. Similarly, the victimization rates reported by women ranged from 27 to 39%, and rates reported by men were from 27 to 56% (Magdol et al., 1997). These findings are primarily from studies by family violence researchers, pioneered and typified by the larger-scale surveys conducted by Strauss and colleagues (Straus & Gelles, 1986). The family violence perspective forms the second major body of work on the topic of physical aggression in couples and is mostly based on results from use of the Conflict Tactics Scale (CTS; Straus, 1979) assessing the prevalence and frequency of acts ranging from pushing and shoving to assaults with a weapon.

As might be expected, the dialogue between researchers from feminist or male-focused versus family violence perspectives regarding the interpretation of these findings has been prolonged and heated. There have been several critiques of the CTS, for example, that it does not adequately take the context and impact of aggression into account (Heyman, Feldbau-Kohn, Ehrensaft, Langhinrichsen-Rohling, & O'Leary, 2001). It has frequently been posited that women's aggression toward a partner is in self-defense (e.g., Makepeace, 1986), that it is infrequent and of low severity (Johnson, 1995), that women experience greater impact of aggression than their partners, including more and more severe injuries (Morse, 1995; Vivian & Langhinrichsen-Rohling, 1994), and also that only women experience fear of their partner's aggression (Cascardi, O'Leary, Lawrence, & Schlee, 1995; Jacobson et al., 1994).

There is now considerable evidence that women's role in aggression toward a partner is more active than depicted in the studies just cited. A substantial amount of violence in intimate relationships is initiated by women, rather than by men (Bland & Orn, 1986; DeMaris, 1992; Morse, 1995; Stets & Straus, 1990). Among the women involved in violent relationships in the National Family Violence Survey, 53.1% reported initiating physical aggression, whereas 42.3% of them reported that their partner initiated such aggression. Several studies have indicated that, regardless of whether the information came from men or women respondents or whether severe and minor assaults were examined separately, findings were robust in indicating at least equal rates of assaults by the women and men partners (Carrado, George, Loxam, Jones, & Templar, 1996; Straus, 1997). Furthermore, a few studies that examined reasons for aggression indicated that a majority of women did not identify their aggression as self-defense or retaliation (Carrado et al.,

1996). Rather, men were more likely to report using physical aggression in the effort to retaliate for being hit first than were women (Follingstad, Wright, Lloyd, & Sebastian, 1991). Archer's (2000) meta-analysis study of sex differences in injuries suggested that studies with samples at younger ages (ages 14–22 years) found almost equal injury rates, whereas studies using older age samples found higher rates of infliction of injuries by men, but still with a significant proportion of injuries sustained by men. These findings are contradictory to the self-defense argument and suggest that, by a conservative estimate, women contribute at least equally to the initiation of physical violence in couples' relationships.

## A DEVELOPMENTAL PERSPECTIVE: ANTISOCIAL GIRLS, ANTISOCIAL PARTNERS

Building on the family violence approaches, a third perspective has emerged that focuses on the developmental origins of partner violence and examines violence and aggression toward a partner within the context of the developmental histories of behaviors and experiences in childhood and adolescence of both young men and women. The developmental approach has surfaced from several longitudinal studies that were originally designed to address aspects of child and adolescent development, particularly the development of antisocial behavior, but had the unique opportunity to assess aggression toward a partner in later adolescence and young adulthood. Findings from these studies indicate that conduct problems or antisocial behavior in childhood or adolescence are predictive of later aggression toward a partner for both young men (Andrews, Foster, Capaldi, & Hops, 2000; Capaldi & Clark, 1998; Ehrensaft, Cohen, Brown, Smailes, & Johnson, 2003; Magdol et al., 1998; Woodward, Fergusson, & Horwood, 2002) and young women (Andrews et al., 2000; Ehrensaft et al., 2003; Giordano, Millhollin, Cernkovich, Pugh, & Randolph, 1999; Magdol et al., 1998; Woodward et al., 2002). Magdol and colleagues (1998) found that problem behavior (i.e., conduct problems, aggressive behavior, and substance use) was the most consistent predictor of physical aggression toward a partner in young adulthood, especially for women. In addition, antisocial behavior during childhood and adolescence was found to be predictive of victimization as well as perpetration for women in young adulthood (Bardone, Moffitt, Caspi, Dickson, & Silva, 1996; Magdol et al., 1998).

The findings from developmental studies have several major implications. The first is that aggression toward a partner by men is associated with a developmental history of antisocial behavior, rather than being a strategy employed by men in general. Second, it appears that there is similarity in the developmental histories of young men and women who engage in aggression toward a partner. Young women who have previously shown higher levels of antisocial behavior are more likely to use aggressive tactics with their partners and to be involved in violent relationships. That there is similarity in men and women in the etiology of this behavior is not consistent with theories which posit, at least for late adolescents and young adults, that this behavior is different in men and women and that aggression toward a partner is predominantly a male phenomenon.

A further contribution of developmental approaches to the area of partner violence is that they provide an important conceptual framework for developing a comprehensive theory of partner violence that is based on the interrelated developmental influences of multiple factors (Capaldi & Clark, 1998). These may include contextual factors (e.g., socioeconomic status), parental behaviors (e.g., antisocial behavior and aggression toward a partner), parenting (e.g., discipline and monitoring), and child development (e.g., history of aggressive behaviors, academic failure). Such developmental models also have profound significance for the development of intervention and prevention programs early on for high-risk individuals. Girls with higher levels of antisocial behavior are also more likely to leave the family-of-origin home early, have multiple cohabitation partners, and experience early childbearing (Bardone et al., 1996). Thus, being in violent relationships also adds to the risk for the offspring of these young women. Findings from these prospective studies are sufficiently compelling to indicate that girls (as well as boys) with behavioral problems should participate in programs to prevent violence in their later romantic relationships.

## A DEVELOPMENTAL SYSTEMS PERSPECTIVE

More recently, the developmental model has been expanded to incorporate a developmental contextual perspective whereby aggression toward a partner is examined within a lifespan, individual–environment interaction framework (Capaldi & Gorman-Smith, 2003; Capaldi & Shortt, 2003). This approach, which is perhaps best characterized as a developmental systems perspective, posits that the manifestation or continuation of individual behavior is an interaction between individual prior dispositions and learning and the environments selected or entered. Given that intimate relationships are dyadic and reciprocal by nature, a partner's characteristics, behaviors, and interactions with the partner constitutes a pivotal environment for an individual, and the couple constitutes a developmental system. Therefore, from this perspective, women (as well as men) play a significant role in partners' aggressive behavior.

One piece of evidence that supports this developmental systems model can be found in studies on assortative partnering. Several studies have found that there is assortative partnering by antisocial behavior and that this contributes to the continuity of personality attributes such as antisocial behavior for both men and women (Caspi & Herbener, 1990; Quinton, Pickles, Maughan, & Rutter, 1993). According to the developmental systems perspective, assortative partnering tends to occur through at least two individual–environment interaction mechanisms. The first mechanism is by active selection of environments (e.g., a young woman who likes to "party" and use substances is likely to meet young men with the same preferences at such activities and is likely to date such young men). Second, engagement in conduct problems and related adjustment failures (Capaldi & Shortt, 2003) leads to unintended restriction of environmental options (e.g., an adolescent who drops out of high school may not attend a 4-year college and is unlikely to date a young woman attending such a college). Once the young man and woman are involved in a relationship, interactions between the partners can also provoke or reinforce aggressive behaviors within dyads (Buss, 1987; Scarr & McCartney, 1983). Aggressive characteristics of the partner may tend to support or to evoke aggressive characteristics of the individual. If the partner accepts aggressive behavior by the individual, rather than expressing dislike, this may encourage the continuance of the behavior. An individual may evoke responses from their partner by verbal aggression (e.g., threats and jealous accusations may be responded to with similarly aggressive responses) or by physical aggression (e.g., if one partner hits, the other may hit back). The likelihood of aggressive exchanges taking place increases when both partners have poor interpersonal skills due to antisocial behavior or depressive symptoms. When aggression does occur during interactions, it is likely to escalate or be prolonged in couples when both partners are high in antisocial behavior or depressive symptoms. Therefore, a strong influence on aggression toward a partner is hypothesized to be the partner's risk characteristics.

## STUDY DESIGN

As implied in the discussions of the developmental systems model, one of the challenges in the study of partner violence involves study designs. Until very recently, relatively little headway was being made in addressing the controversial issues in the field and in understanding the occurrence of physical aggression in young couples because of limitations in the prevailing samples and study designs. These limitations include small samples of convenience, lack of prospective longitudinal designs, surveys asking limited questions of only one partner, overreliance on self-report data, and large-scale surveys that may have been unable to recruit some of the most aggressive and problematic individuals.

There are three critical study design issues that must be addressed in order to further advance our understandings of aggression toward a partner, or domestic violence, and the role of men and women in such behavior. Currently, much of our thinking regarding gender differences in aggression toward a partner is based on studies where data were collected only from women and/or where the same data were not collected for both sexes. Even when both sexes were examined, most often the individuals were not paired couples. However, to examine the behavior of men and women and to draw any conclusions regarding gender differences, the *same* data should be collected on both the men and the women in a relationship, and where possible, the significance of *differences* in findings for the men and women should be tested directly. Another issue is that multimethod, multiagent studies are needed in this area. Observational study of couples' behavior is particularly crucial, as interviews and questionnaires may elicit socially desirable responses and also be affected by gender stereotypes. We find that research on aggression in intimate relationships is one of the areas that is vulnerable to gender stereotypes and that it is important to be forthright in examining the effects of gender stereotyped biases from initial design and to interpretation of results. Finally, it is important to have a prospective longitudinal design to examine changes in aggression over time, including the possibility that the developmental patterns of partner aggression between men and women in adulthood may differ.

## AGE TRENDS IN AGGRESSION TOWARD A PARTNER

The finding that rates of physical aggression toward a partner have been found to be highest at young ages and to decrease with time (Gelles & Straus, 1988) has prompted further study of the prevalence of aggression in younger, dating couples. Prevalence rates of perpetration or victimization among adolescents range from 20 to 60%, and hypothesized age trends in prevalence in men's physical aggression toward a partner estimated from cross-sectional data indicate a sharp rise from ages 15–25 years, a peak prevalence at around age 25 years, and a sharp decline to about age 35 years (O'Leary, 1999). However, it is not clear if the hypothesized rise to age 25 years mainly reflects the fact that many more individuals are engaged in romantic relationships at age 25 years than age 15 years. The relative engagement in aggression toward a partner by men and women may vary by age. In a meta-analysis of sex differences

in aggression between male–female partners (Archer, 2000), a categorical analysis by age showed values in the direction of a higher prevalence
of female than male physical aggression for the younger age group (ages
14–22 years) and a higher prevalence of aggression for men than women
in the older age group (ages 23–49 years), although the shift was relatively small. We begin the second part of the chapter by describing our
research design, including samples and measures, followed by descriptions of findings from our research on aggression in intimate relationships among young adults that illuminates the role of at-risk late adolescent and young adult women in aggression in young couples.

## OREGON YOUTH STUDY AND COUPLES STUDY

Our research on partner violence is based on data from the Oregon
Youth Study (OYS) and the Couples Study of the OYS men and their intimate partners. The OYS is an ongoing community-based longitudinal
study in which 206 boys were recruited through fourth-grade classes in
higher crime areas of a medium-sized metropolitan city in the Pacific
Northwest. Yearly assessments were collected through young adulthood,
including data from multiple sources (e.g., the boy, both parents, teachers, school and official records, peers, romantic partners) and observational data of family, peer, and romantic partner interactions, as well as
interview and questionnaire data. Participation rates in late adolescence
and young adulthood averaged about 98%, or a sample size of just over
200 (Capaldi, Chamberlain, Fetrow, & Wilson, 1997).

The Couples Study is another ongoing longitudinal study of the
OYS young men and their women partners. The first wave of the Couples Study was collected when the OYS men were in late adolescence
(time 1, ages 17–20 years; $n = 118$). The second and third follow-up
data collections were conducted when the men were in young adulthood
(time 2, ages 20–23 years; $n = 159$) and early adulthood (time 3, ages
23–25 years; $n = 148$), respectively. The average length of relationship
increased from 11 months to 2 years and 10 months between time 1 and
time 3, and the proportion of couples that were cohabiting or married
increased from 30 to 72%. The study utilizes the developmental systems
perspective, whereby both partners' individual characteristics (e.g., antisocial behavior and depressive symptoms), several relational aspects
(e.g., conflict, satisfaction, aggression toward a partner), and interactional processes are closely examined.

Aggression toward a partner was measured by both partners' reports of psychological and physical aggression, including both their own
and their partner's behaviors, as well as by coded behavior and coder

ratings of a problem-solving interaction between the young couple where they discussed issues selected from a couples' issues checklist (Capaldi & Clark, 1998; Capaldi & Crosby, 1997). Our study is the first, to our knowledge, that has observed physical aggression in laboratory interactions (for a discussion of safety issues, see Capaldi & Clark, 1998). Physical aggression (and psychological aggression) are coded while couples discuss relationship problems. The microsocial coded variable for physically aggressive behaviors included aversive physical contact that ranged from slight shoves to punches and hard hits, and included a wide variety of acts such as pinching, poking with a pencil, and kicking. Self-report data included interview and questionnaire measures of physical and psychological aggression at each time point and included the CTS from time 2 onward.

Young men and women picked topics for discussion independently. The most frequently picked topic at time 1 (ages 17–20 years for the young man) was partner's jealousy (chosen by 15% of young men and 14% of young women), followed by the issue of where to go when going out together (11% men, 9% women). For the young women, the next three ranked topics were not having enough money for dates/activities; not liking the way her partner drinks, smokes, or uses drugs; and having a hard time talking to each other. The next three ranked topics for the young men included the money and partner's substance use items, and also included not liking some of his partner's friends. At the later time points (time 2 and time 3, ages 20–23 and 23–25 years for the young men), partner's jealousy dropped somewhat lower in the rankings. Not having enough money for activities was the most frequently picked topic by both young women and men at both of these assessments.

Overall, this study design permitted the testing of several hypotheses, including direct comparisons of each partner's violent behavior using both partners' reports and observational data, testing developmental influences of both partners on partner violence, and examining each partner's contribution to aggression within dyads. Findings presented in this chapter are from the subsets of OYS men and their women partners who participated at time 1, time 2, or time 3.

## ASSORTATIVE PARTNERING AND ITS
## ASSOCIATION WITH PARTNER VIOLENCE

As an effort to test effects of both partners' characteristics on aggression within dyads, Kim and Capaldi (2004) examined whether high levels of antisocial behavior and depressive symptoms on the part of the young women were predictive of aggression in their relationship over and above prediction from the young men's antisocial behavior and depressive symptoms (i.e., whether assortative partnering by antisocial behavior and depressive symptoms was associated with increased risk for aggression in the relationship). We found significant evidence of assortative partnering by antisocial behavior and depressive symptoms. Levels of antisocial behavior of both partners' were strongly associated, as were depressive symptoms (Kim & Capaldi, 2004). Both physical and psychological aggression in the dyad were predicted by the young woman's antisocial behavior and depressive symptoms, both concurrently and across time. Furthermore, as hypothesized by the developmental systems model, hierarchical regression analyses, including the young men's antisocial behavior and depressive symptoms, indicated that the women partners' concurrent antisocial behavior and depressive symptoms accounted for a significant amount of variance in the young men's psychological aggression, and her depressive symptoms were predictive of his physical aggression. Furthermore, both her antisocial behavior and depressive symptoms were predictive of her own physical and psychological aggression toward a partner. Longitudinal analyses, controlling for prior levels of aggression, indicated that the women's depressive symptoms were still predictive of the men's psychological aggression and that her own psychological aggression toward a partner was best predicted by her own antisocial behavior and depressive symptoms. Thus, the women's risk characteristics contributed to aggression within the dyads over and beyond the contribution from the men's antisocial behavior. These findings are consistent with the hypothesis that not only men's but also their women partners' characteristics contribute to aggression within dyads and suggest that future research should place a focus on dyadic processes of the couple.

## FREQUENT PHYSICAL AGGRESSION, INJURY, AND FEAR

In an attempt to reconcile the disparate findings of family violence and agency or shelter sample studies, Johnson (1995) posited two theoretically different kinds of violence in couples, namely, common couple violence and patriarchal terrorism. Common couple violence is hypothesized to be due to conflicts between partners that are poorly managed and occasionally escalate to minor violence and, more rarely, to serious violence, and it is posited to be more likely to be mutual, of lower frequency, and less likely to persist. Patriarchal terrorism is patterned male violence against women, and Johnson argues that such violence is likely to be much more frequent, persistent, and almost exclusively perpetrated by men. It follows that a critical question regarding the role of men and women in physical aggression toward a partner is whether the characteristics of such aggression actually differ by gender, particularly the frequency and severity of such aggression. Capaldi and Owen (2001) examined the association of *frequent* physical aggression with the impacts of injury and fear and conducted gender comparisons using time 2 data (ages 20–23 years).

## BIDIRECTIONALITY OF FREQUENT PHYSICAL AGGRESSION

Contrary to Johnson's (1995) thesis that frequent physical aggression in romantic relationships is a male-only phenomena, it was hypothesized that such aggression in couples would be likely to be bidirectional or mutual, given that physical aggression is predicted by antisocial behavior, and women also show antisocial behavior, although at lower levels than men. To test this hypothesis, Capaldi and Owen (2001) identified a group of young men and women with a mean number of aggressive acts of one or more per week in order to provide a close match to mean levels for shelter samples. By either partner's report, 9% of the young men and 13% of the young women were in this frequent group. Frequent physical aggression was significantly likely to be bidirectional in couples—the proportion of such couples was 6 times higher than expected by chance. The proportion of couples in which the man was high and the woman low was 6 times lower than expected by chance. Five percent of women were frequently physically aggressive, but had partners with low levels of aggression. That the proportion of women in the frequently physically aggressive category was somewhat higher than the proportion of men was unexpected, and indicates that antisocial behavior is unlikely to be the full explanation for levels of physical aggression toward a partner. As discussed earlier, depressive symptoms, particularly in women, were predictive of aggression, which could explain the relatively large proportion of women in the frequently physically aggressive category.

## GENDER DIFFERENCES IN INJURY RATES

Capaldi and Owen (2001) also examined gender differences in the prevalence of injuries. Injury was defined as being hurt by a partner and was judged to be on purpose or due to aggression. Thirteen percent of the young men and 9% of the young women indicated that they had been hurt at least once, with 4% of the young men and 3% of the young women indicating that they had been hurt five or more times. Injury was also likely to be mutual, at 3 times higher than expected by chance. The prevalence of injuries for young men and women in the sample was not significantly different. The most common injury for the young men was being cut or bleeding and for the young women was bruising. Descriptions of injury occasions indicated aggressive attacks by partners of both sexes. However, the three most severe injuries were to women. The probability of an injury was surprisingly low, in that even when the partner was frequently physically aggressive with an average of over one occasion of physical aggression toward a partner per week, the probability of any injury was only .40 for the young women and .19 for the young men.

## WOMEN'S PERPETRATION AND THEIR OWN RISK FOR INJURY

When the young woman was frequently aggressive toward her partner, she herself had a 3 times greater likelihood of injury, and also she had a higher probability of more frequent and severe injuries. These findings are in keeping with the contention of Straus and colleagues that one reason why physical aggression toward a partner by women is an important problem is because it may put them in danger of retaliation by their partners that may result in injury (Feld & Straus, 1989; Straus, 1999).

## PHYSICAL AGGRESSION AND FEAR

Jacobson and colleagues (1994) posited that men's violence provokes more fear in women than vice versa; therefore, the impact of violence by a partner for men and women is distinctly different. Jacobson and colleagues argued that if the function of male physical aggression is control of the partner, then only the woman should experience and express fear during arguments. Capaldi and Owen (2001) examined gender differences in the impact of fear and the association of fear with having a frequently aggressive partner and with having sustained an injury. It was predicted that due to mutual fighting and aggression and that because some young men experience injuries, men would show some degree of fear of a partner's behavior, but that young women would be more likely to be frightened by their partner's behaviors than would men.

Findings for distributions on a self-report item regarding whether the young men and women were sometimes frightened by their partner's behavior indicated no significant difference in mean levels for young men and young women on their ratings of how true it was that they were sometimes frightened by their partner's behavior. The association between being in the frequently aggressive group and the partner's report of how fearful he or she felt was significant for men's aggression and women's fear, and approached significance for the young women's aggression and her partner being fearful. For both men and women, there were significant associations between reports of being fearful of a partner and of having sustained any injury.

## STABILITY AND CHANGE IN AGGRESSION TOWARD A PARTNER OVER TIME

A major implication of the developmental systems theoretical perspective is that young men's aggression toward a partner may be expected to show some stability across partners, but also may be expected to show some changes with new partners. If aggression toward a partner was found to be as stable over time for men with new partners as for men with the same partner, but the aggression of the new women partners did not show significant association with that of the prior partners, this would be strong evidence that the aggression was *entirely* associated with something within the man (e.g., patriarchal dominance or antisocial behavior). If aggression toward a partner is more stable over time for men with the same partner than with a different partner, this suggests that characteristics of the partner or the dyadic context and interaction play an influential role in the occurrence of such aggression.

Findings for stability in aggression toward a partner from late adolescence to young adulthood indicated that there was significant stability in both physical and psychological aggression toward a partner by *both* the young man and woman, if the couple remained intact over that period (Capaldi, Shortt, & Crosby, 2003). If the young man was with a new partner, there was no significant association in the aggression construct or in reported aggression across this period. There was some evidence of significant stability in aggression in men across partners from the observational data. Further evidence for the dyadic nature of change over time came from examining the association of the levels of change for both the young men and their partners. Strong associations were found between the partners for change over time in both physical and psychological aggression within both same- and different-partner couples. Aggression thus appears to be predominantly bidirectional, with the direction of change over time for both physical and psychological aggression toward a partner tending to be synchronous.

## INITIATION OF PHYSICALLY AGGRESSIVE
## EPISODES IN YOUNG COUPLES

As discussed earlier, several studies found similar or somewhat higher rates of physical aggression initiated by women than by men (e.g., Carrado et al., 1996). All of these studies, however, used self-reports to assess initiation of violence. In recent work, we examined whether information from observation data at time 1, time 2, and time 3 would replicate the findings from the self-report data. Our observational data consisted of the discussion tasks, including party planning, each partner's chosen issue, and each partner's chosen goal discussions. Observational findings indicated that the young women were consistently more likely to initiate physical aggression than were the young men. The findings across studies on initiation of aggression thus indicate that women are engaged in initiation of aggression and do not only use aggression in self-defense.

## CONCLUSION

Findings from the OYS and Couples Study indicated that both young men and young women contribute to aggression in intimate relationships. Moreover, the role of young women, both in terms of prior developmental risk and in terms of active initiation of and engagement in physical aggression, is much greater than has been generally assumed. Young women were observed to initiate physical aggression toward their partners more frequently than were the young men. Frequent physical aggression was found likely to be bidirectional. In addition, young men, as well as young women, were found to experience negative impacts of aggression in the form of injuries and fear. Overall, the relative prevalence of frequent physical aggression by women and of injury and fear for men was surprisingly high. These findings are consistent with a model of assortative partnering by developmental risk (antisocial behavior and depressive symptoms) and of mutual couple conflict and aggression. Taken together, these findings suggest that the negative impact of women's aggression on men is substantial, rather than negligible, as frequently claimed.

Recent developmental studies on girls' antisocial behavior indicated that girls with conduct disorder or aggressive behavior in adolescence continue to have severe adjustment problems in adulthood, including difficulties in establishing a stable family and involvement in physical aggression in intimate relationships (e.g., Bardone et al., 1996). Due to a lack of attention to women's aggressive behaviors in general, our knowledge of women's role in aggression in intimate relationships is very limited. However, our findings, along with a few developmental studies on antisocial behavior in girls, indicate that the study of aggression toward a partner can be further advanced by careful assessments of women's role in aggression within the dyad. The findings that young women play an active role in aggressive relationships suggest that studying only men is unlikely to advance our understanding of the mechanisms involved in aggression toward a partner.

In conclusion, our main position is that aggression toward a partner should be approached as a process that involves interactions between individual characteristics, contextual factors, and dynamics of the relationship. Women, whether aggressive or not, should be recognized as having influence on aggressive behavior within the intimate relationship. It is believed that research based on such a perspective would help clarify the diverse influences on and pathways of aggression toward a partner and particularly benefit intervention efforts for couples in aggressive relationships. Our findings do suggest that domestic violence prevention and treatment services should include women as well as men.

## ACKNOWLEDGMENTS

Support for the Couples Study was provided by Grant No. RO1 MH 50259 from the Prevention, Early Intervention, and Epidemiology Branch, National Institute of Mental Health (NIMH), U.S. Public Health Service (USPHS). Support for the Oregon Youth Study was provided by Grant No. R37 MH 37940 from the Prevention, Early Intervention, and Epidemiology Branch, NIMH, USPHS. Support for the Intergenerational Study was provided by Grant No. HD 34511 from the National Institute of Child Health and Human Development, USPHS. Additional support was provided by Grant No. MH P30 46690 from the Prevention, Early Intervention, and Epidemiology Branch, NIMH, and the Office of Research on Minority Health, USPHS.

## REFERENCES

Andrews, J. A., Foster, S. L., Capaldi, D. M., & Hops, H. (2000). Adolescent and family predictors of physical aggression, communication, and satisfaction in young adult couples: A prospective analysis. *Journal of Consulting and Clinical Psychology, 68*, 195–208.

Archer, J. (2000). Sex differences in aggression between heterosexual partners: A meta-analytic review. *Psychological Bulletin, 126*, 651–680.

Bardone, A. M., Moffitt, T. E., Caspi, A., Dickson, N., & Silva, P. A. (1996). Adult mental health and social outcomes of adolescent girls with depression and conduct disorder. *Development and Psychopathology, 8*, 811–829.

Bland, R., & Orn, H. (1986). Family violence and psychiatric disorder. *Canadian Journal of Psychiatry, 31*, 129–137.

Brush, L. D. (1990). Violent acts and injurious outcomes in married couples: Methodological issues in the National Survey of Families and Households. *Gender and Society, 4*, 56–67.

Buss, D. M. (1987). Selection, evocation, and manipulation. *Journal of Personality and Social Psychology, 53*, 1214–1221.

Capaldi, D. M., Chamberlain, P., Fetrow, R. A., & Wilson, J. E. (1997). Conducting ecologically valid prevention research: Recruiting and retaining a "whole village" in multimethod, multiagent studies. *American Journal of Community Psychology, 25*, 471–492.

Capaldi, D. M., & Clark, S. (1998). Prospective family predictors of aggression toward female partners for at-risk young men. *Developmental Psychology, 34*, 1175–1188.

Capaldi, D. M., & Crosby, L. (1997). Observed and reported psychological and physical aggression in young, at-risk couples. *Social Development, 6*, 184–206.

Capaldi, D. M., & Gorman-Smith, D. (2003). Physical and psychological aggression in male/female adolescent and young adult couples. In P. Florsheim (Ed.), *Adolescent romantic relations and sexual behavior: Theory, research and practical implications* (pp. 244–278). Mahwah, NJ: Erlbaum.

Capaldi, D. M., & Owen, L. D. (2001). Physical aggression in a community sample of at-risk young couples: Gender comparisons for high frequency, injury, and fear. *Journal of Family Psychology, 15*, 425–440.

Capaldi, D. M., & Shortt, J. W. (2003). Understanding conduct problems in adolescence from a lifespan perspective. In G. R. Adams & M. D. Berzonsky (Eds.), *Blackwell handbook of adolescence* (pp. 470–493). Oxford, UK: Blackwell.

Capaldi, D. M., Shortt, J. W., & Crosby, L. (2003). Physical and psychological aggression in at-risk young couples: Stability and change in young adulthood. *Merrill–Palmer Quarterly, 49*, 1–27.

Carrado, M., George, M. J., Loxam, E., Jones, L., & Templar, D. (1996). Aggression in British heterosexual relationships: A descriptive analysis. *Aggressive Behavior, 22*, 401–415.

Cascardi, M., O'Leary, K. D., Lawrence, E. E., & Schlee, K. A. (1995). Characteristics of women physically abused by their spouses and who seek treatment regarding marital conflict. *Journal of Consulting and Clinical Psychology, 63*, 616–623.

Caspi, A., & Herbener, E. S. (1990). Continuity and change: Assortative marriage and the consistency of personality in adulthood. *Journal of Personality and Social Psychology, 58*, 250–258.

DeMaris, A. (1992). Male versus female initiation of aggression: The case of courtship violence. In E. C. Viano (Ed.), *Intimate violence: Interdisciplinary perspective* (pp. 111–120). Washington, DC: Hemisphere.

Ehrensaft, M. K., Cohen, P., Brown, J., Smailes, E., & Johnson, J. (2003). Intergenerational transmission of partner violence: A 20-year prospective study. *Journal of Consulting and Clinical Psychology, 71*, 741–753.

Elliott, D. S., Huizinga, D., & Morse, B. J. (1985). *The dynamics of delinquent behavior: A national survey progress report.* Boulder: Institute of Behavioral Sciences, University of Colorado.

Feld, S. L., & Straus, M. A. (1989). Escalation and desistance of wife assault in marriage. *Criminology, 27*, 141–161.

Follingstad, D. R., Wright, S., Lloyd, S., & Sebastian, J. A. (1991). Sex differences in motivations and effects in dating violence. *Family Relations, 40*, 51–57.

Gelles, R. J., & Straus, M. A. (1988). *Intimate violence: The causes and consequences of abuse in the American family.* New York: Simon & Schuster.

Giordano, P. C., Millhollin, T. J., Cernkovich, S. A., Pugh, M. D., & Rudolph, J. L. (1999). Delinquency, identity, and women's involvement in relationship violence. *Criminology, 27*, 17–40.

Gottman, J. M. (2001). Crime, hostility, wife battering, and the heart: On the Meehan et al. (2001) failure to replicate the Gottman et al. (1995) typology. *Journal of Family Psychology, 15*, 409–414.

Gottman, J. M., Jacobson, N. S., Rushe, R. H., Shortt, J. W., Babcock, J., La Taillade, J. J., & Waltz, J. (1995). The relationship between heart rate reactivity, emotionally aggressive behavior, and general violence in batterers. *Journal of Family Psychology, 9*, 227–248.

Harned, M. S. (2001). Abused women or abused men? An examination of the context and outcomes of dating violence. *Violence and Victims, 16*, 269–285.

Heyman, R. E., Feldbau-Kohn, S. R., Ehrensaft, M. K., Langhinrichsen-Rohling, J., & O'Leary, K. D. (2001). Can questionnaire reports correctly classify relationship distress and partner physical abuse? *Journal of Family Psychology, 15*, 334–346.

Holtzworth-Munroe, A., Meehan, J. C., Herron, K., Rehman, U., & Stuart, G. L. (2000). Testing the Holtzworth-Munroe and Stuart (1994) batterer typology. *Journal of Consulting and Clinical Psychology, 68*, 1000–1019.

Holtzworth-Munroe, A., & Stuart, G. L. (1994). Typologies of male batterers: Three subtypes and the differences among them. *Psychological Bulletin, 116*, 476–597.

Jacobson, N. S., Gottman, J. M., Waltz, J., Rushe, R., Babcock, J., & Holtzworth-Munroe, A. (1994). Affect, verbal content, and psychophysiology in the arguments of couples with a violent husband. *Journal of Consulting and Clinical Psychology, 62*, 982–988.

Johnson, M. P. (1995). Patriarchal terrorism and common couple violence: Two forms of violence against women. *Journal of Marriage and the Family, 57*, 283–294.

Kim, H. K., & Capaldi, D. M. (2004). The association of antisocial behavior and depressive symptoms between partners and risk for aggression in romantic relationships. *Journal of Family Psychology, 18*, 82–96.

Magdol, L., Moffitt, T. E., Caspi, A., Newman, D. L., Fagan, J., & Silva, P. A. (1997). Gender differences in partner violence in a birth cohort of 21-year-olds: Bridging the gap between clinical and epidemiological approaches. *Journal of Consulting and Clinical Psychology, 65,* 68–78.

Magdol, L., Moffitt, T. E., Caspi, A., & Silva, P. A. (1998). Developmental antecedents of partner abuse: A prospective longitudinal study. *Journal of Abnormal Psychology, 107,* 375–389.

Makepeace, J. A. (1986). Gender differences in courtship violence victimization. *Family Patterns, 35,* 382–388.

Meehan, J. C., Holtzworth-Munroe, A., & Herron, K. (2001). Martially violent men's heart rate reactivity to marital interactions: A failure to replicate the Gottman et al. (1995) typology. *Journal of Family Psychology, 15,* 394–408.

Morse, B. J. (1995). Beyond the Conflict Tactics Scale: Assessing gender differences in partner violence. *Violence and Victims, 10,* 251–272.

O'Leary, K. D. (1999). Developmental and affective issues in assessing and treating partner aggression. *Clinical Psychology: Science and Practice, 6,* 400–414.

Quinton, D., Pickles, A., Maughan, B., & Rutter, M. (1993). Partners, peers, and pathways: Assortative pairing and continuities in conduct disorder. Special Issue: Milestones in the development of resilience. *Development and Psychopathology, 5,* 763–783.

Scarr, S., & McCartney, K. (1983). How people make their own environments: A theory of genotype leading to environment effects. *Child Development, 54,* 424–435.

Stets, J. E., & Straus, M. A. (1990). Gender differences in reporting marital violence and its medical and psychological consequences. In M. A. Straus & R. J. Gelles (Eds.), *Physical violence in American families: Risk factors and adaptations to violence in 8,145 families* (pp. 151–166). New Brunswick, NJ: Transaction.

Straus, M. A. (1979). Measuring intrafamily conflict and violence: The Conflict Tactics (CT) Scale. *Journal of Marriage and the Family, 41,* 75–88.

Straus, M. A. (1997). Physical assaults by women partners: A major social problem. In M. R. Walsh (Ed.), *Women, men and gender: Ongoing debates* (pp. 210–221). New Haven, CT: Yale University Press.

Straus, M. A. (1999). The controversy over domestic violence by women: A methodological, theoretical, and sociology of science analysis. In X. B. Arriaga & S. Oskamp (Eds.), *Violence in intimate relationships* (pp. 17–44). Thousand Oaks, CA: Sage.

Straus, M. A., & Gelles, R. J. (1986). Societal change and change in family violence from 1975–1985 as revealed by two national studies. *Journal of Marriage and the Family, 48,* 465–479.

Straus, M. A., & Gelles, R. J. (1990). *Physical violence in American families: Risk factors and adaptations to violence in 8,145 families.* New Brunswick, NJ: Transaction.

Sugarman, D. B., & Hotaling, G. I. (1989). Dating violence: Prevalence, context, and risk markers. In M. A. Pirog-Good & J. E. Stets (Eds.), *Violence in dating relationships: Emerging social issues* (pp. 3–32). New York: Praeger.

Vivian, D., & Langhinrichsen-Rohling, J. (1994). Are bi-directionally violent couples mutually victimized? A gender-sensitive comparison. *Violence and Victims, 9,* 107–124.

Walker, L. E. (1984). *The battered women syndrome.* New York: Springer.

Woodward, L. J., Fergusson, D. M., & Horwood, L. J. (2002). Romantic relationships of young people with early and late onset antisocial behavior problems. *Journal of Abnormal Child Psychology, 30,* 231–243.

# CHAPTER 12

# Parenting as an Important Outcome of Conduct Disorder in Girls

Mark Zoccolillo, Daniel Paquette, Rima Azar,
Sylvana Côté, and Richard Tremblay

Conduct disorder (CD) is among the most common of psychiatric diagnoses in adolescent girls (Loeber, Burke, Lahey, Winters, & Zera, 2000; Zoccolillo, 1993). According to the criteria of the *Diagnostic and Statistical Manual of Mental Disorders*, fourth edition (DSM-IV; American Psychiatric Association, 1994), it is defined by the presence and persistence of at least 3 of the following 15 behaviors: physical fights, destruction of property, telling lies, running away from home, truancy, stealing (with or without confrontation), bullying, carrying or using a weapon, setting fires, breaking and entering, cruelty to people or animals, staying out late despite parent's prohibitions, and forced sex. An excellent comprehensive study and overview of CD in girls is presented in "Sex Differences in Antisocial Behavior" (Moffitt, Caspi, Rutter, & Silva, 2001).

Common antisocial behaviors in girls with CD include lying, truancy, running away from home, and stealing without confrontation (Zoccolillo & Rogers, 1991). Relative to other girls, girls with CD also report more violent behaviors but are less violent than boys with CD (Loeber et al., 2000; Moffitt et al., 2001). In a clinical sample of adolescent girls from a community psychiatric hospital, half had been arrested but few were convicted of serious offenses (Zoccolillo & Rogers, 1991). Offenses against others in this sample ranged from traffic offenses and shoplifting to suspected murder of a young child.

Girls with conduct disorder have poor adult outcomes (Pajer,

242

1998). Relative to girls without CD, girls with CD have increased mortality, lower educational attainment, criminality, poor job histories, welfare dependence, marital difficulties, substance dependence, depression, and antisocial personality disorder (Bardone et al., 1998; Bardone, Moffitt, Caspi, & Dickson, 1996; Robins, 1966; Serbin, Peters, McAffer, & Schwartzman, 1991; Zoccolillo, Pickles, Quinton, & Rutter, 1992; Zoccolillo & Rogers, 1991).

One adult outcome of CD in girls that has received little attention is that of parenting (Moffitt et al., 2001). There are several reasons why studying parenting in women with a history of conduct disorder is important. First, being a competent parent is a major indicator of mental health. Second, as noted later, children of women with a history of CD are at considerable risk and women with a history of CD are relatively frequent (10%) in the population (Zoccolillo, 1993). Reducing the risk to their children is of considerable importance for the well-being of children in general. Third, CD is a familial disorder with both genetic and shared environment effects (Connell & Goodman, 2002; Rhee & Waldman, 2002). Studying the family environment specific to families where mothers had a history of CD is critical to better understand such intergenerational transmission.

In this chapter we review parenting by mothers with CD and present some recent data from two ongoing studies. Implications for research on girls with CD, prevention of CD, and social policy are discussed.

Three important definitions of terms are in order. First, parenting is defined broadly. Any behavior of the parent that affects the child is defined as parenting. The term "family environment" is used synonymously with parenting. Second, our focus is on mothers with a history of CD rather than mothers with concurrent adult antisocial behaviors. There are two reasons for this. Virtually all mothers will have passed through the age of risk for CD symptoms before having their first child. However, teen or young mothers will not have passed through the age of risk for adult behaviors. Also, CD symptoms can be used to identify girls for intervention programs before they have children. Because of the sparse literature in the area, we have not restricted our definition of conduct disorder to studies using only DSM-IV criteria, but rather have included any useful studies in the area. Third, we use the term "risk factor" broadly to mean any potentially adverse factor for child development that is associated with maternal history of CD. For many of the factors, causality has not been established.

In this chapter, we focus on family environmental influence during the developmental period from conception to preschool. The preschool years represent the earliest age at which children who develop antisocial personality disorder differ from other children (Caspi, Moffitt, Newman, & Silva, 1996), suggesting that critical factors contributing to the onset of these problems occur earlier (e.g., from conception to preschool). As discussed later, studying the early environment of infants of mothers with a history of CD is an excellent way to study potentially causal early risk factors. In addition, the literature in this area is sparse, as opposed to the considerable literature on mother–child interactions during the elementary and later school years (Hinshaw, 2002; Shaw, Owens, Giovannelli, & Winslow, 2001). Hence, a review of this area is timely, with the hope that it will encourage more research in this area.

## PARENTING BY WOMEN
## WITH CONDUCT DISORDER

Only a limited number of studies have examined parenting risk factors in mothers who have a history of CD. Chapter 14 of a recent publication from the Dunedin longitudinal birth cohort study, "Sex, Antisocial Behavior, and Mating: Mate Selection and Early Childbearing," provides an excellent presentation on this subject (Moffitt et al., 2001). In addition to the Dunedin studies, there are two ongoing studies of maternal CD and parenting risk by the authors of this chapter, described later.

The first study is the Longitudinal Study of Child Development in Quebec (LSCDQ). Infants were selected based on birth certificate data in 1998 to be representative of the province of Quebec. They were 5 months of age at the first assessment, and assessments were conducted every 12 months thereafter. At the 5-month assessment, 2,120 infants were studied. Many different variables were assessed by maternal and paternal interview and self-report, and observational data were collected on the infant and the home. A unique aspect of this study is that maternal and paternal antisocial disorder were assessed by self-report questionnaire of five (four in the father) CD symptoms and four adult antisocial symptoms.[1]

The second study is the Montreal Adolescent Mother Study (MAMS). This is an ongoing study of 261 adolescent mothers in Montreal, Quebec, recruited through a pediatric obstetric clinic, a high school for teen mothers, and group homes for delinquent girls. Forty-two percent of the mothers met modified DSM-III-R (American Psychiatric Association, 1987) criteria for CD. Almost all of the mothers were single, most had not finished high school, and most were either supported financially by parents or on welfare. A strength of this sample for assessing parenting risk associated with CD was that all of the mothers (those with and without CD) shared similar backgrounds and current circumstances of considerable adversity. Because of this, differences in parenting risk by CD are more likely to be specific to CD rather than related to adversity itself. Extensive self-report, interview, and observational data are available on this sample.

Clinical observations gleaned from clinical work with females with a history of CD over the past 16 years by the first author (MZ) are also presented. Hard data in this area are limited, and it is hoped that preliminary results and clinical observations will help fill in the gaps and guide future research and interventions. Nonetheless, we have tried to make clear where our conclusions come from so the reader can weigh the strength of the evidence.

The risks associated with maternal history of CD are multiple and occur across different domains. They occur at different points in the development of the child. Some are limited in impact to a specific time period, whereas others persist over time. In order to provide a quick visual summary of known risks associated with maternal CD, a summary table of risk by developmental period through preschool is presented (see Table 12.1). The risks are ordered by the child's development, from conception to entry into school.

Risk to the offspring can be summarized as follows. Risk begins at conception when a mother with CD chooses an antisocial mate and has her child during her teen years (Kessler et al., 1997; Maughan & Lindelow, 1997; Miller-Johnson et al., 1999; Moffitt et al., 2001; Serbin et al., 1991; Wakschlag et al., 2000; Woodward & Fergusson, 1999; Zoccolillo, 2000). The risk continues *in utero*, where the infant is more likely to be exposed to cigarette smoke and other toxins (Wakschlag, Pickett, Cook, Benowitz, & Leventhal, 2002; Zoccolillo, 2000). Mothers with CD are also more likely to be physically abused during pregnancy, and their offspring are more likely to be born preterm (MAMS, unpublished data). After birth, and very early in development, mothers with CD are less sensitive to their infants than are other mothers (Cassidy, Zoccolillo, & Hughes, 1996; Hans, Bernstein, & Henson, 1999; Serbin et al., 1991), and are also more likely to be irritated by normal infant behavior, such as crying (Bosquet & Egeland, 2000; Zoccolillo, 2000). They are also more likely to continue using drugs, alcohol, and cigarettes (Zoccolillo, 2000). It can be inferred that infants of mothers with CD often receive less cognitive stimulation, since the parents are less educated and more likely to be poor and have fewer toys and books in the home (Zoccolillo, 2000). Biological fathers are more likely to be absent from the home, although there may be a succession of antisocial male figures in the household (MAMS, unpublished data; Moffitt et al., 2001;

TABLE 12.1. Risk Factors for Offspring of Mothers with Conduct Disorder

| Risk factors | Time of risk | | | | |
|---|---|---|---|---|---|
| | C | PN | I | T | PS |
| Antisocial biological father | X | * | * | * | * |
| Young or adolescent mother | X | * | * | * | * |
| Exposure to prenatal tobacco smoke | | X | * | * | * |
| Exposure to alcohol and illegal drugs | | X | | | |
| Physical abuse *in utero* | | X | | | |
| Preterm birth | | X | | | |
| Poverty | | X | * | * | * |
| Antisocial males in the home | | X | * | * | * |
| Decreased maternal sensitivity | | | X | * | * |
| Maternal irritability or harsh parenting | | | X | * | * |
| Low maternal educational level | | | X | * | * |
| Absence of father | | | X | * | * |
| Intoxicated mother | | | X | * | * |
| Physical injury; accidents | | | X | * | * |
| Physical abuse/neglect | | | X | * | * |
| Coercive/inconsistent/ineffective parenting | | | | X | * |

*Note.* X, first appearance of risk factor; *, persistence of risk factor; C, conception; PN, prenatal; I, infancy; T, toddler; PS, preschool.

Zoccolillo, 2000). During the first few years of life, these children will also likely experience more accidents and visit the hospital more often (Serbin, Peters, & Schwartzman, 1996; Serbin et al., Chapter 13, this volume). By the beginning of the toddler years, the pattern of harsh and inconsistent parenting seen in later life in families with children with CD has begun (Bosquet & Egeland, 2000; Hinshaw, 2002; Shaw et al., 2001).

## IMPLICATIONS FOR RESEARCH ON THE DEVELOPMENT OF CONDUCT DISORDER IN GIRLS

The roots of many of the parenting risk factors evident in mothers with CD are present before the birth of the child and need to be studied while those mothers-to-be are in their preadolescence and adolescence. Four risk factors in particular will be discussed: assortative mating, adolescent motherhood, maternal sensitivity, and maternal irritability or harsh parenting.

## Assortative Mating

Girls with CD are more likely to mate with antisocial males (Cairns & Cairns, 1994; Kandel, Davies, & Baydar, 1990; Moffitt et al., 2001; Zoccolillo, 2000; Zoccolillo et al., 1992). This has serious implications for their offspring for two reasons (Moffitt et al., 2001). First, in all likelihood, having both parents who share genetic vulnerability to CD increases child risk for biological vulnerability to the disorder. Second, due to their behavior, antisocial fathers negatively impact their children's environment and mother's well-being. Antisocial fathers seriously limit the potential effects of intervention programs. Hence, understanding why girls with CD mate with antisocial men is a major research priority (Moffitt et al., 2001).

Studies of assortative mating suggest that behavioral homophily (e.g., similarity in antisocial behavior) explains much of the association, rather than similarity of social backgrounds more generally (Krueger, Moffitt, Caspi, Bleske, & Silva, 1998). There is very little research, however, on why this occurs. Longitudinal studies following girls from preadolescence to young adulthood are needed to address hypotheses on assortative mating.

Some potential research questions follow: First, to what extent is assortative mating a choice on the part of the girl? Assortative mating could arise due to choices made by antisocial males to select girls with CD and by nonantisocial males to avoid selecting these girls as spouses and mothers, without any active role by the female. While factors other than female choice for antisocial males may well contribute to the assortative mating, in this author's (M.Z.) experience, girls with CD are quite specifically attracted to antisocial males, findings also supported by data from the Dunedin study (Krueger et al., 1998). Nonetheless, this issue needs further clarification. Second, assuming that choice of antisocial males by girls with CD is a significant factor in assortative mating, when does this preference emerge? Little is known about whether this attraction arises only in the context of sexual maturity or is present even before puberty (but see Pepler, Craig, Yule, & Connolly, Chapter 5, this volume, for some preliminary ideas). Third, do girls with CD differ from other girls in what they consider attractive in males? A related question is whether girls with CD differ from others girls in what they consider as necessary qualities for a good father/husband. These are very basic yet unanswered questions. A better understanding of the factors that differentiate girls with and without CD in this area may pave the way for studies examining the developmental precursors of these differences.

## Adolescent Motherhood

A recent quote from the Dunedin study illustrates the issue well: "Antisocial males and females selectively reproduce at a younger age, with an antisocial mate. Conduct-disordered Study members were one-fifth of the cohort, but they produced nearly two-thirds of the offspring born to the Dunedin cohort members as teenage parents" (Moffitt et al., 2001, p. 196). There are little data on *why* girls with CD have their first child at a younger age.

It is important to note, however, that many adolescent mothers do not have CD. Indeed, reviewing the literature on early parenthood, Wakschlag and Hans (2000) suggest two contrasting profiles of young mothers. The first group is one in which young maternal age is part of a "conduct problem" pathway, as noted earlier. The second group is one in which an early transition to parenthood is not a problem behavior per se, but rather represents an adaptation to limited social and economic opportunities. It is important to distinguish between direct effects of CD on childbearing and indirect effects (e.g., CD on educational attainment leading to dropping out of high school, followed by early childbearing, as described later).

It seems unlikely that childbearing in girls with CD is *only* an accidental consequence of promiscuity and lack of birth control, because were these children unwanted, their mothers could opt for either abortion or adoption. In the author's (M.Z.) experience in Montreal, where birth control and abortion are easily accessible to adolescent mothers, it is striking how many teen mothers with CD become pregnant despite access to contraception and choose to keep and raise their infants themselves. Many girls with CD who become young mothers appear to want to have children; it is not solely an accidental outcome.

A second, testable hypothesis is that girls with CD, who often do poorly academically and drop out of high school, move forward with child rearing as the "natural" next step in their life course. Because many adolescent mothers do not have CD, and because the timing of pregnancy and end of schooling can be easily ascertained, it would be relatively simple to test this hypothesis as a determinant of teen motherhood in girls with CD. An alternative or additional hypothesis is that girls with CD think about having children or desire to have children at an earlier age than other girls, due perhaps to a need to feel connected and loved. It may also be that the deficits in self-control, planning, and organization that may contribute to CD risk and to academic difficulties are also reflected in a failure of these girls to plan birth control or to organize effectively for alternatives to child rearing (e.g., abortion or adoption). Research on childbearing should clearly distinguish among factors that influence sexual activity, contraception, pregnancy, and childbearing, in order to better unpack the interacting influences that increase teen parenthood among girls with CD.

## Maternal Sensitivity

A consistent finding is that women with a history of CD or antisocial personality disorder show decreased levels of maternal sensitivity to their infants (Cassidy et al., 1996; Hans et al., 1999; Serbin et al., 1991). For example, in the MAMS, a significant negative relationship emerged between the number of CD symptoms in the mother's history and her maternal sensitivity to her 4-month-old infant. Little is known about why mothers with CD are less sensitive, although there is some evidence that the social skill deficits and emotional immaturity associated with CD may continue into late adolescence and early adult relationships. Our limited experience suggests that mothers with a history of CD respond positively to interventions aimed at improving their maternal sensitivity prenatally and postnatally, a finding noted in other studies of adolescent mothers (Barnet, Duggan, Devoe, & Burrell, 2002; Letourneau, 2001). This raises the issue of whether the poor sensitivity is more due to an absence of good role models for normal mother–infant relationships (remediable by teaching) as opposed to fixed personality traits, which may not be as amenable to change. Because low levels of maternal sensitivity have been found as early as 4 months among mothers with CD (Cassidy et al., 1996), predictor and prevention studies of maternal sensitivity should start early, ideally before the infant is born.

## Maternal Irritability

In the LSCDQ, mothers with histories of CD symptoms showed increased irritability in reaction to normal infant behavior when their babies were 5 months old. Other research suggests that, by the time the infants reach toddlerhood (18 months and older), these mothers will likely show elevated levels of harsh and punitive parenting (Bosquet & Egeland, 2000). It is important to note that increased irritability to infant behavior does not necessarily reflect rejection or dislike of the infant, because on questions reflecting maternal warmth mothers do not differ by the number of conduct problems (LSCDQ) (Zoccolillo, 2000).

Why are mothers with CD more irritable? One possibility is that is part of the same underlying core disorder that leads to increased conflict with their own parents, peers, and male companions. Another possibility is that the expectations of mothers with CD regarding their infants are not in keeping with infant development. In our limited experience one striking finding is that adolescent mothers with CD (or with a history of CD) believe their infant's behaviors (e.g., crying, urinating on the mother while diapers are being changed), even at 1 or 2 months of age, are intentional and directed at that mother. Educating the mother about normal infant development may decrease this irritability. As with maternal sensitivity, developing and testing hypotheses regarding the factors contributing to maternal irritability is critical, not only with regard to understanding intergenerational transmission but also for devising rational, effective interventions.

The issues of assortative mating, early childbearing, and maternal sensitivity and irritability illustrate the importance for researchers studying antisocial behavior in girls to think of them as future mothers and to plan research accordingly.

## IMPLICATIONS FOR RESEARCH ON THE DEVELOPMENT OF CONDUCT DISORDER

There are several implications from these findings for research on the development of CD, including issues regarding the timing of risk, the multiplicity of risk, the strong correlation of genetic and environmental risk, and the intergenerational transmission of risk.

### The Timing of Risk

Risk begins at conception and accumulates rapidly. Few studies have looked at the prenatal or infancy period with regard to risk factors for later CD (Hinshaw, 2002; Shaw et al., 2001). However, the evidence is clear that risk begins at conception. Research that begins with samples of toddlers or older children may overestimate "child effects." For example, a toddler may be "difficult" at 18 months due to poor maternal responsiveness from birth onwards. If maternal sensitivity prior to 18 months is not measured, then it is easy to ascribe the toddler behavior to temperament or genetics (Aguilar, Sroufe, Egeland, & Carlson, 2000; Belsky, Hsieh, & Crnic, 1998). A striking impression from following infants of mothers with CD, and supported by research conducted by Serbin and colleagues examining hospital records (Serbin et al., 1996; Serbin et al., Chapter 13, this volume), is that these infants are also at elevated risk for various brain insults, such as minor head injuries and inadequate feeding.

It is our impression that while intensive prospective studies miss some risk, retrospective studies of infancy and the prenatal period will miss a good deal more. More prospective research studies are needed, starting prenatally or at birth. Furthermore, researchers investigating older samples should always bear in mind the unmeasured risk during early life.

## The Multiplicity of Risk and the Development of Causal Models

The presence of multiple risk factors poses a challenge to the researcher. An association between a risk factor and an outcome may well be spurious and due to any number of other co-occurring factors.

The presence of multiple, highly associated risk factors poses a major difficulty for hypothesis-driven research. The reason is that not enough is known about all the potential risk factors associated with maternal CD and how they are interconnected to adequately control for all possible confounds and interactions while testing any particular hypothesis. Furthermore, significant interactions may exist among multiple risk factors. More descriptive studies examining the family environments of mothers with a history of CD are needed in order to develop hypothesis-driven research that is plausible and in keeping with the complexity of these families. It is also clear that the risk factors associated with maternal CD and intergenerational transmission cut across many domains of research; hence, researchers cannot limit themselves to their own narrow areas of specialization when trying to unravel the causes of CD.

The association between multiple risk factors and maternal CD should also make researchers cautious with regard to a cumulative risk approach (e.g., adding up the number of risk factors). Studies on the adult outcome of CD have found that it is specifically a poor outcome across *multiple* domains that is associated with CD and not any one specific poor outcome (Zoccolillo et al., 1992). A cumulative risk model that does not control for this strong association with maternal and paternal CD cannot be considered causal.

Despite the complexity of the many potential risk factors associated with CD, it is critical to develop testable causal models for the impact of maternal CD on intergenerational transmission. One good candidate as a causal factor is low maternal sensitivity. There are several reasons why this variable may be causally linked to later CD. First, it is associated with maternal CD and antisocial personality disorder (Cassidy et al., 1996; Hans et al., 1999; Serbin et al., 1991). Second, low maternal sensitivity is present at 4 months of age, and preliminary studies suggest that this association is mother-, not infant-, driven. Third, it is a variable that is very proximal to the infant. Fourth, it fits with developmental theory with regard to the findings that link child aggression with insecure attachment (Hinshaw, 2002; Shaw et al., 2001). Fifth, one study that controlled for a number of other risk variables has found that low maternal sensitivity predicted CD at age 10 (Wakschlag & Hans, 1999). As both a model to follow when considering causal models for CD and as a potential causal risk factor in its own right, maternal sensitivity is a good candidate for comprehensive and well-designed prospective studies of the development of CD.

## Gene–Environment Correlations and Interactions

Genetically informative studies (twin and adoption studies) have consistently suggested a heritable component to various forms of antisocial behavior, including CD (Cadoret, Yates, Troughton, Woodworth, & Stewart, 1995; Eley, Lichtenstein, & Stevenson, 1999; Langbehn, Cadoret, Yates, Troughton, & Stewart, 1998; Rutter, 1997; Rutter, Silberg, O'Connor, & Simonoff, 1999). This poses major difficulties in interpreting the association between a risk factor and CD if this same risk factor is associated with CD in either biological parent (Rutter, 1997). Since maternal CD is associated with a plethora of risk factors, any suspected risk factor for CD must be assessed to see if it is also associated with a parental diagnosis of CD and then controlled for appropriately.

Controlling for parental CD requires assessing it in both biological parents. This can be difficult because biological fathers are often missing, and the more antisocial the mother, the greater the chance the father will be missing (Zoccolillo, 2000). In addition, it is not clear how parental CD is best assessed in terms of its potential impact on offspring (Loeber et al., 2000). That is, even one symptom of parental CD may increase the probability of poor child outcomes (Robins & Regier, 1991). Multiple measures of parental history and functioning, in addition to the categorical diagnosis of CD, are therefore desirable in order to test various models concerning the biological, caregiving, and lifestyle factors that may contribute to the intergenerational transmission of CD. Studies examining the impact of various risk factors in parents with no history at all of CD may not shed much light on this question, as they do not provide opportunities to examine the impact of the multiple risk factors that typically exist for mothers with histories of CD, nor do they allow for the examination of gene–environment interactions (Caspi et al., 2002).

Another option is to hope that genetic studies will identify genes associated with CD, which can then be used as true indicators of genetic risk (Caspi et al., 2002). However, the same problems of missing fathers, unclear pedigrees, and unclear phenotype make setting up appropriate designs difficult.

At present, modeling strategies that account for maternal and paternal disorder, missing fathers, genetic relatedness, and parenting risk factors need to be further developed. It is critical for such models to incorporate measures of genetic relatedness in their models and to test alternatives to identify the best-fitting models. Appropriate controls for both genetic and environmental risk associated with parental CD are needed to compare various causal models. If a potential risk variable is no longer associated with offspring outcome of CD, it would be very useful to know if it is because of controlling for "genes" or unmeasured environmental risk factors. While not perfect, such models can test alternative hypotheses for the best-fitting models.

## IMPLICATIONS FOR PREVENTION AND INTERVENTION

Viewing parenting risk as an outcome of maternal CD has several important implications for prevention and intervention.

### Preventive Intervention Targeting Risk at Conception

Prevention or intervention programs that begin in the preschool years are working uphill against genetic risk, possible behavioral teratogenic risk (e.g., prenatal exposure to cigarette smoke), and against several years of poor mother–infant interactions. Risk-reduction programs may be more effective if they begin reducing risk at conception and during the prenatal period. The nurse home visitation program developed by Olds and colleagues (1998) is a good example of a successful program in this area, although evidence of effectiveness with mothers who have a history of CD is needed.

### Tailoring Interventions

In the design of interventions, it may be critical to conceptualize risk and protection in the context of the development and natural history of maternal CD. Two examples of this are maternal educational attainment and single parent status. In general, providing mothers with the opportunity for further education and for obtaining a high school degree may appear a useful strategy to promote economic stability and self-sufficiency. However, viewed within the development of CD, where low educational attainment may be the consequence of early cognitive delays and years of truancy and school discipline problems, the provision of supplementary educational opportunities may not be straightforward. These women may be less responsive to educational interventions than women without such a history, given both learning delays and difficulties, as well as low levels of self-efficacy and motivation. A second example concerns participation of the absent father in the care of the child. This may make sense in many cases. However, for many of the mothers with a history of CD, the "absent father" may be highly antisocial and a danger to the mother and infant. Hence, such interventions may be ineffective or counterproductive.

## Preventive Intervention Prior to Pregnancy

Some of the key risk factors to children of mothers with CD occur long before the birth of the child and may best be addressed in the mother's childhood or adolescence. Two examples are prenatal smoking and assortative mating.

In the MAMS, CD predicts whether a mother is a smoker at the time of conception but not whether she continues to smoke during pregnancy. Other studies on persistence of smoking during pregnancy (Kirkland, Dodds, & Brosky, 2000) and the low success rates of smoking reduction programs during pregnancy (Lumley, Oliver, & Waters, 2000) suggest that efforts to prevent teenage girls from smoking or encouraging them to stop long before pregnancy are needed.

Preventing association with antisocial males may also be more easily targeted prior to motherhood, for several reasons. One reason is that, in our experience, these mothers want a father for the baby and make repeated efforts to encourage involvement by the father, even when it is clear that he does not want to be involved or he is a danger to the mother and of infant. This makes it very difficult to convince mothers to try to set even modest limits on the antisocial fathers of their infants (e.g., that he is not to be drunk or high when around the infant, etc.). Second, antisocial males, whether the infant's father or current boyfriend, can (and do) disrupt any intervention by encouraging the mother to drop out of the intervention. Even the successful home intervention program of Olds and colleagues had no effect in families where there was marital conflict (Eckenrode et al., 2000), underlining the difficulty of working with both an antisocial mother and antisocial father.

Helping girls with CD make better decisions regarding the men in their lives is not only important with regard to their offspring but also for the well-being of the girl. Association with antisocial males is a major contributor to mortality in girls with CD and also to their overall outcome (Moffitt et al., 2001; Zoccolillo & Rogers, 1991). Furthermore, it is well accepted that preventing association with deviant peers in general, for both boys and girls, is a legitimate goal of treatment and management of CD.

## Maternal History of Conduct Disorder as a Screening Factor and Moderator of Intervention

A history of CD (which is easily ascertained) (Zoccolillo, 2000) is a useful indicator of hidden risk and the need for careful follow-up. A valid question is whether screening for risk should focus on all the risk factors associated with maternal CD rather than a mother's own history of CD. There are several reasons why it is important to screen based on a mother's history of CD. First, maternal CD itself may make it necessary to adapt interventions designed for mothers without CD. Second, CD may be an optimal predictor of future difficulties in parenting. For example, poor maternal responsivity is specifically associated with maternal CD (Cassidy et al.,1996; Hans et al. 1999; Serbin et al., 1991). To prevent this pattern from beginning it is important to start prenatally; using maternal CD as a screen may thus identify those mothers most at risk. Another example is that associating with antisocial males places a woman (and her baby) at risk for being physically abused during and after pregnancy. Knowing that a mother has CD, even if there is no current boyfriend, is a warning of the increased likelihood that she may consort with antisocial males. Third, screening for risk in real-life situations, such as obstetric and pediatric settings, requires brief and efficient instruments. Maternal CD is easily assessed by questionnaire or interview, and identifies a very high-risk population for further evaluation and monitoring.

In addition, it may be important to examine maternal history of CD as a moderator of the efficacy of interventions, given the multiplicity of risks associated with such a history. It is possible that the impact of interventions may differ depending upon maternal history of CD and associated risk factors, such as smoking during pregnancy or having an antisocial father.

## Need for Research on Effective Interventions

At present, effective interventions for most risk factors associated with maternal CD are not available, and much more research is needed. Several factors account for the dearth of research in this area. The first is the absence (until relatively recently) of interest in CD in girls (Zoccolillo, 1993). A second factor stems from the gap in the intervention literature focused on parenting of infants among mothers with a history of CD. This is due in part to the fact that precursors to aggression or CD can be measured in the late toddler or preschool years but not in infancy. Hence, most CD research begins in the preschool years, and few infant researchers have focused specifically on the impact of maternal CD on child rearing and infant development. A third factor is that understanding and intervening effectively is made difficult by the complexity of CD and the multifaceted nature of intergenerational transmission, involving poorly understood transactions between genes and environment. Conversely, researchers are trained within narrow areas of specialization and tend to focus less on a comprehensive view of the disorder and more on specific factors. These barriers need to be addressed in order to develop a comprehensive research agenda examining the intergenerational transmission of conduct disorder, and corresponding intervention approaches.

## SOCIAL POLICY CONSIDERATIONS

In the absence of studies on interventions with mothers with CD, it is not possible to make strong recommendations for social policy with regard to effective and efficient programs. Nonetheless, it is possible to suggest some modifications to existing practices and to clarify some important issues with regard to parenting and maternal CD.

### Promoting Healthy Parenting versus Monitoring for Child Abuse and Neglect

A potential concern raised with regard to promoting parenting in mothers with CD is the issue of child abuse and neglect. Based on the first author's (MZ) experience in the MAMS, and as a clinician working with this same population, several points can be made.

First, CD is a relatively broad construct, with a population prevalence of up to 10% in adolescent girls (Zoccolillo, 1993). However, very few girls with CD are violent offenders. At least with adolescent mothers, many mothers with CD accept help with parenting and make real efforts to be a good parent. The physically abusive, uncaring, or hateful mother is fortunately uncommon, even in mothers with CD.

Second, it is important to distinguish between increased risk to the infant and child abuse or neglect, which must be reported to the authorities. Much suboptimal parenting is not reportable abuse or neglect; examples include maternal smoking during pregnancy and choice of male companions.

Third, it is critical in working with this population to have a clear understanding of what is healthy, normal development and to avoid making comparisons based on socioeconomic status or idealized parenting. When parenting is reduced to the essentials, many mothers with CD are not abusive or neglectful but do need help.

Fourth, during pregnancy and the first 2 years of life, health and development issues (e.g., poor weight gain) are salient and often indicators of poor parenting. Furthermore, most mothers with CD will be found at obstetric, pediatric, and family medicine clinics. Services for these mothers may therefore be best based at obstetric, pediatric, and family clinics. Working closely with medical providers may enhance access to the population of mothers with CD, and may provide a more appealing source of assistance than intervention provided via social services (Olds et al., 1998).

## Stigma and Labeling

Both research and interventions on parenting in mothers with a history of CD carry some risk of stigmatizing these mothers. The ultimate goal of both research and interventions should be to reduce (or avoid) parental breakdown, child abuse and neglect, and removal of the infant from the home. These goals need to be emphasized.

## Providing Parenting Support in Service Settings

One important direction for future policy is to increase relevant intervention services to adolescent girls who are already in criminal justice, mental health, or social service facilities. A large proportion of adolescent girls in institutions (including foster care) have CD and will become young mothers. However, services for these girls often do not include parenting support. In some instances, the lack of services in this area results from adolescent mothers achieving adult status and thus the end of the mandate for services or reaching the end of a juvenile justice sentence. In other instances, parenting is seen as an unwanted outcome. Nonetheless, identifying these girls as high risk and helping them to find appropriate services to ensure a healthy outcome for the child is critical for both the mother and the child.

## Routine Screening for Maternal Conduct Disorder

In current practice, maternal depression and substance abuse are well-established mental health risk factors that are routinely assessed in health care settings, such as obstetric and newborn baby clinics. Maternal history of CD should be added to the list of mental health problems included in routine screenings to identify potential problems in parenting and the need for preventive intervention and parenting support.

## Including Conduct Disorder as a Risk Factor for Adolescent Motherhood

There is now good evidence that CD in girls is a major risk factor for adolescent pregnancy, and a significant proportion of all adolescent mothers have CD (Kessler et al., 1997; Maughan & Lindelow, 1997; Miller-Johnson et al., 1999; Moffitt et al., 2001; Serbin et al., 1991; Wakschlag et al., 2000; Woodward & Fergusson, 1999; Zoccolillo, 2000). Programs that target adolescent pregnancy and child bearing need to take this association into account.

## CONCLUSION

The striking finding that childhood behavior problems of the mother very much determine the risk for her yet-unconceived child emphasize the importance of taking into account multiple generations when looking at risk factors. The disorder itself creates the very conditions necessary for the disorder to arise again in the next generation. Breaking the cycle of intergenerational transmission of CD remains an elusive goal. Understanding the determinants of parenting risk in girls with CD is a critical step in finding ways to break this cycle. However, much more interest is needed by both researchers and by clinicians who work with these girls. New conceptual models of intergenerational transmission of risk that focus on the interplay of genetic and environmental factors are also needed.

## NOTE

1. Publications available on the World Wide Web in English at *www.stat.gouv.qc.ca/publications/liste_an.htm*. In the section on the Longitudinal Study of Child Development in Québec (ÉLDEQ 1998–2002), details of the study are available, including the relationship among parental conduct problems and parenting risk (Zoccolillo, 2000).

## REFERENCES

Aguilar, B., Sroufe, L. A., Egeland, B., & Carlson, E. (2000). Distinguishing the early-onset/persistent and adolescence-onset antisocial behavior types: From birth to 16 years. *Development and Psychopathology, 12*, 109–132.

American Psychiatric Association. (1987). *Diagnostic and statistical manual of mental disorders* (3rd ed.). Washington, DC: Author.

American Psychiatric Association. (1994). *Diagnostic and statistical manual of mental disorders* (4th ed.). Washington, DC: Author.

Bardone, A. M., Moffitt, T. E., Caspi, A., Dickson, N., Stanton, W. R., & Silva, P. A. (1998). Adult physical health outcomes of adolescent girls with conduct disorder, depression, and anxiety. *Journal of the American Academy of Child and Adolescent Psychiatry, 37*, 594–601.

Bardone, A., Moffitt, T., Caspi, A., & Dickson, N. (1996). Adult mental health and social outcomes of adolescent girls with depression and conduct disorder. *Development and Psychopathology, 8*, 811–829.

Barnet, B., Duggan, A. K., Devoe, M., & Burrell, L. (2002). The effect of volunteer home visitation for adolescent mothers on parenting and mental health outcomes: A randomized trial. *Archives of Pediatrics and Adolescent Medicine, 156*, 1216–1222.

Belsky, J., Hsieh, K. H., & Crnic, K. (1998). Mothering, fathering, and infant negativity as antecedents of boys' externalizing problems and inhibition at age 3 years: Differential susceptibility to rearing experience? *Development and Psychopathology, 10*, 301–319.

Bosquet, M., & Egeland, B. (2000). Predicting parenting behaviors from Antisocial Practices content scale scores of the MMPI-2 administered during pregnancy. *Journal of Personality Assessment, 74*, 146–162.

Cadoret, R. J., Yates, W. R., Troughton, E., Woodworth, G., & Stewart, M. A. (1995). Genetic–environmental interaction in the genesis of aggressivity and conduct disorders. *Archives of General Psychiatry, 52*, 916–924.

Cairns, R. B., & Cairns, B. D. (1994). *Lifelines and risks: Pathways of youth in our time.* Cambridge, UK: Cambridge University Press.

Caspi, A., McClay, J., Moffitt, T. E., Mill, J., Martin, J., Craig, I. W., Taylor, A., & Poulton, R. (2002). Role of genotype in the cycle of violence in maltreated children. *Science, 297*, 851–854.

Caspi, A., Moffitt, T. E., Newman, D. L., & Silva, P. A. (1996). Behavioral observations at age 3 years predict adult psychiatric disorders: Longitudinal evidence from a birth cohort. *Archives of General Psychiatry, 53*, 1033–1039.

Cassidy, B., Zoccolillo, M., & Hughes, S. (1996). Psychopathology in adolescent mothers and its effects on mother–infant interactions: A pilot study. *Canadian Journal of Psychiatry [Revue Canadienne de Psychiatrie], 41*, 379–384.

Connell, A. M., & Goodman, S. H. (2002). The association between psychopathology in fathers versus mothers and children's internalizing and externalizing behavior problems: A meta-analysis. *Psychological Bulletin, 128*, 746–773.

Eckenrode, J., Ganzel, B., Henderson, C. R., Jr., Smith, E., Olds, D. L., Powers, J., Cole, R., Kitzman, H., & Sidora, K. (2000). Preventing child abuse and neglect with a program of nurse home visitation: The limiting effects of domestic violence. *Journal of the American Medical Association, 284*, 1385–1391.

Eley, T. C., Lichtenstein, P., & Stevenson, J. (1999). Sex differences in the etiology of aggressive and nonaggressive antisocial behavior: Results from two twin studies. *Child Development, 70*, 155–168.

Hans, S. L., Bernstein V. J., & Henson L. G. (1999). The role of psychopathology in the parenting of drug-dependent women. *Development and Psychopathology, 11*, 957–977.

Hinshaw, S. P. (2002). Process, mechanism, and explanation related to externalizing behavior in developmental psychopathology. *Journal of Abnormal Child Psychology, 30*, 431–446.

260

Kandel, D., Davies, M., & Baydar, N. (1990). The creation of interpersonal contexts: Homophily in dyadic relationships in adolescence and young adulthood. In L. N. Robins & M. Rutter (Eds.), *Straight and devious pathways from childhood to adulthood* (pp. 182–204). Cambridge, UK: Cambridge University Press.

Kessler, R. C., Berglund, P. A., Foster, C. L., Saunders, W. B., Stang, P. E., & Walters, E. E. (1997). Social consequences of psychiatric disorders: II. Teenage parenthood. *American Journal of Psychiatry, 154,* 1405–1411.

Kirkland, S. A., Dodds, L. A., & Brosky, G. (2000). The natural history of smoking during pregnancy among women in Nova Scotia. *Canadian Medical Association Journal, 163,* 281–282.

Krueger, R. F., Moffitt, T. E., Caspi, A., Bleske, A., & Silva, P. A. (1998). Assortative mating for antisocial behavior: Developmental and methodological implications. *Behavior Genetics, 28,* 173–186.

Langbehn, D. R., Cadoret, R. J., Yates, W. R., Troughton, E. P., & Stewart, M. A. (1998). Distinct contributions of conduct and oppositional defiant symptoms to adult antisocial behavior: Evidence from an adoption study. *Archives of General Psychiatry, 55,* 821–829.

Letourneau, N. (2001). Improving adolescent parent–infant interactions: A pilot study. *Journal of Pediatric Nursing, 16,* 53–62.

Loeber, R., Burke, J. D., Lahey, B. B., Winters, A., & Zera, M. (2000). Oppositional defiant and conduct disorder: A review of the past 10 years, part I. *Journal of the American Academy of Child and Adolescent Psychiatry, 39,* 1468–1484.

Lumley, J., Oliver, S., & Waters, E. (2000). Interventions for promoting smoking cessation during pregnancy. *Cochrane Database of Systematic Review* (2), CD001055.

Maughan, B., & Lindelow, M. (1997). Secular change in psychosocial risks: The case of teenage motherhood. *Psychological Medicine, 27,* 1129–1144.

Miller-Johnson, S., Winn, D. M., Coie, J., Maumary-Gremaud, A., Hyman, C., Terry, R., & Lochman, J. (1999). Motherhood during the teen years: A developmental perspective on risk factors for childbearing. *Development and Psychopathology, 11,* 85–100.

Moffitt, T. E., Caspi, A., Rutter, M., & Silva, P. (2001). *Sex differences in antisocial behaviour.* Cambridge, UK: Cambridge University Press.

Olds, D., Henderson, C. R. J., Cole, R., Eckenrode, J., Kitzman, H., Luckey, D., Pettitt, L., Sidora, K., Morris, P., & Powers, J. (1998). Long-term effects of nurse home visitation on children's criminal and antisocial behavior: 15-year follow-up of a randomized controlled trial. *Journal of the American Medical Association, 280,* 1238–1244.

Pajer, K. A. (1998). What happens to "bad" girls? A review of the adult outcomes of antisocial adolescent girls. *American Journal of Psychiatry, 155,* 862–870.

Rhee, S. H., & Waldman, I. (2002). Genetic and environmental influences on antisocial behavior: A meta-analysis of twin and adoption studies. *Psychological Bulletin, 128,* 490–529.

Robins, L. N. (1966). *Deviant children grown up.* Baltimore: Williams & Wilkins.

Robins, L. N., & Regier, D. A. (1991). *Psychiatric disorders in America: The epidemiologic catchment area study.* New York: Free Press.

Rutter, M. (1997). Nature–nurture integration. The example of antisocial behavior. *American Psychologist, 52,* 390–398.

Rutter, M., Silberg, J., O'Connor, T., & Simonoff, E. (1999). Genetics and child psychiatry: II. Empirical research findings. *Journal of Child Psychology and Psychiatry and Allied Disciplines, 40,* 19–55.

Serbin, L., Peters, P., McAffer, V., & Schwartzman, A. (1991). Childhood aggression and withdrawal as predictors of adolescent pregnancy, early parenthood, and environmental risk for the next generation. *Canadian Journal of Behavioural Science, 23,* 318–331.

Serbin, L. A., Peters, P. L., & Schwartzman, A. E. (1996). Longitudinal study of early childhood injuries and acute illnesses in the offspring of adolescent mothers who were aggressive, withdrawn, or aggressive–withdrawn in childhood. *Journal of Abnormal Psychology, 105,* 500–507.

Shaw, D. S., Owens, E. B., Giovannelli, J., & Winslow, E. B. (2001). Infant and toddler pathways leading to early externalizing disorders. *Journal of the American Academy of Child and Adolescent Psychiatry, 40,* 36–43.

Wakschlag, L. S., Gordon, R., Lahey, B. B., Loeber, R., Green, S., & Leventhal, B. L. (2000). Maternal age at first birth and boys' risk for conduct disorder. *Journal of Research on Adolescence, 10,* 417–441.

Wakschlag, L. S., & Hans, S. L. (1999). Relation of maternal responsiveness during infancy to the development of behavior problems in high-risk youths. *Developmental Psychology, 35,* 569–579.

Wakschlag, L. S., & Hans, S. L. (2000). Early parenthood in context: Implications for development and intervention. In C. Zeanah (Ed.), *Handbook of infant mental health* (2nd ed., pp. 129–144). New York: Guilford Press.

Wakschlag, L. S., Pickett, K. E., Cook, E., Jr., Benowitz, N. L., & Leventhal, B. L. (2002). Maternal smoking during pregnancy and severe antisocial behavior in offspring: A review. *American Journal of Public Health, 92,* 966–974.

Woodward, L. J., & Fergusson, D. M. (1999). Early conduct problems and later risk of teenage pregnancy in girls. *Development and Psychopathology, 11,* 127–141.

Zoccolillo, M. (1993). Gender issues in conduct disorder. *Development and Psychopathology, 5,* 65–78.

Zoccolillo, M. (2000). Parents' health and social adjustment: Part II. Social adjustment. In M. Jette, H. Desrosiers, R. E. Tremblay, & J. Thibault (Eds.), *Longitudinal study of child development in Quebec (ELDEQ 1998–2002).* Québec: Institut de la statistique du Québec. Available at www.stat.gouv.qc.ca/publications/liste_an.htm

Zoccolillo, M., Pickles, A., Quinton, D., & Rutter, M. (1992). The outcome of childhood conduct disorder: Implications for defining adult personality disorder and conduct disorder. *Psychological Medicine, 22,* 971–986.

Zoccolillo, M., & Rogers, K. (1991). Characteristics and outcome of hospitalized adolescent girls with conduct disorder. *Journal of the American Academy of Child and Adolescent Psychiatry, 30,* 973–981.

# CHAPTER 13

# When Aggressive Girls Become Mothers

## Problems in Parenting, Health, and Development across Two Generations

Lisa A. Serbin, Dale M. Stack, Natacha De Genna,
Naomi Grunzeweig, Caroline E. Temcheff,
Alex E. Schwartzman, *and* Jane Ledingham

For many years, aggression in girls was a relatively neglected topic in the research literature. Until recently, girls were routinely excluded from longitudinal research designs on childhood aggression for several reasons. First, relatively few girls are referred, either within the mental health or juvenile justice systems, for problems related to aggression. Consequently, there were often too few aggressive girls available to study within a particular subject pool; thus girls were either omitted or simply combined with boys for purposes of analysis. Second, from a policy perspective there seemed to be little justification for studying the long-term developmental trajectories of aggressive girls, or to examine the pathways to adolescent and adult violence among females, since it was well known among decision makers that women did not commit many violent crimes.

Over the past several years, studies have begun to emerge showing that childhood aggression can be reliably identified and assessed in girls within community-based samples (Moskowitz & Schwartzman, 1989; Serbin, Moskowitz, Schwartzman, & Ledingham, 1991; Stack, Serbin,

Schwartzman, & Ledingham, in press). It became clear that aggression in girls may predict patterns of negative adolescent and adult outcomes that are distinct from the overt delinquency and other long-term outcomes typical of aggressive boys (Schwartzman & Mohan, 1999; Schwartzman, Verlaan, Peters, & Serbin, 1995; Serbin, Peters, McAffer, & Schwartzman, 1991). Longitudinal data revealed that aggression in girls was fairly stable over time, at least from childhood to adolescence (Coie & Dodge, 1998; Serbin, Peters, et al., 1991; Serbin et al., 1998; Stack et al., in press). Additionally, longitudinal studies began to show that the developmental trajectories of highly aggressive girls were generally problematic, in terms of both "homotypic" outcomes, such as juvenile delinquency and criminal offending, as well as "heterotypic" outcomes, such as school dropout, smoking, substance abuse, early-onset, high-risk sexual activity during the teen years, and mental health problems (Huesmann, Eron, Lefkowitz, & Walder, 1984; Moskowitz, Schwartzman, & Ledingham, 1985; Olweus, 1984). Increased interest in domestic violence (including spousal, child, and elder abuse and victimization) has also led to an increase in studies of women's aggression and an interest in its developmental antecedents during childhood.

Recent findings suggest that aggressive behaviour in girls may be a key element of a complex, transgenerational social pattern. The developmental trajectories of aggressive girls are interwoven with the histories of their parents, their own children, and their extended families. As with aggression in boys, particularly those who begin their antisocial behavior in early childhood, the risk equation for early-onset, persistent aggression in girls may also include genetic, neurocognitive, neuroendocrine, and other biologically based risk factors. However, in part because aggression has traditionally been characterized as a primarily male phenomenon with stability of gender differences observed across the lifespan, research attention has been largely directed toward physical and overt manifestations of aggression. As a result, indirect and covert expressions of aggression have been relatively neglected. However, the fact that males are considered to be more physically aggressive than females does not imply that females engage in fewer conflictual relations or experience decreased hostility (Bjorkqvist, 1994; Crick & Grotpeter, 1995). Possibly due to the fact that females are generally physically weaker than males, and perhaps also due to social constraints, women may develop alternative strategies to achieve their desired ends, engaging in more verbal or indirect forms of aggression rather than outright physical coercion. These indirect forms of aggression are often referred to as "relational aggression," and include attempts to harm others by means of causing damage to others' friendships or sense of inclusion in the associated peer group. Developmental change also characterizes girls' aggression; while continuing to use direct confrontation, emerging adolescent women also tend to exhibit social ostracism as a central feature of their expression of aggression (Cairns, Cairns, Neckerman, Ferguson, & Gariepy, 1989).

Another way researchers have studied manifestations or expressions of aggression over time is to examine "risk-taking" behavior. For example, a pattern of high-risk sexual behavior in adolescence has been documented in a number of prospective longitudinal studies of aggressive girls, including the age of onset of sexual activity and early pregnancy (e.g., Cairns & Cairns, 1994; Scaramella, Conger, Simons, & Whitbeck, 1998; Serbin, Peters, et al., 1991). Although it may be the case that early aggression is predictive of high-risk sexual activity for both genders (Capaldi, Crosby, & Stoolmiller, 1996), the established pattern of childhood aggression in boys as a predictor of ongoing delinquency and crime has been of primary interest in that literature (Capaldi, 1992; Conger, Elder, Lorenz, Simons, & Whitbeck, 1994; Farrington, 1991; Magnusson, 1988). Furthermore, while risk-taking behavior is one avenue to study heterotypic expressions of aggression, the effects of continued aggression may also manifest themselves in parenting behavior, the social and physical environment, and even the developmental and health outcomes of parent and child.

In the present chapter, we focus on a Canadian study of long-term trajectories and sequelae of girlhood aggression in the context of a broad range of negative psychosocial and health outcomes, including maternal and child health, difficulties in parenting, and the intergenerational transfer of risk to offspring. In general, we address the following three questions. First, what are the trajectories and pathways by which childhood aggression places a successive generation at risk for negative developmental outcomes? Second, are the risk factors and pathways from childhood aggression to problematic parenthood the same for men and women? Third, how do the offspring of parents with a history of childhood aggression fare in early childhood, and what are their prospects for the future?

## THE CONCORDIA LONGITUDINAL RISK PROJECT

### Overview: Design and Early Findings

The participants in the studies reviewed in this chapter come from a large, community-based research sample of disadvantaged families whose average income level and occupational status, for the most part, are significantly below the average levels for Canada and Quebec. This ongoing intergenerational study was begun by Jane Ledingham and Alex

Schwartzman (Ledingham, 1981; Schwartzman, Ledingham, & Serbin, 1985) in 1976–1978, when the parents of the current young participants were themselves elementary school-age children.

## Identification of the Original Sample

The Concordia Longitudinal Risk Project (CLRP) began in the school years 1976–1977 and 1977–1978 with the screening of 4,109 French-speaking school children attending regular grade 1, 4, and 7 classes in inner-city schools located in lower socioeconomic, inner-city neighborhoods of Montreal, Canada. Participation in the screening was voluntary, with over 95% of students consenting to participate. In total, 1,770 children met the criteria for inclusion (described later), including approximately equal numbers of boys ($n$ = 861) and girls ($n$ = 909) from each grade level.

The screening process involved the classification of children along the dimensions of aggression and social withdrawal by means of a French translation of the Pupil Evaluation Inventory (PEI; Pekarik, Prinz, Liebert, Weintraub, & Neale, 1976), a peer nomination instrument. The PEI consists of 34 items that load onto three factors: Aggression, Withdrawal, and Likeability. Scale items assess not only the behavior of the child, but also the reactions of peers toward the child. For the purpose of the Concordia project, children were screened only on the Aggression and Withdrawal factors.[1] Approximately half of the original participants had elevated risk profiles due to extreme patterns of atypical behavior, while the other half of the sample was normative in terms of social behavior, but came from the same inner-city schools in disadvantaged neighbourhoods.

Percentile cutoffs were established to identify children who exhibited extreme scores on the Aggression and/or Withdrawal scales, while enabling adequate sample sizes for statistical analysis. Children who scored above the 95th percentile on Aggression and below the 75th percentile on Withdrawal, relative to same-sex classmates, were selected for the aggressive group ($n$ = 101 girls, 97 boys); the reverse criteria were used to select the withdrawn group ($n$ = 112 girls, 108 boys). As a function of the low probability of achieving extreme scores on both dimensions, more liberal criteria were used to identify a sufficient number of children to form the aggressive–withdrawn group. $z$ scores equal to or above the 75th percentile on both Aggression and Withdrawal were criteria for membership in this group ($n$ = 129 girls, 109 boys). Finally, age-matched children for whom $z$ scores on Aggression and Withdrawal scales fell in the average range (i.e., between the 25th and 75th percentile) were selected for the contrast group ($n$ = 567 girls, 547 boys). For a

more extensive description of the original methodology, see Schwartzman and colleagues (1985; Ledingham, 1981; Ledingham & Schwartzman, 1981).

There are several unique features that characterize the CLRP. Unlike
most longitudinal studies of childhood aggression or other childhood
behavior problems, this is a community-based (rather than a clinical)
sample. Use of a community sample not only avoids the selection biases
inherent in clinic-referred samples, but is also more representative of the
population of Quebec. However, unlike many longitudinal studies of
disadvantaged children, specific atypical patterns of social behavior (i.e.,
aggression and withdrawal) were initially identified and could be followed as predictors within a population at high risk for psychosocial
problems. Another unique feature of the original design was the inclusion of an approximately equal number of girls and boys within each of
the risk profiles, based on comparisons to their same-sex peers. Consequently, the Concordia study is one of the few longitudinal studies
worldwide that has followed a large sample of aggressive girls into
adulthood. Due to the nature of the design, with some participants
showing patterns of atypical behavior and others with normative patterns of behavior, we are able to observe those factors that are predictive
of positive adaptation, an important focus of recent research on risk and
resiliency.

Now that the original participants are in their late 20s to early 30s,
many have become parents. This reality provides us with a unique opportunity to examine the sequelae of an aggressive behavioral style within the context of familial relations and the risk to the next generation.
Given this important and rare opportunity, intergenerational studies of
the offspring of the Concordia sample were underway virtually as soon
as children began to be born in the late 1980s (Serbin, Peters, et al.,
1991). The results to date strongly suggest that psychosocial risk may be
transferred across generations, via the behavior, functioning, environment, and social and economic circumstances of the participants as they
become parents (Serbin, Moskowitz, et al., 1991; Serbin, Peters, &
Schwartzman, 1996; Serbin et al., 1998, 2002; Stack et al., in press).

Children growing up under disadvantaged conditions are likely to
become the parents of another disadvantaged generation who, like their
parents, are born with a high risk of serious psychosocial and health
problems. However, longitudinal studies reveal that psychosocial risk is,
as the term denotes, probabilistic. Many children from "high-risk" backgrounds grow up to have reasonably prosperous and productive lives,
despite their poor prospects at birth (Elder & Caspi, 1988; Furstenberg,
Brooks-Gunn, & Morgan, 1987; Hardy et al., 1997; Rutter, 1987;
Werner & Smith, 1992).

The remaining sections of the chapter underscore some of the risk and protective factors (i.e., those factors that predict maladaptive and adaptive adjustment, respectively) in our prospective longitudinal study of two generations, and describe how girls' aggression is manifested across the lifespan, particularly highlighting the psychosocial, lifestyle, developmental, and health sequelae of girls' aggression. Other important foci include the pathways through which aggression develops and the transfer of risk for aggression across generations.

## Trajectories of Highly Aggressive Girls in the Concordia Longitudinal Risk Project through Middle Childhood, Adolescence, and Early Adulthood

Although many similarities exist between the risk trajectories of aggressive girls and aggressive boys, the path followed by many aggressive girls has proved to be rather distinctive. Recall that the highly aggressive girls in the sample were defined according to gender-based norms: That is, according to peer ratings they were more aggressive than the other girls in their class. However, it was the highly aggressive boys who were described by peers in terms of a profile underlining public, disruptive behavior perceived as intrusive, uncontrolled, and immature (Schwartzman et al., 1995).

At the time of identification, the highly aggressive children of both sexes were likely to have lower IQs and lower standardized academic achievement test scores than either the comparison or the socially withdrawn groups of children (Ledingham, 1981; Schwartzman et al., 1985). In other words, aggression was associated with cognitive and academic difficulties in both sexes, beginning as early as first grade. The joint constellation of aggression and withdrawal was particularly problematic, and this group of children high on both dimensions had the lowest average IQ and school achievement scores in the sample.

In a first follow-up study of academic outcomes 3 years after identification, few gender differences emerged in terms of the school progress of highly aggressive children; both aggressive girls and boys were more likely to have repeated a grade, or to have been placed in a special class for children with behavioral or learning problems (Schwartzman et al., 1985). These failure rates continued into high school, with the original aggression scores predicting elevated rates of high school dropout for both sexes, and the aggressive–withdrawn group failing at the highest rates. Aggression was clearly a negative predictor of academic success within both short-term and long-term time frames, especially if combined with other social and academic problems.

Aggression in elementary school-age girls was not solely problematic in terms of its association with lower cognitive or academic ability. Even when academic ability scores were controlled statistically, girls' aggression in elementary school continued to predict high school dropout (Serbin et al., 1998). Moreover, beginning in elementary school, the social and behavioral pathways to academic failure for girls and boys were somewhat different.

In an observational study of a sample of 174 fifth- and sixth-grade children on the playground (a younger group identified from among the same schools and using the same methods as the original CLRP project; Lyons, Serbin, & Marchessault, 1988; Serbin, Lyons, Marchessault, Schwartzman, & Ledingham, 1987; Serbin, Marchessault, McAffer, Peters, & Schwartzman, 1993), we found that peer-nominated aggressive girls and boys were more physically aggressive during play than nonaggressive children of either sex. In general, relatively few episodes of explicit or extreme aggression or violence were observed during this study of social interaction during recess periods. Most aggressive events were incorporated into episodes of "rough-and-tumble" play: for example, tackling, pushing, hitting, or kicking during games or lining up, and so forth. The peer-identified aggressive girls spent much of their time playing with boys engaged in "rough-and-tumble" play behavior (an atypical behavior pattern for girls at this age), and most of their observed aggressive acts were directed at boys (rather than other girls).

Girls' aggression in the later elementary school grades was associated with a preference for male playmates who were likely to reciprocate the "rough-and-tumble" play style, whereas other girls disliked this rough physical style of play. This pattern of associating with boys, especially those with aggressive play styles, and being avoided by girls may be a core element in the subsequent development of aggressive girls. Girls who are drawn to peer groups that engage in aggression and other types of risk-taking behavior in elementary school may expand their repertoire of deviant behavior as they mature, following the norms and values of their peer subgroup.

In early and mid-adolescence, girls' aggression was associated with elevated rates of self-reported smoking, alcohol, and illegal drug usage, suggesting that these girls continue to seek out behaviorally compatible peer groups, probably comprised of boys and girls with similar aggressive or "predelinquent" behavioral styles, if not those peers actively engaging in delinquent behavior. The aggressive girls, in general, report far less overt criminal or violent behavior than the aggressive boys during adolescence, as reflected in their much lower arrest records (Schwartzman & Mohan, 1999). However, they do have a higher arrest rate in their late teens than other girls, and along with their self reported "risktaking" behavior (such as smoking and drug use), it is highly likely that this is indicative of a pattern that will promote continuity in their negative life trajectories.

Another aspect of the risk-taking behavior and peer relations typical of the highly aggressive girls in the Concordia sample relates to their sexual behavior during adolescence. Using the relative risk ratio, a statistic which is widely used in epidemiological research (RR; Rothman, 1986), examination of adolescent health care records of 853 women revealed elevated risks for a variety of gynecological problems for aggressive girls throughout the teen years (Serbin, Peters, et al., 1991). A risk ratio permits comparison between the prevalence of a specific outcome within a risk population and the prevalence in a comparison group. For example, a risk ratio of 1 indicates an equivalence of this outcome in the risk and comparison groups, while a value greater than 1 indicates an increased prevalence of the outcome in the risk group. If the confidence interval created surrounding the observed RR (typically a 95% confidence interval) includes the value of 1, then the difference between the two groups cannot be considered a "true" difference. If, however, the confidence interval falls above the value of 1, then the difference is statistically significant and is considered meaningful. Calculations of the risk ratios revealed that childhood aggression predicted elevated rates of gynecological problems (RR = 2.55) and birth control use (RR = 2.04) between 11 and 17 years of age. Girls high in aggression were also found to have elevated incidence of sexually transmitted diseases (STDs) between the ages of 14 and 20 (RR = 1.54) and were more likely to have been pregnant before the age of 23 (RR = 1.36; Serbin, Peters, et al., 1991). The pattern observed in girls who were both aggressive and withdrawn in middle childhood was found to be even more dramatic. In addition to similar risk patterns found among the aggressive group, girls high in both of these risk dimensions were also found to have a teen pregnancy rate of 48% between the ages of 14 and 20 years (RR = 2.05). In other words, girlhood aggression seems to have predicted early, unprotected sexual activity during the teen years. This pattern continued into late adolescence and early adulthood, when teen parenthood, multiparity (defined as having more than one child by age 23), close spacing of successive births (less than 2 years apart), and obstetric and delivery complications were elevated risks for girls with childhood histories of aggression, and especially those with a combined history of aggression and withdrawal (Serbin et al., 1998).

These fertility patterns are associated with problematic subsequent histories for both parents and children, as opportunities for continuing education and achieving higher occupational status are curtailed, along with a probability of lower income across the life course (Furstenberg et al., 1987; Furstenberg, Brooks-Gunn, & Chase-Lansdale, 1989). For offspring, the risks extend to physical health and lack of social and economic support during the important prenatal period and continuing throughout childhood. As discussed later in the sections on health and the description of outcomes for offspring, these concerns for the health of offspring of highly aggressive women, especially those born to teen mothers, were confirmed in an examination of their pediatric medical records.

Finally, mental health outcomes for highly aggressive girls were examined in late adolescence and early adulthood. Interestingly, and consistent with the relatively low rates of criminal behavior in late adolescence and early adulthood by the women in the aggressive and aggressive–withdrawn groups, these peer-identified patterns of psychosocial risk were not associated with conduct disorder per se, but were predictive of elevated rates of depression and anxiety disorders (Schwartzman et al., 1995). In other words, aggression in girls appears to predict "internalizing" disorders in early adulthood, along with histories of adolescent risk-taking behavior (including smoking and alcohol and substance use) and unprotected sexual activity, as well as school dropout and early parenthood. We are currently studying the mental health status of the Concordia project participants as they complete the "vulnerability" period for major mental illness in early adulthood (i.e., mid-30s), and we will have more information on rates of specific disorders within the next few years.

The stress associated with the lifestyle suggested by these histories is no doubt considerable, involving incremental social, economic, and educational disadvantage across adolescence, as well as the likelihood of early parenthood with inadequate social, emotional, and financial support. This cumulative and acute stress may, in part, account for the elevated rates of mental health problems in these women. The long-term problems of aggressive girls cannot, however, be entirely attributed to their elevated risk for school dropout, early parenthood, and other stressful socioeconomic conditions. As we discuss in a later section, childhood aggression seems to reflect a stable behavioral style that continues to influence social relations into adulthood, including marital interaction patterns and parent–child relationships.

## MATERNAL HEALTH

Health behaviors and symptoms in adults may vary as a function of childhood risk status, indicating that childhood social behavior may help predict their future health outcomes as well as transmission of risk to the next generation via parenting. Girls who are seen as very aggressive by their peers may develop different health habits and physical ailments, which may in turn affect the physical environments (beginning *in utero*) of their future children. For example, mothers who were aggressive in childhood were more likely to have smoked during their pregnancies (De Genna, 2001; De Genna, Stack, Serbin, Schwartzman, & Ledingham, 2004), which suggests continuity of adolescent "risktaking" health behaviors into the main childbearing years. Current maternal smoking in mothers of young children, which may have an impact both on mothers' and children's current and future health, was also predicted by maternal childhood aggression and by previous use of controlled substances (De Genna, 2001; De Genna et al., 2004). Since smokers are also more likely to have partners who smoke (Walsh, Redman, Brinsmead, & Fryer, 1997), this has serious implications for the effects of secondhand smoke on the offspring of mothers who were aggressive as girls.

Moreover, there is evidence that childhood aggressive behavior in girls is related to poorer physical health in adulthood, even in these relatively young women. For example, maternal childhood aggression predicted respiratory complaints, including at least one experience of asthma, bronchitis, pneumonia, or sinusitis 3 months prior to our evaluation. Although roughly 20% of the mothers who were low on childhood aggression reported chronic respiratory problems, 26% of the mothers who were both aggressive and withdrawn and 44% of the mothers who were aggressive in childhood reported such health problems. The deleterious effects of maternal childhood aggression on maternal respiratory health were above and beyond the effects attributable to maternal education as well as current maternal smoking, which were controlled for in regression analysis. Previous alcohol and drug use predicted overall number of recent maternal symptoms (De Genna, 2001). Finally, mothers high on both childhood aggression and social withdrawal were more likely to have risk factors for chronic disease such as obesity as defined by body mass index (BMI), anemia, high blood pressure, and diabetes (De Genna et al., 2004; Stack, Serbin, De Genna, Schwartzman, & Ledingham, 2004).

Taken together, our findings suggest that when becoming parents, girls' health is ultimately affected by the trajectories followed by their aggression, as well as the combination of aggression and withdrawal. Moreover, this process can be explained in part by the girls' lifestyles, with negative patterns of fertility and poor health habits emerging in adolescence. That is, risk-taking behavior in aggressive teenage girls (e.g., timing of sexual activity, early pregnancy, tobacco dependence) was shown to adversely affect their health as young mothers. These health problems subsequently affect their offspring's chances for healthy lifestyles, in that mothers' health lifestyles affect their offspring's developmental outcomes and health, and they contribute to the quality of the home environment, discussed in the next section.

## CHILD HEALTH

We now turn to the health of the offspring of the Concordia sample. As anticipated, these children showed a variety of elevated risks from birth onward. However, it should be noted that risk is by definition probabilistic in the offspring generation, as it is for the previous one. Although a greater number of Concordia project offspring may have a given problem than the general population, many of the children, even those with multiple risk indicators in their histories and current situations, will not develop serious health, developmental, or behavioral problems. Nonetheless, the potential for a transfer of risk to the next generation via health is present in these families, whether through hereditary vulnerability or the modeling of poor health habits, and it is therefore important to monitor multiple outcomes in this generation.

We first examined the medical records of 94 children who were the offspring of teenage girls from the Concordia study (Serbin et al., 1996). These children's complete histories of emergency room (ER) visits between the time of their birth and age 4 were obtained from the provincial records office. We found that maternal childhood aggression was predictive of annual rates of visits to the ER, more specifically for treatment of injuries, acute infections, and asthma. Rates of emergency hospitalizations and emergency surgeries followed a similar pattern. For the children of women with histories of both aggression and withdrawal (the most elevated risk group), the average annual rate of ER visits for treatment by age 4 was three, compared with a modal rate of zero in the children of women from the comparison group. Clearly, the young offspring of the aggressive and aggressive–withdrawn women who had had children at a younger age were at elevated risk compared with the offspring of teen mothers who did not have high levels of aggression in their childhood behavioral histories.

Although we do not know the exact reasons for these group differences, the health data have implications for both behavioral and environmental explanations. First, the injury patterns in the children of mothers who were aggressive as children raise the serious possibility of child abuse and neglect. We could not investigate this directly from the medical records available to us at the time, which were intended to record service usage, but we are currently examining this possibility in an ongoing study. Similarly, the high rate of infections might suggest inadequate or unbalanced diets, weakened immune systems due to stress, and/ or poor hygiene in the home. It is fairly clear, however, that these results do not simply reflect family disorganization or inappropriate use of ER services (i.e., in lieu of regular medical care). Emergency hospitalization rates (with admission determined by medical staff) were consistent with patterns of walk-in ER visits (which may depend primarily on parental judgment and decision making; Serbin et al., 1996).

In a more recent study of the outcomes of 175 families (114 of whom were mothers with childhood histories of aggression or aggression–withdrawal) with offspring ages 1–6 years (Serbin, Stack, & Schwartz-man, 2000; Stack et al., in press), a number of common childhood health problems emerged. Almost a third of mothers reported chronic and recurrent respiratory illness in their children (asthma, bronchitis, upper respiratory infections, nasal allergies); 31% reported frequent middle ear infections (otitis media); and 10% reported severe illnesses (such as cancer, epilepsy, heart problems, kidney problems, thyroid problems, and lupus). Consistent with the literature on gender differences in early childhood health outcomes (Gissler, Jarvelin, Louhiala, & Hemminki, 1999; Siegel, 1982), boys in this intergenerational sample had more physical health problems in their medical histories than girls. For example, they had more overall illnesses as well as more respiratory problems, even after controlling for neonatal health status and maternal smoking in regression analyses (De Genna, 2001; Serbin et al., 2000; Stack et al., 2003, in press).

Physical health problems in children were predicted by a variety of historical and current factors including neonatal health status, current maternal tobacco use, and high levels of parenting stress, as well as mothers' childhood histories of aggression (which predicted mothers' smoking and children's respiratory problems) and social withdrawal (which predicted frequency of both pre- and perinatal health problems as well as infantile colic). Therefore, the effects of maternal childhood risk on offspring's health may be both direct and indirect. Not only do children inherit their parents' predispositions to particular illnesses, but they are also exposed to environments of their parents' choosing, as well as learning patterns of health behaviors such as poor nutrition, less consistent or effective use of preventative health services, and use of tobacco, alcohol, and controlled substances.

## PREDICTING PARENTING AND ENVIRONMENT

In specifically considering the trajectories of women's lives, longitudinal studies must consider the importance of motherhood and parenting.

Early parenthood, which is a major risk for girls from economically and socially disadvantaged backgrounds (Hechtman, 1989; Musick, 1993), has the potential to change young girls' lives in substantial and lasting ways. Teen parenthood is related to lower occupational status and a variety of psychosocial problems for women across their subsequent life course (Furstenberg et al., 1989). Negative long-term outcomes for teen mothers are particularly likely if these young women are prevented from completing high school or continuing their education because of successive, closely spaced pregnancies and ensuing family responsibilities (Layzer, St. Pierre, & Bernstein, 1996). Becoming mothers before completing high school and being socially and economically prepared to raise children constitutes an important aspect of the life difficulties facing aggressive girls as young adults.

The potential negative consequences of early parenthood are not restricted to young mothers, but include their offspring as well (Conger et al., 1994). Circumstances of birth play a major role in determining the child's future (Baldwin & Cain,1980; Hardy et al., 1989; Hechtman, 1989; Layzer et al., 1996; Whitman, Borkowski, Schellenbach, & Nath, 1987). Mothers' health, physical and emotional maturity, education, and family support are all important predictors of the health and development of their children. As the child confronts challenges throughout infancy and early childhood, the mother's resources and parenting ability will have an ongoing impact on developmental outcomes for her offspring. In a longitudinal context of prediction from earlier events, four important points of transition and intergenerational transfer of risk can be conceptualized: prenatal health, birth circumstances, postnatal health of mother and infant, and parenting. Each of these points of transition has implications for the future health and functioning of the entire family.

In considering whether childhood aggression might interfere with mothers' abilities to effectively parent their young children, we explored unresponsive parenting toward infants, toddlers, and school-age offspring to see whether these would be apparent in observations of mother–child interactions. In one study (Cooperman, 1996; Serbin et al., 1998), 84 women from the original sample participated with their eldest children (5–12 years of age) in four videotaped laboratory tasks. Both childhood aggression and maternal education proved to be independent predictors of maternal behavior. Aggression was predictive of unresponsive maternal behavior, while lower education predicted mothers' aggressive behavior toward offspring, lack of supportive behavior, and unresponsiveness. We also examined whether mothers' psychosocial difficulties during childhood would predict maladaptive behavior patterns to offspring during the observed interactions. Mothers' childhood aggression was predictive of offspring's restlessness. In the prediction of aggressivity in offspring (i.e., verbal and/or physical behavior, including hostility and defiance), a trend was observed for the children of aggressive mothers. That is, the more aggressive a mother was as a child, the more aggressive her child was observed to be. Finally, there was a significant relationship between girlhood aggression and unresponsive behavior in offspring, such that the more aggressive the mother was in childhood, the more likely her child was to engage in unresponsive behavior during the observed interaction period. Education appeared to be the major pathway identified for the relationship between mothers' childhood aggression and children's current behavior; however, mothers' childhood behavior also predicted parental and child behavior when education levels were controlled statistically. In addition to its independent predictive ability, childhood aggression was associated with low levels of school performance, which is a well-documented risk factor for problems in parent and child functioning (Milling Kinard & Reinherz, 1987; Velez, Johnson, & Cohen, 1989).

In a further study of parents and offspring, (Bentley, 1997, 2002; Bentley, Stack, & Serbin, 1998; Bentley, Stack, Serbin, Schwartzman, & Ledingham, 2002), we assessed the quality of the mother–child relationship during a 15-minute free-play session using the Emotional Availability Scales (Biringen, Robinson & Emde, 1988). Our results revealed that the quality of emotional availability may be compromised by mother's childhood risk status. In particular, mothers who were identified in childhood as being both aggressive and socially withdrawn demonstrated higher levels of hostility when interacting with their children. Moreover, mothers with higher stress levels were less sensitive and more hostile with their children during the free play.

In other studies with the Concordia sample we have examined specific forms of parenting (such as teaching styles) as well as contextual variables that might be considered pathways or mechanisms for the transfer of risk. For example, in one study we found that parents' childhood histories of aggression negatively predicted the provision of cognitive stimulation to their preschool-age offspring (Saltaris, 1999; Saltaris et al., in press). Cognitive stimulation was measured in two contexts: (1) maternal scaffolding during a structured teaching task with puzzles, and (2) the quality of the home environment, measured by the HOME scales (Bradley & Caldwell, 1984). Furthermore, these measures of cognitive stimulation were demonstrated to be mediators of offspring's cognitive competence. In another words, it appears that mothers' aggressive interpersonal style also affects their offspring's cognitive development via an understimulating home environment and less than optimal interpersonal teaching styles.

Finally, based on path models of the childhood and adolescent histories of 450 parents from the Concordia sample, four threats to parenting were identified: (1) school failure/dropout, (2) early parenthood, (3) single parenthood, and (4) poverty (Cooperman et al., 2002; Serbin, 2002). Results indicated that these threats to parenting were predicted by childhood aggression and withdrawal, academic achievement, and school dropout. In addition, separate models for men and women highlighted some differences, effectively demonstrating the negative impact of single parenthood on outcomes for women and children.

## CHILD OUTCOMES

In the aforementioned study of the 175 families with offspring between ages of 1 and 6, 60% of the children were found to have moderate to severe developmental, cognitive, or behavioral problems and 20–30% required urgent attention (e.g., speech/language therapy, behavioral treatment, stimulation programs). Thirty percent of the children studied had IQ scores below 85, which suggests the likelihood of ongoing cognitive delays and has serious implications for future school achievement and completion of high school. The rate of behavioral problems in delayed children doubled from toddler to preschool-age cohorts. That is, behavioral problems were twice as prevalent in children between the ages of 4 and 6 years, compared to those between the ages of 1 and 3, climbing to over 50% in the older cohort. This study also revealed important results regarding the comorbidity of developmental and behavioral problems. More specifically, 35% of the children had both cognitive and behavioral problems; this figure increased to 75% in 4- to 6-year-old boys. Finally, as mentioned earlier, there were elevated health risks (relative to population base rates), especially for respiratory-related illnesses (asthma, bronchitis) and ear infections.

Taken together, the main predictors of risk to offspring were parental history of aggression, current poverty, and parental smoking (predicting respiratory illnesses, asthma, bronchitis, etc.). There were also some "microprocesses" within the parenting and home environments that placed the children at additional risk. These include parenting stress, lack of satisfaction with social support, and quality of the home environment. Together, these environmental and parenting factors predicted children's IQ scores. However, it is also clear that maternal education served as a powerful buffer in these high-risk families, and may help explain why some women with negative psychosocial histories are better able to meet the challenges of adulthood and parenting.

## SUMMARY

Girls' aggression is a risk factor for a variety of circumstances that "threaten" the quality of their parenting and the home environment. These circumstances include school dropout, early parenthood, single parenthood, and poverty. Low academic ability (specifically in the areas of language arts and math), co-varying with aggression, is directly implicated in this profile. Gender differences with regard to the life trajectories of mothers and fathers were also found. In particular, research findings have underscored the importance of single parenthood as a risk factor for poverty, particularly for women and children. Moreover, academic ability moderates school success for aggressive girls (i.e., aggression does not directly predict dropout for girls).

During early childhood, risk to offspring can be conceived as "heterotypic," with cognitive and language development especially vulnerable. With respect to socioemotional functioning, both internalizing and externalizing problems are more likely in sons, whereas adaptive behavior is threatened in daughters. Physical health is also implicated in this course; parental smoking predicts upper respiratory illness, bronchitis, and asthma in children, particularly in boys. Our results suggest that the process through which risk is incurred is at least fourfold. First, socioeconomic status and the environment (i.e., poverty) provide a physical and cultural context for children's development, beginning in the prenatal period. Second, mothers' levels of distress (social support, parenting stress, and mental health symptoms) may also play an important role in the transfer of risk. Third, mothers' behavioral styles can influence the transfer of risk, specifically those styles that can be described as being conflictual/punitive, self-absorbed, and/or neglectful. Finally, risk can be incurred because mothers are not able to provide developmentally appropriate cognitive stimulation (as evidenced during a structured teaching task, maternal scaffolding, and scores on the HOME; for example, see Bentley, 2002; Saltaris et al., 2003; Serbin, Peters, et al., 1991).

## CONCLUSIONS AND RECOMMENDATIONS

The problematic life course of aggressive girls is the focus of an increasing number of longitudinal studies currently being carried out in many different countries, including ongoing projects in Canada, the United States, Britain, Scandinavia, Germany, and New Zealand. It is now acknowledged that this pattern of behavior is likely to be indicative of serious social and academic difficulties for the child herself, and is liable to have important negative consequences (such as victimization and bully-ing) for peers and others living in the girls' social environment. The long-term effects of girlhood aggression are just beginning to be understood in terms of life trajectories for aggressive girls themselves, as well as in terms of the impact on family members, on society at large, and, most recently, on the next generation: children born to girls with histories of aggressive behavior.

The women in the Concordia sample have pursued a wide variety of life trajectories. Early aggression appears to have had negative conse-quences via at least two distinct routes (i.e., a direct path and an indirect path). First, the aggressive behavioral patterns visible to peers in the chil-dren's elementary school classes seem to reflect a distinct interpersonal style that has been shown to be fairly stable across age. This style is echoed in successive social relationships, including those with peers, partners, and spouses, and, eventually, their young offspring. The nega-tive impact of this pattern in girls may be most obvious in continuing or even lifelong violent, neglectful, or coercive interpersonal relations in successive stages of the life course (e.g., bullying and coercive peer rela-tions, dating and spousal violence, child neglect and abuse, elder abuse). This pattern is also demonstrated in terms of associated health risks (e.g., smoking, substance abuse, early and unprotected sexual activity) and violations of legal and social conventions (e.g., traffic infractions and other "nonviolent" crime, school dropout, early parenthood, unem-ployment, welfare dependence). Such activities are related to modeling and support from the peer group with which aggressive girls associate. These subsequent difficulties doubtlessly perpetuate the negative trajec-tories of highly aggressive girls.

On the more positive side, however, protective factors (notably aca-demic ability and educational achievement) were also identified within the Concordia sample. Income (closely related to educational attain-ment) was also a powerful predictor and contextual modulator of the long-term outcomes associated with girlhood aggression. Many of the women (and their offspring) are now doing relatively well, despite their poor prospects in childhood or early adolescence. The ongoing chal-lenges for researchers in this field are to (1) pinpoint the processes whereby risk and protective factors operate; (2) isolate the amount of risk associated with distinct negative outcomes that may be quantita-tively attributed to specific predictors; (3) develop and evaluate para-digms for the reduction or elimination of these negative predictors in the context of research and social, educational, and health policy; and (4) conversely, the potential positive effects of maximizing the "buffers" and protective factors identified in longitudinal studies also needs to be ex-plored.

With regard to specific implications for future research directions, the following issues are underscored:

1. The need to continue to follow aggressive girls across their life course, looking at outcomes such as mental and physical health, social and occupational functioning, and family relations as important domains in middle adulthood and beyond.
2. The need to understand the direct and indirect processes whereby these children and their families remain at risk over time.
3. The need for a better understanding of social, environmental, cultural, economic, and other contextual factors as modulators of the risk process.
4. The need for a better understanding of the biological and health factors involved in aggressive behavioral styles in girls, both in terms of the origins and maintenance of aggressive behavior, and its consequences for women over the life course.
5. The need for parallel studies of aggressive boys in the research contexts of family, health, academic, and occupational outcomes, as most of the research on aggression and conduct disorder in boys has focused on risk for delinquency, crime, substance abuse, and the like.

## POLICY IMPLICATIONS

Some implications of these findings from the Concordia Project for social and health policy can be summarized as follows:

1. Aggression in girls is a predictor of long-term social, academic, and health problems, which can be identified as early as grade 1. Accordingly, it is crucial to identify high-risk children early and to provide appropriate and comprehensive intervention to families. A need for educational, economic, mental health, and medical services from birth onwards are all implicated in these results as essential for the healthy development of young children from high-risk backgrounds.

2. By the time children reach elementary school with patterns of aggression, social withdrawal, and poor cognitive and language skills, it may already be late to prevent academic and social problems. In elementary school-age populations, intensive and continuing programs are necessary to identify children with these problems, and then intervene appropriately.

3. Girls with both aggressive behavior and learning problems are at highest risk.

4. These results also support the urgent need for academic, social, and health support for high-risk girls in high school, in order to help them complete their education and to prevent early parenthood. Intervention programs to support high school completion may be crucial, not only for the trajectories of girls, but also for the health and development of their offspring.

5. Young parents, especially those with high-risk profiles, require economic and social support to successfully stimulate the development of their young children, and to promote their physical health.

6. Finally, these results strongly support the need to provide education, in addition to social and economic support, to high-risk parents with young children.

## CLOSING

There has been a great deal of progress in recent years in our knowledge and understanding of the complex ways in which an aggressive behavioral style places women at risk for ongoing problems across the life course. Aggression in girls is now acknowledged as a stable indicator of risk for continuing social, emotional, occupational, and health difficulties, both for the aggressive girls themselves as well as their families. The relation between girlhood aggression and intergenerational risk is also being clarified. Girls' aggression is clearly a risk factor for a variety of circumstances that may "threaten" the quality of their parenting and the home environment, which has serious implications for health and social policy. The developmental trajectories of girls and boys obviously intersect, particularly in adolescence and during parenthood. If we are to understand the origins and sequelae of aggression in general, we need to include both females and males within our conceptual and empirical frameworks.

## ACKNOWLEDGMENTS

The research described in this chapter was partially supported by grants from Child Care Visions (HRDC Canada), Child and Youth Mental Health and Wellbeing (Health Canada), the Canadian Institute for Health Research (CIHR), FQRSC/NATEQ Québec (Fonds québécois de la recherche sur la société e la culture / Le fonds nature et technologies), and the Social Sciences and Humanities Research Council of Canada (SSHRC). The Concordia Longitudinal Risk Research Program originated in 1976 under the direction of Jane Ledingham and Alex Schwartzman. The intergenerational project is currently directed by Lisa A. Serbin, Dale M. Stack, and Alex E. Schwartzman.

We thank Claude Senneville, Irfan Yaqub, and Zhang Ming Wang for their assistance in data analysis. We also thank Vivianne Bentley, Jessica Cooperman, Jennifer Karp, Valerie McAffer, Patricia Peters, and Christina Saltaris, who contributed to various stages of the Concordia Inter-generational Project. We are also appreciative for the help of research assistants Julie Brousseau, Dany Lacroix, Cheryl-Lynn Rogers, Manon St-Germain, Sandra Thibault, Nathalie Vaudry, and Diane Viau. We are particularly grateful to the Commission des écoles catholiques de montréal (CÉCM), Commission d'accès à l'information (CAI), Régie de l'assurance-maladie du Québec (RAMQ), Centre des services sociaux du Montréal métropolitain (CSSMM), Centre des services sociaux Richelieu (CSSR), and the Régie de l'assurance-automobile du Québec (RAAQ). Finally, we are most indebted to the participants in the study.

## NOTE

1. Aggression items measure constructs including relational, verbal, and physical aggression; for example, "Those who try to get other people in trouble," "Those who get mad when they don't get their way," "Those who tell other children what to do," and "Those who start a fight over nothing." Social withdrawal items tap concepts such as sadness, shyness, and social isolation; for example, "Those who are too shy to make friends easily," "Those who never seem to be having a good time," "Those who are upset when called on to answer questions in class," and "Those who are usually chosen last to join in group activities."

## REFERENCES

Baldwin, W., & Cain, V. S. (1980). The children of teenage parents. *Family Planning Perspectives, 12,* 34–43.

Bentley, V. (1997). *Maternal childhood risk status as a predictor of emotional availability and physical contact in mother–child interactions: An intergenerational study.* Unpublished master's thesis, Department of Psychology, Concordia University.

Bentley, V. (2002). *The influence of parental and contextual factors on the quality of the mother–child relationship and child cognitive and behavioural outcomes: Implications for the intergenerational transfer of risk.* Unpublished doctoral dissertation, Department of Psychology, Concordia University.

Bentley, V. M., Stack, D. M., & Serbin, L. A. (1998, April). *Maternal childhood risk status as a predictor of emotional availability in mother–child interactions.* Poster presented at the meeting of the International Conference on Infant Studies, Atlanta, GA.

Bentley, V. M., Stack, D. M., Serbin, L. A., Schwartzman, A. E., & Ledingham, J. (2002, August). *The influence of parental and contextual factors on the quality of the mother–child relationship: Implications for the intergenerational transmission of risk.* Poster presented at the International Society for the Study of Behavioural Development Biennial Conference, Ottawa, ON, Canada.

Biringen, Z., Robinson, J. L., & Emde, R. N. (1988). *The Emotional Availability Scales*. Unpublished manuscript, University of Colorado Health Sciences Center, Denver.

Bjorkqvist, K. (1994). Sex differences in physical, verbal, and indirect aggression: A review of recent research. *Sex Roles, 30*, 177–188.

Bradley, R. H., & Caldwell, B. M. (1984). The Home Inventory and family demographics. *Developmental Psychology, 20*, 315–320.

Cairns, R. B., & Cairns, B. D. (1994). *Lifelines and risks: Pathways of youth in our time*. New York: Cambridge University Press.

Cairns, R. B., Cairns, B. D., Neckerman, H. J., Ferguson, L. L., & Gariepy, J. L. (1989). Growth and aggression: I. Childhood to early adolescence. *Developmental Psychology, 25*, 320–330.

Capaldi, D. M., Crosby, L., & Stoolmiller, M. (1996). Predicting the timing of first sexual intercourse for at-risk adolescent males. *Child Development, 67*, 344–359.

Capaldi, E. J. (1992). The organization of behavior. *Journal of Applied Behavior Analysis, 25*, 575–577.

Coie, J. D., & Dodge, K. A. (1998). Aggression and antisocial behavior. In W. Damon & N. Eisenberg (Eds.), *Handbook of child psychology: Vol. 3. Social, emotional and personality fevelopment* (5th ed., pp. 779–863). New York: Wiley.

Conger, R. D., & Elder, G. H., Jr., with Lorenz, F. O., Simons, R. L., & Whitbeck, L. B. (1994). *Families in troubled times: Adapting to change in rural America* (Social institutions and social change). New York: de Gruyter.

Cooperman, J. M. (1996). *Maternal aggression and withdrawal in childhood: Continuity and intergenerational risk transmission*. Unpublished master's thesis, Concordia University.

Cooperman, J. M., Serbin, L. A., Schwartzman, A. E., Stack, D. M., Saltaris, C., & Karp, J. (2002, September). *The inter-generational carousel of disadvantage: Parenting conditions that foster another "go around" and those that stop the ride*. Paper presented at the Life History Research Society Meeting, New York.

Crick, N. R., & Grotpeter, J. K. (1995). Relational aggression, gender and social psychological adjustment. *Child Development, 66*, 710–722.

De Genna, N. (2001). *An investigation of physical health in high-risk mothers and their preschoolers: An inter-generational study*. Unpublished master's thesis, Department of Psychology, Concordia University.

De Genna, N. M., Stack, D. M., Serbin, L. A., Schwartzman, A. E., & Ledingham, J. E. (2004, May). *Maternal aggression and withdrawal, health-risk behaviours, and health in offspring: An intergenerational study*. Paper presented at the biennial meeting of the International Society for Infant Studies, Chicago.

Elder, G. H., Jr., & Caspi, A. (1988). Human development and social change: An emerging perspective on the life course. In N. Bolger, A. Caspi, G. Downey, & M. Moorehouse (Eds.), *Persons in context: Developmental processes*. New York: Cambridge University Press.

Farrington, D. P. (1991). Psychological contributions to the explanation of offending. *Issues in Criminological and Legal Psychology, 1*(17), 7–19.

Furstenberg, F. F., Jr., Brooks-Gunn, J., & Chase-Lansdale, L. (1989). Teenaged pregnancy and childbearing. *American Psychologist, 44*, 313–320.

Furstenberg, F. F., Jr., Brooks-Gunn, J., & Morgan, S. P. (1987). *Adolescent mothers in later life.* New York: Cambridge University Press.

Gissler, M., Jarvelin, M. R., Louhiala, P., & Hemminki, E. (1999). Boys have more health problems in childhood than girls: Follow-up of the 1987 Finnish birth cohort. *Acta Paediatrica, 88*, 310–314.

Hardy, J. B., Shapiro, S., Mellits, E. D., Skinner, E. A., Astone, N. M., Ensminger, M. E., & Hechtman, L. (1989). Teenage mothers and their children: Risks and problems. A review. *Canadian Journal of Psychiatry, 34*, 569–575.

Hardy, J. B., Shapiro, S., Mellits, E. D., Skinner, E. A., Astone, N. M., Ensminger, M., LaVeist, T., Baumgardner, R. A., & Starfield, B. H. (1997). Self-sufficiency at ages 27 to 33 years: Factors present between birth and 18 years that predict educational attainment among children born to inner-city families. *Pediatrics, 99*, 80–87.

Hechtman, L. (1989). Teenage mothers and their children: Risks and problems. A review. *Canadian Journal of Psychiatry, 34*, 569–575.

Huesmann, L. R., Eron, L. D., Lefkowitz, M. M., & Walder, L. D. (1984). The stability of aggression over time and generations. *Developmental Psychology, 20*, 1120–1134.

Layzer, J., St. Pierre, R., & Bernstein, L. (1996). *Early life trajectories of teenage mothers vs. older mothers.* Paper presented at the annual meeting of the Society for Research on Adolescence, Boston.

Ledingham, J. E. (1981). Developmental patterns of aggressive and withdrawn behavior in childhood: A possible method for identifying preschizophrenics. *Journal of Abnormal Child Psychology, 9*(1), 1–22.

Ledingham, J. E., & Schwartzman, A. E. (1981). L'identification de nouvelles populations a risque élevé: Le risque du chercheur [Identification of new populations at high risk: Risk to the researcher]. In G. Lauzon (Ed.), *Actes du Colloque sur la Recherche Sociale.* Quebec: Ministere des Affaires Sociales.

Lyons, J., Serbin, L. A., & Marchessault, K. (1988). The social behaviour of peer-identified aggressive, withdrawn, and aggressive/ withdrawn children. *Journal of Abnormal Child Psychology, 16*(5), 539–552.

Magnusson, D. (1988). *Paths through life* (Vol. 1). Hillsdale, NJ: Erlbaum.

Milling Kinard, E., & Reinherz, H. (1987). School aptitude and achievement in children of adolescent mothers. *Journal of Youth and Adolescence, 16*, 69–87.

Moskowitz, D. S., & Schwartzman, A. E. (1989). Painting group portraits: Studying life outcomes for aggressive and withdrawn children. *Journal of Personality, 57*(4), 723–746.

Moskowitz, D. S., Schwartzman, A. E., & Ledingham, J. E. (1985). Stability and change in aggression and withdrawal in middle childhood and early adolescence. *Journal of Abnormal Psychology, 94*(1), 30–41.

Musick, J. S. (1993). *Young, poor, and pregnant: The psychology of teenage motherhood.* New Haven, CT: Yale University Press.

Olweus, D. (1984). Stability in aggressive and withdrawn, inhibited behavior patterns. In R. M. Kaplan, V. J. Konecni, & R. W. Novaco (Eds.), *Aggression in children and youth* (pp. 104–137). Netherlands: Martinus Nijhoff.

Pekarik, E. G., Prinz, R. J., Liebert, D. E., Weintraub, S., & Neale, J. M. (1976). The Pupil Evaluation Inventory: A sociometric technique for assessing children's social behavior. *Journal of Abnormal Psychology*, 4(1), 83–97.

Rothman, K. J. (1986). *Modern epidemiology*. Toronto: Little, Brown.

Rutter, M. (1987). Psychosocial resilience and protective mechanisms. *American Journal of Orthopsychiatry*, 57(3), 316–331.

Saltaris, C. (1999). *The influence of intellectual stimulation on the cognitive functioning of high-risk preschoolers: Implications for the transmission of risk across generations* Unpublished master's thesis, Department of Psychology, Concordia University.

Saltaris, C., Serbin, L. A., Stack, D. M., Karp, J. A., Schwartzman, A. E., & Ledingham, J. (in press). Nurturing cognitive competence in preschoolers: A longitudinal study of intergenerational continuity and risk. *International Journal of Behavioral Development*.

Scaramella, L. V., Conger, R. D., Simons, R. L., & Whitbeck, L. B. (1998). Predicting risk for pregnancy by late adolescence: A social contextual perspective. *Developmental Psychology*, 34(6), 1233–1245.

Schwartzman, A. E., Ledingham, J., & Serbin, L. A. (1985). Identification of children at risk for adult schizophrenia: A longitudinal study. *International Review of Applied Psychology*, 34(3), 363–380.

Schwartzman, A. E., & Mohan, R. (1999, June). *Gender differences in the adult criminal behavior patterns of aggressive and withdrawn children*. Presented at the ninth scientific meeting of the International Society for Research in Child and Adolescent Psychopathology, Barcelona, Spain.

Schwartzman, A. E., Verlaan, P., Peters, P., & Serbin, L. (1995). Sex roles as coercion. In J. McCord (Ed.), *Coercion and punishment in long-term perspectives* (pp. 362–375). New York: Cambridge University Press.

Serbin, L. A. (2002, May). *When aggressive girls become mothers: Problems in parenting, health, and development across two generations*. Paper presented at the Conference on Aggression, Antisocial Behavior, and Violence among Girls: A Developmental Perspective, Sanford Institute of Public Policy, Duke University, Durham, NC.

Serbin, L. A., Cooperman, J. M., Peters, P. L., Lehoux, P. M., Stack, D. M., & Schwartzman, A. E. (1998). Inter-generational transfer of psychosocial risk in women with childhood histories of aggression, withdrawal or aggression and withdrawal. *Developmental Psychology*, 34, 1246–1262.

Serbin, L. A., Lyons, J., Marchessault, K., Schwartzman, A. E., & Ledingham, J. (1987). Observational validation of a peer nomination technique for identifying aggressive, withdrawn and aggressive-withdrawn children. *Journal of Consulting and Clinical Psychology*, 55(1), 109–110.

Serbin, L. A., Marchessault, K., McAffer, V., Peters P., & Schwartzman, A. E. (1993). Patterns of social behavior on the playground in 9- to 11-year- old girls and boys: Relation to teacher perceptions and to peer ratings of aggression, withdrawal and likability. In C. Hart (Ed.), *Children on playgrounds: Research perspectives and applications* (pp. 162–183). Albany: State University of New York Press.

Serbin, L. A., Moskowitz, D. S., Schwartzman, A. E., & Ledingham, J. E. (1991).

Aggressive, withdrawn, and aggressive/withdrawn children in adolescence: Into the next generation. In D. Peplar & K. A. Rubin (Eds.), *The development and treatment of childhood aggression* (pp. 55–70). New York: Guilford Press.

Serbin, L. A., Peters, P. L., McAffer, V. J., & Schwartzman, A. E. (1991). Childhood aggression and withdrawal as predictors of adolescent pregnancy, early parenthood, and environmental risk for the next generation. *Canadian Journal of Behavioural Science, 23*(3), 318–331.

Serbin, L. A., Peters, P. L., & Schwartzman, A. E. (1996). Longitudinal study of early childhood injuries and acute illnesses in the offspring of adolescent mothers who were aggressive, withdrawn, or aggressive-withdrawn in childhood. *Journal of Abnormal Psychology, 105*(4), 500–507.

Serbin, L. A., Stack, D. M., & Schwartzman, A. E. (2000). *Identification and prediction of risk and resiliency in high-risk preschoolers: An intergenerational study* (Final Report No. 6070-10-5/9515). Ottawa, ON, Canada: Child, Youth and Family Health Unit, Child and Youth Division, Health Canada.

Serbin, L. A., Stack, D. M., Schwartzman, A. E., Cooperman, J. Bentley, B., Saltaris, C., & Ledingham, J. (2002). A longitudinal study of aggressive and withdrawn children into adulthood: Patterns of parenting and risk to offspring. In R. J. McMahon & R. Peters (Eds.), *The effects of parental dysfunction on children* (pp. 43–69). New York: Kluwer Academic/Plenum Press.

Siegel, L. (1982). Reproductive, perinatal and environmental factors as predictors of the cognitive and language development of preterm and fullterm infants. *Child Development, 53*, 963–973.

Stack, D. M., Serbin, L. A., De Genna, N., Schwartzman, A. E., & Ledingham, J. (2004). *From mother to child: An intergenerational study of maternal high risk behaviors and physical health in offspring of mothers with histories of aggression and social withdrawal.* Manuscript in preparation.

Stack, D. M., Serbin, L. A., Schwartzman, A. E., & Ledingham, J. (in press). Girls' aggression across the life course: Long-term outcomes and intergenerational risk. In D. Peplar, K. Madsen, C. Webster, & K. Levene (Eds.), *Development and treatment of girlhood aggression.* Mahwah, NJ: Erlbaum.

Velez, C. N., Johnson, J., & Cohen, P. (1989). A longitudinal analysis of selected risk factors for childhood psychopathology. *Journal of the American Academy of Child and Adolescent Psychiatry, 28*, 861–864.

Walsh, R. A., Redman, S., Brinsmead, M. W., & Fryer, J. L. (1997). Predictors of smoking in pregnancy and attitudes and knowledge of risks of pregnant smokers. *Drug and Alcohol Review, 16*(1), 41–67.

Werner, E., & Smith, R. (1992). *Overcoming the odds: High-risk children from birth to adulthood.* Ithaca, NY: Cornell University Press.

Whitman, T. L., Borkowski, J. G., Schellenbach, C. J., & Nath, P. S. (1987). Predicting and understanding development delay of children of adolescent mothers: A multidimensional approach. *American Journal of Mental Deficiency, 92* (1), 40–56.

# PART V

# IMPLICATIONS FOR POLICY AND INTERVENTION

# Future Directions and Priorities for Prevention and Intervention

Marion K. Underwood *and* John D. Coie

As the contributions to this volume make abundantly clear, girls behave aggressively in a variety of ways, and their aggressive behavior has serious negative consequences during childhood, in adolescence, as they enter romantic relationships, and as they become parents. Rapidly accumulating research evidence documenting the dire outcomes associated with girls' aggression demands that prevention and intervention efforts begin in earnest to address girls' needs. These excellent chapters offer many important clues as to what might be the optimal design, timing, and content of programs to prevent and interrupt girls' aggression. This commentary will attempt to integrate the many useful suggestions for intervention that follow from the work in this volume, beginning with approaches for intervening to reduce physical aggression and disruptive behavior, then continuing with strategies for reducing more common, subtle forms of hurtful behavior. Because programs to reduce girls' aggression must be tailored to their needs at specific developmental periods, much of this commentary will be organized developmentally. The focus here will be understanding girls' aggression in its own right and closely examining the processes by which it unfolds (Maccoby, Chapter 1, this volume), so that our efforts to prevent or interrupt it will be maximally effective.

## REDUCING GIRLS' PHYSICAL AGGRESSION
## AND DISRUPTIVE BEHAVIOR

All of the longitudinal data presented in this book clearly demonstrate that girlhood aggression contributes to a cascading set of negative outcomes as young women move into adolescence and adulthood. Young girls who engage in disruptive behavior and fight are at risk for being rejected by peers, feeling alienated and unsupported in their relationships with peers and adults, struggling academically, affiliating with other peers prone to deviant behavior, becoming involved in more serious antisocial behaviors, choosing antisocial romantic partners, initiating and receiving partner violence, becoming adolescent mothers, having children with more health problems, and being less sensitive and responsive as parents (see especially Capaldi, Kim, & Shortt, Chapter 11; Pepler, Craig, Yuile, & Connolly, Chapter 5; Serbin et al., Chapter 13; and Zoccolillo, Paquette, Azar, Côté, & Tremblay, Chapter 12). Some few aggressive girls become sufficiently antisocial and even violent that they are incarcerated; if they are also mothers, many lose custody of their children, and opportunities for stable employment and relationships diminish substantially (Giordano, Cernkovich, & Lowery, Chapter 9).

Given the low base rates of girls engaging in physical aggression and violence (see Coie & Dodge, 1998, for a review), identifying girls at risk is a critically important step for prevention and intervention programs. The contributions in this volume offer important clues as to risk factors. Understanding more about how biological factors relate to girls' aggression will likely help us understand at what point in development intervention efforts are most likely to succeed (Susman & Pajer, Chapter 2). For example, some girls who are temperamentally overactive as toddlers and preschoolers may be at risk. Another biological factor associated with increased risk for aggressive behavior is early pubertal development (Susman & Pajer, Chapter 2). Interestingly, girls report engaging in high levels of bullying as they enter puberty (Pepler, Craig, Yuile, & Connolly, Chapter 5), and early-developing girls may be likely targets as well as perpetrators. Still another group of girls at special risk for developing aggression may be sexually abused girls, particularly those abused by their biological fathers over a long period of time (Trickett & Gordis, Chapter 8).

Longitudinal studies suggest that aggression and disruptive behavior in early childhood predict a host of later problems for girls (Bierman et al., Chapter 7; Serbin et al., Chapter 13). A broad screening strategy considering oppositional–defiant and attentional difficulties in addition to early aggression is more effective in identifying girls at risk for aggression and peer problems in fourth grade and antisocial behavior in seventh grade than is one that just targets physical aggression (Bierman et al., Chapter 7). Evidence suggests that active and disruptive girls are every bit as much at risk as disruptive boys, even if there are fewer of them or if the level of physical aggression drops off, relative to boys, during the school years.

Contributors agree that successful interventions will need to offer services for high-risk girls at every developmental stage (see especially Serbin et al., Chapter 13; Zoccolillo et al., Chapter 12). However, it is much less clear what the content of these interventions should be and whether gender-specific interventions are required to help aggressive girls.

We concur with several of these authors that prevention of aggressive behavior will require intervening prenatally with programs for high-risk expectant mothers, especially young adolescent mothers and those who were themselves aggressive or disruptive as children (see especially Serbin et al., Chapter 13; Zoccolillo et al., Chapter 12). As aggressive girls become parents, research suggests they will need a variety of types of services to augment their skills in parenting. Given that children of young mothers with histories of girlhood aggression may be more prone to infections and injuries (Serbin et al., Chapter 13), these young women may benefit from basic training in practical skills such as the hygienic care of young children, childproofing, nutrition and meal planning, and household management. Young mothers with a history of conduct disorder have also been observed to be low on maternal sensitivity (Serbin et al., Chapter 13), and prone to maternal irritability and harsh parenting (Zoccolillo et al., Chapter 12). One reason for this may be that they are prone to making hostile attributions for normal infant behaviors, such as viewing crying or urinating during diaper changing as intentional. Young mothers with a history of girlhood aggression may especially benefit from basic instruction in normal child development and strategies for responding to difficult infant behaviors (Zoccolillo et al., Chapter 12). Helping young mothers respond optimally to challenging behaviors of infants and toddlers may help the children be more compliant and responsive to socialization attempts, and the young mothers less likely to engage in coercive parenting practices that set the stage for the child to become aggressive and antisocial (Patterson, 1982).

Regardless of the mother's history of girlhood aggression, prevention programs should target preschool-age girls who are becoming disruptive and noncompliant. The few girls who have these behavior problems are at risk just as much as boys are. Intervening early to give these girls basic skills in attending and relating to people may augment their abilities to respond to adult suggestions, to make the transition to formal schooling, and to succeed in forming early peer relationships. Basic skills in modulating angry and distressed emotions are acquired during the infant and toddler years (Saarni, Mumme, & Campos, 1998), and training parents in the kinds of soothing and emotion labeling skills that promote this development may be important for very young girls. Girls who struggle to form relationships and regulate emotions are at risk for beginning a developmental trajectory toward serious problems in adolescence, and these basic problems, left unaddressed, will decrease the likelihood of their responding well to later intervention attempts.

For girls who persist in showing disruptive and aggressive behavior as they move through elementary school, it will be important to focus programs on building particular skills. In childhood, girls high on aggression tend to engage in high levels of rough-and-tumble play with boys (Serbin et al., Chapter 13). This rough play might be desensitizing them to physically aggressive behavior and setting the stage for early affiliations with males. Thus, a worthwhile goal of intervention might be encouraging and strengthening relationships with other young girls, especially girls with low rates of deviant behavior. However, it may be more practical and realistic to encourage highly active, physically adept girls to engage in team sports, as a less aggressive alternative to informal rough-and-tumble play with boys.

As girls move through middle childhood, it seems particularly likely that girls' episodes of physical aggression are preceded by relational aggression. Understanding how relational aggression leads to physical violence for some girls will be helpful in understanding and predicting which girls are most at risk for violence. Successful interventions for physically aggressive girls will likely need to focus on relational aggression as well (strategies for reducing relational aggression will be discussed in the next section).

During adolescence, successful interventions for aggressive girls will need to address their propensities for affiliating with antisocial males (Zoccolillo et al., Chapter 12) and for becoming adolescent mothers (Serbin et al., Chapter 13; Zoccolillo et al., Chapter 12). That aggressive girls partner with antisocial males increases the girls' risk of being involved in domestic violence (Capaldi et al., Chapter 11), and may be related to girls' involvement in other types of antisocial behavior, including smoking (Zoccolillo et al., Chapter 12) and likely other much more risky activities. Clinical experience suggests that girls with histories of conduct disorder seem determined to actively seek out antisocial males (Zoccolillo et al., Chapter 12); thus, this attraction will likely be difficult to interrupt. On the other hand, programs designed to improve the social skills of these girls in elementary school may enable them to join less deviant peer networks and thus have a broader range of males with whom to form relationships.

Given that assortative mating has dire consequences, including but not limited to domestic violence (Capaldi et al., Chapter 11), adolescent motherhood (Serbin et al., Chapter 13; Zoccolillo et al., Chapter 12), and a serious genetic risk to offspring (Zoccolillo et al., Chapter 12), it may be time to devise clever, strategic interventions that help aggressive girls desire and form relationships with less antisocial men. Public information campaigns may be helpful, to educate girls about romantic violence and the long-term implications for themselves and their children of being involved with aggressive males. Television movies on this topic proliferate in venues such as the Lifetime television network, but media such as these will be unlikely to reach the target audience. The time is ripe for getting film and perhaps even computer/video game creators interesting in developing presentational and interactive games that would engage young women on these topics.

Clearly, interventions with aggressive adolescent girls should include components to prevent pregnancy, but this will likely not be straightforward. Antisocial teen girls have high rates of motherhood even in regions where contraception and abortion are widely available (Zoccolillo et al., Chapter 12). Preventing aggressive girls from wanting to have babies may require inspiring them to want to stay in school (Serbin et al., Chapter 13), to have plans and goals for the future, and to have reasonable employment opportunities (Giordano et al., Chapter 9).

As aggressive girls enter romantic relationships, intervention programs will need to target their propensity for being involved in relationship violence, not just as victims, but also as initiators (Capaldi et al., Chapter 11). When young couples were observed in the laboratory, young women were actually more likely to initiate violence than young men were (Capaldi et al., Chapter 11). Girls as well as boys who report high levels of bullying are more likely to engage in sexual harassment and dating aggression (Pepler et al., Chapter 5). At the very least, these findings suggest that a component of intervention with aggressive girls must be focused on preventing domestic violence, by teaching girls skills in anger control, more appropriate responses to feeling rejected or threatened, and conflict resolution strategies. Here again, the timing for this kind of intervention may need to begin earlier in life for them to be available when they are needed in life with a partner.

The preceding discussion reflects our strong belief that young aggressive, disruptive girls will likely benefit from help in relating to others and managing strong emotions, just as aggressive, disruptive boys do.

How have aggressive girls responded to gender-neutral, large-scale interventions? Does girls' aggression decline as a result of interventions that have been shown to be helpful for boys? The Fast Track intervention project screened both kindergarten boys and girls into high-risk groups for intervention (about one-third of them being girls, based on common selection criteria). These gender-mixed groups were offered social skill training from first grade through fifth grade, with the sessions becoming less frequent each year. Evidence from outcomes assessed at the end of grades 1 and 3 (Conduct Problems Prevention Research Group, 1999, 2002) suggests that boys and girls benefited equally from the program, with early social status improvement being accompanied by more positive social behavior and, eventually, less aggressive and disruptive behavior. For both boys and girls in the intervention group, the developmental trajectories showed a diminishing pattern of multiple forms of serious conduct problem behavior from first to fifth grade, relative to boys and girls in the control group. However, it is also true that as children in the project moved into preadolescence and adolescence, more of the group activities were conducted separately with boys and girls, in response to gender differences in the nature of the issues demanding attention.

Other evidence suggests that older girls may respond poorly to programs designed primarily for boys. Girls in a treatment foster care program actually got worse over 6 months of treatment whereas boys' behavior improved, perhaps because girls were engaging in high levels of relational aggression that was unaddressed by the program (Leve & Chamberlain, in press). In 1998, the Office of Juvenile Justice and Delinquency Prevention offered suggestions for best practices for programs to help antisocial girls: enhancing self-esteem, fostering positive body image, teaching empowerment, and enhancing interpersonal relationships. However, experts in criminology have noted that some of what are touted as optimal characteristics of treatment programs for adolescent girls are really optimal for all youth: supportive therapeutic environments, consideration of developmental issues, training in skills for independent living, and broad-based, long-lasting interventions (Kempf-Leonard & Sample, 2000).

Whether gender-specific intervention is required to help aggressive girls is in large part a developmental question. When intervening to help young aggressive, disruptive children, it may be sensible to work with girls and boys together, because both groups can likely benefit from basic skills training in forming relationships and managing emotions. As children move toward adolescence and gender-specific issues emerge, then it may be critically important to develop programs that focus on girls' relational aggression, propensity for affiliating with antisocial males, sexual decision making, and parenting.

In designing prevention and intervention programs that meet the specific needs of aggressive girls, it will likely be helpful to remember that not all aggressive girls grow up to have serious problems, and to understand what factors might be protective for this particular group. Longitudinal studies suggest that intelligence and educational attainment are protective factors for aggressive girls (Serbin et al., Chapter 13); intelligence may be less amenable to intervention, but helping girls to stay in school should continue to be a priority for programs to help aggressive girls. Just as men may be helped to desist from crime by marriage and employment stability (Sampson & Laub, 1993), girls' desistance may be supported by having stable relationships and job opportunities (Giordano et al., Chapter 9). However, because antisocial women may be even more marginalized and deviant than antisocial men, and may have more associated mental health problems, it will be challenging to help young women have access to what Giordano and colleagues aptly call the full "respectability package." Helping antisocial young women work toward this goal will require offering them treatment for psychological problems, assistance in staying in school, reasonable job opportunities, affordable childcare and support in their parenting, and social services to support them when they falter. Physically aggressive, violent girls will likely respond better to programs that also address their propensity to engage in subtle forms of hurtful behaviors, behaviors that undermine their ability to form relationships and make aggressive girls vexing for caregivers and professionals alike.

## PREVENTING AND INTERRUPTING SUBTLE FORMS OF AGGRESSION

In the last 15 years, scholarship on girls' aggression has moved from a paucity of studies justified by the lower base rates of physical aggression in girls to an explosion of research on the more subtle ways that girls may hurt one another: indirect aggression (Buss, 1961; Feshbach, 1969; Lagerspetz, Bjorkqvist, & Peltonen, 1988), social aggression (Cairns, Cairns, Neckerman, Ferguson, & Gariepy, 1989; Galen & Underwood, 1997), and relational aggression (Crick & Grotpeter, 1995). Efforts to reduce aggression in girls must address these more subtle behaviors, because they are hurtful in their own right, they may lead to episodes involving serious violence, and subtle, manipulative behaviors may make physically aggressive girls difficult to help.

What do the contributions in this volume suggest for the design and content of interventions to reduce indirect/relational/social aggression in girls? Children engage in relational aggression as early as the preschool years, in fairly overt and unsophisticated forms (Crick, Ostrov, Appleyard, Jansen, & Casas, Chapter 4). Preschool children view relational aggression as more acceptable than verbal or physical aggression (Goldstein, Tisak, & Boxer, 2002). Together, these findings suggest that preschool may be a window of opportunity during which adults might have occasions to witness more overt forms of relational aggression and intervene directly *in vivo*, by helping children know adults are aware of the behavior, it hurts people's feelings, and it will have negative consequences.

Although conducting focus groups with teachers may be one approach for devising strategies for reducing relational aggression (Crick et al., Chapter 4), existing research already offers important clues for how social aggression might be prevented or reduced as children mature and forms of these behaviors become more sophisticated. Such strategies might include sensitizing parents to how children might learn social aggression by being triangulated in marital conflicts (Kerig, Brown, & Patenaude, 2001), providing multiple opportunities for more girls to belong so girls may have less intense needs to confirm their own acceptance by excluding others (Adler & Adler, 1995), engaging girls in more structured activities so they have less time for gossip (Larson, Wilson, Brown, Furstenberg, & Verma, 2002), and helping girls to become more comfortable with appropriate competition (Benenson et al., 2002). More skill-focused activities might include social-cognitive interventions to help children make fewer hostile attributions in relationally provoking situations (Crick, Grotpeter, & Bigbee, 2002); assertiveness training; harnessing girls' distaste for social aggression (French, Jansen, & Pidada, 2002) and their considerable empathy (Zahn-Waxler & Polanichka, Chapter 3) to help them refrain; teaching girls to actively defend peer victims, as some are naturally prone to doing (Salmivalli, Lagerspetz, Bjorkqvist, Osterman, & Kaukiainen, 1996); and teaching girls to interrupt malicious gossip by immediately challenging negative evaluation statements (Eder & Enke, 1991; see Underwood, 2003, for a discussion of how already available research evidence might guide specific strategies).

However, adults will need to proceed cautiously in intervening to reduce subtle forms of aggression; adolescent girls believe that adult intervention in situations involving indirect aggression not only is unhelpful, it often makes matters worse (Owens, Shute, & Slee, 2000). The most effective intervention strategies will likely be guided by precise information about how relational aggression unfolds.

Given that girls believe that adult intervention in relational aggression is unhelpful, it may be fruitful to direct intervention efforts not only toward perpetrators of relational aggression, but also to try to reduce the behavior by helping victims respond optimally. Helping victims learn to respond more effectively is not to blame them for being the target of bad behavior, but it is a potential avenue for interrupting subtle behavior that often ignites quickly and wounds deeply before adults know what has happened. This kind of help may be equally necessary for aggressive, socially incompetent girls as for more passive and helpless victims. In a microanalytic study of aggression in girls' playgroups, Putallaz, Kupersmidt, Coie, McKnight, and Grimes (Chapter 6) found that victims of aggression responded by ignoring (60% of the time), confronting or challenging (15%), reactive aggression (13%), and de-escalating by compromising or using humor (12%). When they examined the effectiveness of each of these responses in leading to the episode ending or to the aggressor backing down, as expected, responding with reactive aggression was ineffective (leading to continued aggression 77% of the time). However, Putallaz et al. found that the strategies most often endorsed by adults, either ignoring or confronting, were also quite ineffective, leading to subsequent aggression in 59% of episodes. The most effective victim response in terminating the aggression was also the least common, de-escalating, which led to a positive outcome in 57% of episodes. This close examination of how relational aggression unfolds among girls leads to specific strategies for intervention, teaching victims to de-escalate by changing their behavior, compromising, defending themselves, or using self-deprecating humor. Here again, though, victims might also benefit from help in forming relationships and managing emotions, because without these basic skills, victimized girls will likely have great difficulty learning strategies for de-escalation.

As important as it has been to understand the subtle yet hurtful forms of girls' aggression, it is important to remember that girls' aggression is not entirely relational (Putallaz et al., Chapter 6). Some few girls do engage in physical aggression and serious violence, and high correlations between social and physical aggression in childhood suggest that girls who aggress likely do so in multiple ways (for reviews, see Crick et al. [1999]; Underwood [2003]). A girl who is high on both physical and relational aggression may be difficult to help. Evidence suggests that girls' propensity for "relational hypocrisies" (Zanarini & Gunderson, 1997) might result in adjudicated girls responding poorly to treatment foster care (Leve & Chamberlain, in press) and in many juvenile justice workers trying to avoid working with young female offenders (Chesney-Lind & Belknap, Chapter 10). We know little about the specific social processes by which relational aggression might lead some few girls, perhaps those who lack skills in emotional regulation, to engage in physical aggression, and examining this question could be helpful in identifying girls at risk for violence.

## CONCLUSION

In closing, we wish to emphasize that simply admonishing girls to stop behaving aggressively will likely be ineffective for three fundamental reasons. First, some girls likely behave aggressively because they have deficits in basic skills needed for relating to other people, initiating and maintaining relationships, and managing emotions. Successful interventions for girls at all developmental stages will need to augment these foundational abilities. Second, although these basic skills must be addressed in all intervention programs, specific developmental stages will demand additional strategies to reduce aggressive behavior (for example, reducing relational aggression for girls in middle childhood, and helping adolescent aggressive girls refrain from becoming involved with antisocial men). Third, we must not lose sight of the fact that, at times, girls' aggression can be adaptive for them in important ways. Subtle forms of aggression may sometimes serve important developmental functions for girls; for example, some forms of gossip may serve to maintain group boundaries, join with peers, negotiate identity and moral boundaries, and confirm one's own sense of belonging and acceptance (Putallaz et al., Chapter 6). Girls may even engage in physical violence for adaptive reasons, to defend themselves against abuse, by caregivers as well as romantic partners. Understanding the adaptive functions that aggressive behavior serves for girls is important not only for intellectual but also for practical reasons. If we seek to interrupt aggression, we might do well to consider how girls can meet these needs in other ways.

In considering how to help aggressive and antisocial girls, it may also be helpful to remember that even highly aggressive young women may have strengths by virtue of being female that can be harnessed in interventions. Most girls are likely protected from becoming violent by powerful socialization processes that lead them to care deeply for others (Zahn-Waxler & Polanichka, Chapter 3); even aggressive girls may have some remnant of this strong interpersonal orientation that might help them respond to interventions. Even girls incarcerated for delinquent offenses desire a broad range of services more than boys do: sex education; drug education; anger management; skills in forming positive relationships; help in coping with sexual abuse, physical abuse, and emotional abuse; family therapy; individual therapy; treatment for depression; and general health education (Chesney-Lind & Belknap, Chapter 10).

Understanding more about the specific processes by which girls' aggression unfolds will likely be critically important in interrupting girls' aggressive behavior. How exactly does "girl talk" ignite into hurtful relational aggression (Maccoby, Chapter 1)? How precisely does relational aggression lead to physical violence for some girls, toward peers, adults, and romantic partners? When is girls' aggression adaptive, as a means of social ascendancy or standing up to abuse? Answering these questions might help us intervene early, forcefully, and precisely, to prevent the heartbreaking consequences of girls' aggression and violence, for themselves and for their children.

## REFERENCES

Adler, P. A., & Adler, P. (1995). Dynamics of inclusion and exclusion in pre-adolescent cliques. *Social Psychology Quarterly, 58*(3), 145–162.

Benenson, J. F., Roy, R., Waite, A., Goldbaum, S., Linders, L., & Simpson, A. (2002). Greater discomfort as a proximate cause of sex differences in competition. *Merrill-Palmer Quarterly, 48,* 225–247.

Buss, A. H. (1961). *The psychology of aggression.* New York: Wiley.

Cairns, R. B., Cairns, B. D., Neckerman, H. J., Ferguson, L. L., & Gariepy, J. (1989). Growth and aggression: 1. Childhood to early adolescence. *Developmental Psychology, 25,* 320–330.

Coie, J. D., & Dodge, K. A. (1998). Aggression and antisocial behavior. In N. Eisenberg (Ed.), *Handbook of Child Psychology* (pp. 779–862). New York: Wiley.

Coie, J. D., & Dodge, K. A. (1998). The development of aggression and antisocial behavior. In W. V. Damon & N. Eisenberg (Eds.), *Handbook of child psychology: Vol. 3. Social, emotional, and personality development* (5th ed., pp. 779–862). New York: Wiley.

Conduct Problems Prevention Research Group. (1999). Initial impact of the Fast Track prevention trial for conduct problems: I. The high-risk sample. *Journal of Consulting and Clinical Psychology, 67,* 631–647.

Conduct Problems Prevention Research Group. (2002). Evaluation of the first three years of the Fast Track prevention trial with children at high risk for adolescent conduct problems. *Journal of Abnormal Child Psychology, 30,* 19–35.

Crick, N. R., & Grotpeter, J. K. (1995). Relational aggression, gender, and social-psychological adjustment. *Child Development, 66,* 710–722.

Crick, N. R., Grotpeter, J. K., & Bigbee, M. A. (2002). Relationally and physically aggressive children's intent attributions and feelings of distress for relational and instrumental provocations. *Child Development, 73,* 1134–1142.

Crick, N. R., Wellman, N. E., Casas, J. F., O'Brien, M. A., Nelson, D. A., Grotpeter, J. K., & Markon, K. (1999). Childhood aggression and gender: A new look at an old problem. In D. Bernstein (Ed.), *Nebraska Symposium on Motivation* (pp. 75–140). Lincoln: University of Nebraska Press.

Eder, D., & Enke, J. L. (1991). The structure of gossip: Opportunities and constraints on collective expression among adolescents. *American Sociological Review*, *56*, 494–508.

Feshbach, N. (1969). Gender differences in children's modes of aggressive responses toward outsiders. *Merrill-Palmer Quarterly*, *15*, 249–258.

French, D. C., Jansen, E. A., & Pidada, S. (2002). US and Indonesian children's and adolescent's reports of relational aggression by disliked peers. *Child Development*, *73*, 1143–1150.

Galen, B. R., & Underwood, M. K. (1997). A developmental investigation of social aggression among children. *Developmental Psychology*, *33*, 589–600.

Goldstein, S. E., Tisak, M. S., & Boxer, P. (2002). Preschoolers' normative and prescriptive judgments about relational and overt aggression. *Early Education and Development*, *13*, 23–39.

Kempf-Leonard, K., & Sample, L. L. (2000). Disparity based on sex: Is gender-specific treatment warranted? *Justice Quarterly*, *17*, 89–128.

Kerig, P. K., Brown, C., & Pantenaude, R. (2001, April). Ties that bind: Coparenting, parent–child relations, and triangulation in post-divorce interpersonal conflicts. In M. El-Shiekh (Chair), *Marital conflict and child outcomes: Processes, risk variables, and protective factors*. Symposium presented at the biennial meeting of the Society for Research in Child Development, Minneapolis, MN.

Lagerspetz, K. M. J., Bjorkqvist, K., & Peltonen, T. (1988). Is indirect aggression typical of females? Gender differences in aggressiveness in 11- to 12-year-old children. *Aggressive Behavior*, *14*, 403–414.

Larson, R. W., Wilson, S., Brown, B. B., Furstenberg, F. F., & Verma, S. (2002). Changes in adolescents' interpersonal competence: Are they being prepared for adult relationships in the 21st century? *Journal of Research on Adolescence*, *12*, 31–68.

Leve, L. D., & Chamberlain, P. (in press). Girls in the juvenile justice system: Risk factors and clinical implications. I D. J. Pepler, K. Madsen, C. Webster, & K. Levene (Eds.), *The development and treatment of girlhood aggression*. Mahwah, NJ: Erlbaum.

Office of Juvenile Justice and Delinquency Prevention (OJJDP). (1998). *Guiding principles for promising female programming: An inventory of best practices*. Washington, DC: Author.

Owens, L., Shute, R., & Slee, P. (2000). "Guess what I just heard!": Indirect aggression among teenage girls in Australia. *Aggressive Behavior*, *26*, 67–83.

Patterson, G. R. (1982). *Coercive family process*. Eugene, OR: Castalia.

Saarni, C., Mumme, D. L., & Campos, J. J. (1998). Emotional development: Action, communication, and understanding. In W. V. Damon & N. Eisenberg (Eds.), *Handbook of child psychology: Vol. 3. Social, emotional, and personality development* (5th ed., pp. 779–861). New York: Wiley.

Salmivalli, C., Lagerspetz, K., Bjorkqvist, K., Osterman, K., & Kaukiainen, A. (1996). Bullying as a group process: Participant roles and their relations to social status within the group. *Aggressive Behavior*, *22*, 1–15.

Sampson, R. J., & Laub, J. H. (1993). *Crime in the making: Pathways and turning points through life.* Cambridge, MA: Harvard University Press.

Underwood, M. K. (2003). *Social aggression among girls.* New York: Guilford Press.

Zanarini, M. C., & Gunderson, J. G. (1997). Differential diagnosis of antisocial and borderline personality disorders. In D. M. Stoff, J. Breiling, & J. D. Maser (Eds.), *Handbook of antisocial behavior* (pp. 83–91). New York: Wiley.

# Public Policy and the "Discovery" of Girls' Aggressive Behavior

Kenneth A. Dodge

Time is well past due. Research discoveries and secular trends over the past decade, as reported in this volume, lead overwhelmingly to the conclusion that public policy reform in youth violence must be directed toward the special circumstances of girls.

In the past, deviant girls were relatively ignored, perhaps because the numbers of girls who were overtly physically aggressive were small and their outcomes rarely included serious violence. The findings reported in this volume reveal a different picture: When a broader array of childhood aggressive behaviors (including covert, indirect, and relational aggressive acts) and adult outcomes (including marital assault, drug use, sexually transmitted diseases, welfare dependence, and progeny deviance) are considered, the number of deviant girls is striking and their long-term outcomes are costly for themselves and society. As Giordano, Cernkovich, and Lowery (Chapter 9) found, 83% of adolescent female offenders will not graduate from high school and 55% will end up in the lowest quartile in income.

The policy solutions, however, are not obvious. Although rates of arrest and detention of girls have skyrocketed (Stahl, 2001), self-reports of deviant behavior indicate no such epidemic of problem behavior, suggesting that the secular trends might represent public practice changes more than changes in youth behavior (Huizinga, 1997). It is plausible that these practice changes represent an awakening of the public mind to the realities of deviant girls. Yet another plausible hypothesis is that to-

302

day's policing tactics have become stricter in general, and the problems that are being picked up today are the ones that are disproportionately committed by deviant girls. Trends in policing practices and even some legislatively mandated reforms indicate growing likelihood that police will make an arrest for problems that in the past had been treated as status offenses (e.g., running away, prostitution, and shoplifting) or ignored, including romantic-partner violence, assault by a minor on a parent, and theft of items having low cash value (Harms, 2002). Although these crimes are committed by both males and females, they represent a relatively high proportion of the crimes committed by females (Chesney-Lind & Belknap, Chapter 10). So if the secular trends indicate the *discovery* of girls' problem behavior, rather than its new emergence, what policies are most needed?

Recent research findings also present a conundrum for practice. Even though studies indicate different causal factors for girls and boys (Susman & Pajer, Chapter 2; Zahn-Waxler & Polanichka, Chapter 3), only 5% of the total variance in aggressive behavior defined broadly can be accounted for by sex (Bjorkqvist & Niemela, 1992). Even though the profiles of aggressive behavior differ markedly for girls and boys (Crick, Ostrov, Appleyard, Jansen & Casas, Chapter 4), it is not clear whether different criteria should apply in the psychiatric diagnosis of conduct disorder. Nonetheless, it is clear that squeezing girls into treatment facilities and programs designed for boys is unacceptable public policy. Returning to a practice of ignoring the plight of deviant girls is equally unacceptable, especially as recent studies reveal the large costs that aggressive girls bring to society as they grow into adult criminals who disproportionately utilize government assistance and bear children who grow up to perpetuate the cycle of deviance across generations (Zoccolillo, Paquette, Azar, Côté, & Tremblay, Chapter 12).

This commentary highlights several important policy issues that must be addressed to attend to the needs of deviant girls and points toward the domains for which further research and policy analysis are needed, including developmental theory, screening practices, interventions, and justice policies.

## GIRLS MUST BE INCLUDED

Although the dramatic secular increases in arrests and detentions of adolescent females noted earlier are reason enough to take greater notice of girls' aggression problems, a broader body of research and practice buttresses the case for increased attention to the circumstances of today's girls. Past researchers, practitioners, and policymakers had attended pri-

marily to problems of overt, physical aggression among early-starting
conduct problem cases, which have been and continue to be an overwhelmingly male phenomenon. Arrests for physical violence remain the
domain of boys at a ratio exceeding 4 to 1. Even prevention programming continues to target problems of early-starting overt aggression,
leading to the overidentification of boys at a 3 to 1 ratio (Conduct Problems Prevention Research Group, 1992). Elementary school teachers are
biased toward attention to overt aggression and ignore relational aggression and psychological abuse of peers when they identify children for intervention (Leff, Kupersmidt, Patterson, & Power, 1999). But a variety
of sources indicates that these practices are short-sighted.

Chapters 4 and 7 point out that an exclusive reliance on acts of
overt aggression to identify conduct problems will underdetect some deviant girls who merit intervention. Girls engage in a range of disruptive
and oppositional acts that are indirect and harm others' social relationships. These behaviors are destructive and signal enduring adjustment
problems in girls; however, in the past they went underdetected. Over
the past decade, deviant behaviors by adolescent girls have been increasingly detected for arrest and detention, but early screening efforts have
not focused on the factors that predict these outcomes, and thus girls are
still left out of prevention efforts. To the extent that screening efforts require early-starting deviant behavior, girls might be left out because a
higher proportion of their overt deviance starts in adolescence. Puberty
itself is a risk factor for deviance in girls to a greater extent than in boys
(Susman & Pajer, Chapter 2), as are involvement in a romantic relationship and pregnancy. Thus, screening might also be directed at adolescents.

Girls with serious conduct problems merit intervention because
many grow up to become costly users of government services, their outcomes are destructive to themselves and others, and they bear children
who perpetuate a cycle of deviance (see Zoccolillo et al., Chapter 12,
and Serbin et al., Chapter 13). Although their outcomes do not frequently involve homicidal violence, physical violence in their romantic
relationships (Capaldi, Kim, & Shortt, Chapter 11) and abusive behavior toward their offspring are common (Giordano et al., Chapter 9).
Giordano and colleagues reported that 62% of African American and
41% of European American female adolescent offenders who had been
convicted of a serious felony as adolescents eventually lost custody of a
child by age 30. These girls often grow up to become dependent on
welfare (Zoccolillo & Rogers, 1991), to have low lifetime incomes
(Furstenberg, Brooks-Gunn, & Chase-Lansdale, 1989), and to have a
variety of physical health problems that cost society (e.g., obesity, diabetes, anemia, and high blood pressure; Serbin et al., Chapter 13).

Conduct problem girls are likely to become romantically involved with antisocial men (Moffitt, Caspi, Rutter, & Silva, 2001), to acquire sexually transmitted diseases (Serbin, Peters, McAffer, & Schwartzman, 1991), and to become pregnant multiple times during adolescence. During pregnancy, they expose their offspring to cigarette smoke and physical abuse (Zoccolillo, 2000). As parents, these girls are likely to be relatively insensitive to their infant, be easily irritated, expose their infant to a series of antisocial males (Zoccolillo, 2000), and display harsh and inconsistent parenting (Bosquet & Egeland, 2000). Their infants will experience physical health problems at a high rate (Serbin et al., Chapter 13), have accidents at a relatively high rate, and are at risk for developing conduct problems themselves, thus perpetuating the cycle of deviance (Serbin, Peters, & Schwartzman, 1996). Preventive intervention programs might capture these women by screening during pregnancy to identify new mothers at high risk for perpetuating the cycle of deviance with their children. Although no comprehensive study has been completed of the economic costs that girls with conduct disorder bring to society, it is clear that the costs are great and are larger than past policy would imply.

Thus, the first policy recommendation is that efforts to identify high-risk youth for inclusion in preventive intervention program should expand the range of targeted behaviors and time points to include those behaviors that will capture a higher proportion of high-risk females.

## GIRLS ARE DIFFERENT

Although girls should be included in preventive intervention efforts, Reitsma-Street and Offord (1991) have noted that available "policies and services for female offenders are propelled, as well as legitimized, by truncated theories and incorrect assumptions" (p. 12). The same errors hold for prevention efforts. Both current intervention practice and developmental theory indicate that girls will not be served well by being placed into programs that had been designed for boys.

### Intervention Practice

Even though the 1992 Act reauthorizing the Office of Juvenile Justice and Delinquency Prevention (OJJDP) requires that states establish and track distinct treatment programs for females, by 1998, judges continued to lament the inadequate options and services available for delinquent girls (Holsinger, Belknap, & Sutherland, 1999). The Dade County, Miami, Florida, Juvenile Court Judge Cynthia Lederman blamed the lack of research knowledge at the national level about which programs and services may be effective for girls, as well as the lack of attention and resources to girls at the local level. Within individual detention centers, staff members report three kinds of problems in treating delinquent girls: (1) The still-small numbers of girls make it difficult financially to justify resources that require a critical mass (e.g., gender-specific recreational programming and counselors trained to work with girls); (2) The lack of knowledge about what works with girls makes treatment challenging; and (3) Staff members abhor working with girls because they present many problems.

Framed in this manner, the second policy recommendation is that the national research agenda needs to move toward improving the efficacy of interventions with high-risk girls. The services system needs to fill in the continuum of care for girls by developing programs for girls of different ages with different needs. Perhaps recent efforts such as those suggested by the Office of Juvenile Justice and Delinquency Prevention (OJJDP, 1998) to develop study groups to review the literature and guide customized intervention efforts for girls will be successful. Alternatively, and unfortunately, the time appears ripe for a class-action lawsuit on behalf of high-risk girls to force the juvenile justice and human services systems to provide the comprehensive interventions and resources that are now mandated by law. Class action lawsuits have been a vehicle for reform in the mental health and juvenile justice systems in the past (e.g., Willie M. v. Hunt et al., 1979) and may continue to be a last-resort option to motivate government action.

## Developmental Theory

Models of conduct disorder articulate a primary path of early-starting conduct problems that grow and last across the lifespan and a secondary time-limited path that is related to adolescence (Moffitt, 1993). The growing consensus model of the development of the early starter posits interactions among biological and early-environment factors that place a young child at risk at the time of school entry, with exacerbation of these problems across development through problematic interaction with peers, teachers, parents, and authorities (Conduct Problems Prevention Research Group, 1992). The typical early-starting child is impulsive and has problems with delay of gratification as a toddler (Coie & Dodge, 1998). Although this model is broad enough to accommodate a variety of paths toward chronic deviance, it has evolved to place emphasis on children who are at temperamentally or genetically based high risk and who begin their overt problems early in life (Moffitt & Caspi, 2001).

Empirical studies identify very few females who fit the early-starting pattern of overt deviance (Moffitt & Caspi, 2001; Silverthorn & Frick, 1999). Longitudinal studies of outcomes have suffered in reaching conclusions about females partly because they have identified so few early-starting deviant females for long-term follow-up (Moffitt et al., 2001). Crick and colleagues (Chapter 4) and Bierman and colleagues (Chapter 7) suggest that a broader assessment of emotionally charged nonphysical and relational aggression problems (e.g., whining, stubbornness, teasing) will identify a larger group of girls who may start their behavior problems early in life and who grow in deviance over time. Sophisticated observation and analysis of girls' behavior in contrived play groups (Putallaz, Kupersmidt, Coie, McKnight, & Grimes, Chapter 6) reveal that aggressive behavior by girls does occur at high rates, if broader definitions and milder forms are included. Although the proposal to include a broader definition of aggression in the study of social behavior is entirely appropriate, its implication is that the primary developmental model of early-starting conduct disorder, which emphasizes high rates of overt physical aggression during early childhood, may not be apt for girls. Biological factors such as inattention and impulsivity are much more common for boys than girls (Moffitt et al., 2001) and hence may not play as central a role for girls as for boys.

The early-starter model implies that the early-starting child is biologically disposed toward impulsive deviant behavior and that the environment's reaction to this temperamental style shapes the course of his or her development. Temperamental and biological factors such as impulsivity are rarely the primary components of conduct problems in girls. Rather, a critical component seems to be problems in important social relationships with parents, peers, and romantic partners (Underwood, 2003). Furthermore, studies of girls with criminal histories indicate that the vast majority have suffered trauma in an early relationship, such as physical or sexual abuse (Chesney-Lind & Belknap, Chapter 10; Trickett & Gordis, Chapter 8). Ellis and colleagues (2003) identified father absence during the first 5 years of life as a crucial predictor of adolescent promiscuity and pregnancy among girls in both the United States and New Zealand. Similarly, longitudinal studies indicate that a lack of family support is a stronger predictor of adolescent problem behaviors for girls than boys (Windle, 1992).

One important implication of this research is that relatively more of girls' aggression and deviance occurs as a reaction to a traumatic experience or abusive early environment, whereas relatively more of boys' aggression is related to biological disposition. Although the magnitude of these relative differences is still unknown and might be modest, this conclusion may require us to realign our theories of the relative roles of genes and the environment in deviant behavior or to articulate gender-specific theories. Given that these different pathways are found in both boys and girls, it does not make sense to generate entirely distinct theories for males and females, but rather it does make sense to accommodate gender-linked pathways and forms in a general model.

It is crucial that this assertion leads us to realize that interventions that are designed for high-risk boys may be implicitly oriented toward helping the boy (and the environment) cope with a "chronic illness" (Kazdin, 1993) of difficult temperament that must be accommodated by finding optimal outlets for impulsive behavior, by structuring the environment to limit the boy's possible destructiveness, and by building skills in the boy to help him succeed in spite of an unspoken "disability." To the extent that conduct problems in girls are related to a history of trauma or to ongoing stressful relationships, the successful preventive intervention might be targeted toward resolution of that trauma and stress, both in the child's psychological apparatus and in the external environment.

One way in which interventions might differ, given these two orientations, concerns parenting practices. McFadyen-Ketchum, Bates, Dodge, and Pettit (1996) found that a parenting style of authoritative support led to improvements in behavior problems for young girls but not boys, with the authors concluding that parenting interventions for boys might emphasize strict rules and contingent discipline practices to a greater extent. During early adolescence, at a high-risk time when pubescent girls desire more freedom and independence, effective parenting interventions for girls might well be those that increase the closeness of family ties and reduce the chance for girls to overextend their freedom with misbehavior (Zahn-Waxler & Polanichka, Chapter 3). Griffin, Botvin, Scheier, Diaz, and Miller (2000) found that family dinners and parents' checking of daily homework were protective factors in resisting the development of delinquency in girls but not boys.

Another gender-specific intervention might occur in the emphasis on emotional control versus emotional resolution. Most preventive interventions now emphasize the development of emotional control over impulses through skill building (e.g., Conduct Problems Prevention Research Group, 1999; Tremblay, Pagani-Kurtz, Masse, Vitaro, & Pihl, 1995). These interventions might well be more appropriate for boys than girls. To the extent that conduct problem girls suffer from posttraumatic effects or are embroiled in emotionally stressful relationships, interventions need to address girls' sense of security and understanding of their own relationships. Girls might be less likely to benefit from general social-skill-building intervention programs and more from interventions tailored to their particular life history and circumstances. As yet another example, Giordano and colleagues (Chapter 9) identified the lack of social capital (e.g., a network of supportive relationships) as an impediment to successful outcomes for adolescent female offenders, suggesting that interventions for these girls might be directed toward building this capital.

In sum, the general discoveries that interpersonal relationship trauma plays a major role in the etiology of girls' conduct problems and that relationship support can protect girls' development have important implications for the development of gender-specific interventions that focus on preventing such trauma, intervening quickly and comprehensively to resolve trauma, and providing a system of interpersonal support to protect girls during development. *Thus, the third policy recommendation is that a full continuum of care is needed that provides support for girls both sequentially across time and horizontally across the domains of their lives (e.g., family, peers, school).*

## FUTURE DIRECTIONS IN RESEARCH, PRACTICE, AND POLICY

Now that the door is open to the possibility that long-term prediction of serious antisocial outcomes may differ for males and females, a major research agenda item will be to revisit numerous prediction and screening studies to identify optimal predictor paths for girls and boys separately. Not only might the specific behavioral indicators of risk vary across genders, the optimal age of prediction (and therefore, age of intervention) might differ. Following from these studies, of course, will be a more precise understanding of the mechanisms of development that lead to antisocial outcomes in girls.

One area of future controversy, no doubt, will be whether the criteria for the psychiatric diagnosis of conduct disorder should differ for girls and boys. Given the different patterns of behavior that are associated with costly outcomes for girls and boys, the options for diagnostic practice will be to create separate disorders for the two gender groups, to assign different criteria to the diagnosis of conduct disorder for girls and boys, or to create subtypes of conduct disorder that are correlated with gender. It is plausible that the trauma-related problems in interpersonal relationships that characterize some conduct problem girls constitute a separate subtype of conduct disorder that is distinct from the more biologically based, life-persistent pattern that characterizes some conduct problem boys.

As the knowledge about development becomes more precise, interventions must grow increasingly specific for girls and boys. The implementation and evaluation of interventions specifically for girls awaits the next generation of research and practice in this domain.

## REFERENCES

Bjorkqvist, K., & Niemela, P. (1992). New trends in the study of female aggression. In K. Bjorkqvist (Ed.), *Of mice and women: Aspects of female aggression* (pp. 1–16). San Diego, CA: Academic Press.

Bosquet, M., & Egeland, B. (2000). Predicting parenting behaviors from Antisocial Practices content scale scores of the MMPI-2 administered during pregnancy. *Journal of Personality Assessment, 74,* 146–162.

Coie, J. D., & Dodge, K. A. (1998). Aggression and anti-social behavior. In W. Damon & N. Eisenberg (Eds.), *Handbook of child psychology: Vol. 3. Social, emotional, and personality development* (5th ed., pp. 779–862). New York: Wiley.

Conduct Problems Prevention Research Group. (1992). A developmental and clinical model for the prevention of conduct disorders: The Fast Track Program. *Development and Psychopathology, 4,* 509–527.

Conduct Problems Prevention Research Group. (1999). Initial impact of the Fast Track Prevention Trial for Conduct Problems: I. The high-risk sample. *Journal of Consulting and Clinical Psychology, 67,* 631–647.

Ellis, B. J., Bates, J. E., Dodge, K. A., Fergussen, D. M., Horwood, L. J., Pettit, G. S., & Woodward, L. (2003). Does father absence place daughters at special risk for early sexual activity and teenage pregnancy? *Child Development, 74,* 801–821.

Furstenberg, F. F., Jr., Brooks-Gunn, J., & Chase-Lansdale, L. (1989). Teenaged pregnancy and childbearing. *American Psychologyist, 44,* 313–320.

Griffin, K. W., Botvin, G. J., Scheier, L. M., Diaz, T., & Miller, N. L. (2000). Parenting practices as predictors of substance use, delinquency, and aggression among urban minority youth: Moderating effects of family structure and gender. *Psychology of Addictive Behaviors, 14*(2), 174–184.

Harms, P. (2002). *Detention in delinquency cases, 1989–1998* (OJJDP Fact Sheet, No. 1). Washington, DC: U.S. Department of Justice.

Holsinger, K., Belknap, J., & Sutherland, J. L. (1999). *Assessing the gender specific program and service needs for adolescent females in the juvenile justice system* (Report) Columbus, OH: Office of Criminal Justice Services.

Huizinga, D. (1997). *Over-time changes in delinquency and drug use: The 1970's to the 1990's.* Unpublished report, Office of Juvenile Justice and Delinquency Prevention.

Kazdin, A. E. (1993). Treatment of conduct disorder: Progress and directions in psychotherapy research. *Development and Psychopathology, 7,* 715–726.

Leff, S. S., Kupersmidt, J. B., Patterson, C. J., & Power, T. J. (1999). Factors influencing teacher identification of peer bullies and victims. *School Psychology Review, 28,* 505–517.

McFadyen-Ketchum, S. A., Bates, J. E., Dodge, K. A., & Pettit, G. S. (1996). Pattern of change in early childhood aggressive-disruptive behavior: Gender differences in predictions from early coercive ad affectionate mother–child interactions. *Child Development, 67,* 2417–2433.

Moffitt, T. E. (1993). The neuropsychology of conduct disorder. *Development and Psychopathology, 5,* 135–152.

Moffitt, T. E., & Caspi, A. (2001). Childhood predictors differentiate life-course persistent and adolescence-limited antisocial pathways among males and females. *Development and Psychopathology, 13*(2), 355–375.

Moffitt, T. E., Caspi, A., Rutter, M., & Silva, P. A. (2001). *Sex differences in antisocial behaviour: Conduct disorder, delinquency, and violence in the Dunedin longitudinal study.* Cambridge, UK: Cambridge University Press.

Office of Juvenile Justice and Delinquency Prevention. (1998). *What about girls? Females in the juvenile justice system* [Flyer]. Washington, DC: Department of Justice.

Reitsma-Street, M., & Offord, D. R. (1991). Girl delinquents and their sisters: A challenge for practice. *Canadian Social Work Review, 8*(1), 11–27.

Serbin, L. A., Peters, P. L., McAffer, V. J., & Schwartzman, A. E. (1991). Childhood aggression and withdrawal as predictors of adolescent pregnancy, early parenthood, and environmental risk for the next generation. *Canadian Journal of Behavioural Science, 23*(3), 318–331.

Serbin, L. A., Peters, P., & Schwartzman, A. E. (1996). Longitudinal study of early childhood injuries and acute illnesses in the offspring of adolescent mothers who were aggressive, withdrawn, or aggressive-withdrawn in childhood. *Journal of Abnormal Psychology, 105,* 500–507.

Silverthorn, P., & Frick, P. J. (1999). Developmental pathways to antisocial behavior: The delayed-onset pathway in girls. *Development and Psychopathology, 11,* 101–126.

Stahl, A. (2001, August). *Delinquency cases in juvenile courts, 1998* (OJJDP Fact Sheet, No. 31). Washington, DC: U.S. Government Printing Office.

Tremblay, R. E., Pagani-Kurtz, L., Masse, L. C., Vitaro, F., & Pihl, R. O. (1995). A bi-modal preventive intervention for disruptive kindergarten boys: Its impact through mid-adolescence. *Journal of Consulting and Clinical Psychology, 63,* 560–568.

Underwood, M. (2003). *Social aggression among girls.* New York: Guilford Press.

Windle, M. (1992). A longitudinal study of stress buffering for adolescent problem behaviors. *Developmental Psychology, 28,* 522–530.

Zoccolillo, M. (2000). Parents' health and social adjustment: Part II. Social adjustment. In M. Jette, H. Desrosiers, R. E. Tremblay, & J. Thibault (Eds.), *Longitudinal study of child development in Quebec (ELDEQ 1998–2002).* Quebec: Institut de la statistique du Quebec.

Zoccolillo, M., & Rogers, K. (1991). Characteristics and outcome of hospitalized adolescent girls with conduct disorder. *Journal of the American Academy of Child and Adolescent Psychiatry, 30,* 973–981.

# Index

Page numbers followed by an *f* indicate figure, *t* indicate table.